Additional Praise for *The End of Epidemics*

"Dr. Jonathan Quick has written an insightful, accessible, and personal history of modern epidemics, including such killers as smallpox and Ebola, and their dramatic impact on our lives and world. More important, Dr. Quick is not merely wringing his hands about the infectious catastrophes that are surely facing us, he focuses on the important actions needed to prevent social, economic, and health consequences of inattention. Governments, international institutions, the private sector, and civil society had better take heed: prepare and plan now—or pay the price, in dollars and lives, tomorrow."   —Rear Admiral Kenneth Bernard, former senior official for
Biodefense and Health Security under presidents
George W. Bush and Bill Clinton

"Infectious disease outbreaks rival natural disasters and wars in their capacity to endanger human health, cripple economies, and disrupt societies. *The End of Epidemics* shows us that by learning from the past we can build a world more resilient to infectious disease. But we must act quickly."   —Dr. Jeremy Farrar, Director, Wellcome Trust

"Quick is an internationally recognized leader in global health—his focus on innovation and new technologies is vital to pandemic threat prevention and preparedness to save lives around the globe."   —Dr. Rajiv Shah, President, Rockefeller Foundation

"Dr. Quick has written a fascinating book. Following decades of working in some of the world's most epidemic-prone countries, he argues for scientific and public health developments that can save humanity from deadly microorganisms."
—Dr. David Heymann, Professor, Infectious Disease Epidemiology,
London School of Hygiene and Tropical Medicine

"A well-documented and gripping account of the peril posed by pandemics. Dr. Quick, a global health leader from the front lines of the AIDS and Ebola [epidemics], weaves rich historical facts and decades of personal experience to ring the alarm over the pandemic threat."   —Dr. Ariel Pablos-Méndez, former head of Global Health,
U.S. Agency for International Development

THE END OF EPIDEMICS

THE END
OF
EPIDEMICS

The Looming Threat to Humanity
and How to Stop It

Jonathan D. Quick, MD,
with Bronwyn Fryer

St. Martin's Press ♨ New York

www.stmartins.com

Designed by Patrice Sheridan

Book illustrations by Mia Roca Alcover

LIBRARY OF CONGRESS CATALOGING-IN-PUBLICATION DATA

Names: Quick, Jonathan D., author. | Fryer, Bronwyn, author.
Title: The end of epidemics : the looming threat to humanity and how to stop
   it / Jonathan D. Quick and Bronwyn Fryer.
Description: New York : St. Martin's Press, 2018. | Includes bibliographical
   references and index.
Identifiers: LCCN 2017037542| ISBN 9781250117779 (hardcover) |
   ISBN 9781250117786 (ebook)
Subjects: | MESH: Epidemics—prevention & control
Classification: LCC RA651 | NLM WA 105 | DDC 614.4—dc23
LC record available at https://lccn.loc.gov/2017037542

Our books may be purchased in bulk for promotional, educational, or business use.
Please contact your local bookseller or the Macmillan Corporate and
Premium Sales Department at 1-800-221-7945, extension 5442, or
by email at MacmillanSpecialMarkets@macmillan.com.

First Edition: January 2018

10 9 8 7 6 5 4 3 2 1

To the memories of

Dr. D. A. Henderson, a tenacious and ultimately victorious

leader in the battle to end the scourge of smallpox.

and

Nurse Salome Karwah, an Ebola survivor who saved many lives

and later was left to die in childbirth, a victim of stigma.

Unless otherwise specified, all dollar amounts are U.S. currency.

CONTENTS

PART II. STOPPING PANDEMICS BEFORE THEY START

ACRONYMS

ACLU	American Civil Liberties Union
ACT UP	AIDS Coalition to Unleash Power
ADDO	Accredited Drug Dispensing Outlet
AIDS	Acquired Immune Deficiency Syndrome
BSE	bovine spongiform encephalopathy
BSL	Biosafety Level
CAFO	Concentrated Animal Feeding Operations
CDC	Centers for Disease Control and Prevention (U.S.)
DDT	dichlorodiphenyltrichloroethane
DNA	deoxyribonucleic acid
EIS	Epidemic Intelligence Service
FAO	Food and Agriculture Organization of the United Nations
G7	Group of 7
G20	Group of 20
GAO	United States Government Accountability Office
GDP	gross domestic product
GHSA	Global Health Security Agenda
GPHIN	Global Public Health Intelligence Network
GRID	Gay Related Immune Deficiency
HIV	human immunodeficiency virus
IHR	International Health Regulation
ISIS	Islamic State in Iraq and Syria
MERS	Middle East Respiratory Syndrome
MBM	meat and bone meal
MMR	measles mumps rubella
MRSA	Methicillin-resistant *Staphylococcus aureus*
MSF	Médecins Sans Frontières (in English, Doctors Without Borders)
MSH	Management Sciences for Health

NGO	nongovernmental organization
NIH	National Institutes of Health (U.S.)
PEF	Pandemic Emergency Financing
PEPFAR	President's Emergency Plan for AIDS Relief (U.S.)
PHEIC	Public Health Emergency of International Concern
R&D	research and development
SARS	severe acute respiratory syndrome
SMAC	Social Mobilization Action Consortium
TAC	Treatment Action Campaign
UNAIDS	Joint United Nations Programme on HIV/AIDS
UNICEF	United Nations Children's Fund
USAID	United States Agency for International Development
USDA	U.S. Department of Agriculture
vCJD	Creutzfeldt–Jakob (mad cow) disease
WHO	World Health Organization

PROLOGUE

A FEAR I'D NEVER FELT BEFORE

What can be done to stop the next killer virus from destroying millions of lives?

Following a frightening meeting with my staff at the peak of the West Africa Ebola crisis, I asked myself, "What would it take to prevent such devastating epidemics?" A new pandemic could kill more than 300 million people worldwide. It could also reduce global GDP by 5 to 10 percent—an impact equivalent to the financial crisis of 2008. There will always be new outbreaks of infectious diseases. But as a medical doctor and a global health leader, I know that by following the prescriptions laid out in this book, it is within the power of modern public-health leaders to keep such outbreaks from exploding into catastrophic epidemics that kill thousands or millions.

I was more alarmed than I had ever been in my 35 years of working in public health. The world was facing a potentially global catastrophe unlike anything I, or any of my colleagues, had ever seen. In response to the fears of my far-flung staff, I knew I had to be straightforward and talk frankly and calmly about the crisis.

It was a rainy Thursday morning, October 9, 2014, and 100 of us were stuffed into a classroom-sized room where I was hosting a videoconference for the global health nonprofit that I led, Management Sciences for Health (MSH). More than 500 staff members from our home office near Boston, and those in field offices in Africa, Asia, and Latin America, were huddled around our various communication devices, listening intently. We had all read or heard appalling reports from medical teams on the ground in West Africa, where the Ebola virus was spinning out of control, condemning thousands of people—including some of our own beloved colleagues—to horrific deaths. At this moment, some team members were reporting in from ground zero in Liberia, where the epidemic was rampaging.

"The treatment facilities are overrun with cases," they told us. "Whole parts of the health system are at a standstill. Staff and patients are scared away. Patients refuse to go to community health centers; they see them as places to die. Corpses are lying in the streets." Women were delivering babies without trained help. Malaria cases were going untreated, adding to the death toll. In defiance of ancient traditions in which families lovingly touch and swaddle the dead, villagers were being instructed by strange people in alien-looking plastic moon suits not to hug each other, shake hands, or touch their loved ones.

"With the risk to our staff, why are we there?" someone sitting near me asked.

It was an obvious question. And we all wondered about the follow-on: Where would Ebola travel next, given all the remote places MSH operated in around the planet? Thomas Duncan, the first Ebola patient in the U.S., had died just the day before at Texas Health Presbyterian Hospital in Dallas. Which city would be next? Paris? Tokyo? Moscow? Mexico City? Right here, where some of us were sitting, in Boston? Symptoms didn't show up for several days. Unknowingly infected people who had been in West Africa could be coming to our offices.

I was especially worried for our staff in the hot zone. Ian Sliney, our stiff-upper-lipped British colleague, candidly admitted that, despite taking all pre-cautions, he was worried. What could I tell him and the others? Ian and hundreds like him were real heroes, first responders on the front lines of the outbreak. They were taking their temperatures constantly and dousing their hands, arms, feet, and everything else in chlorine.

"I know there is a lot of fear out there and also among you," I said. "But, in good conscience, we can't not be involved." I then read a letter from Niniola Soleye, a staff member in Nigeria. Her aunt, a doctor, had died trying to stop the spread of the disease. "My aunt's death is painful," she had written, "but it comforts me to know that I'm part of an organization that's truly committed to saving lives." I hoped her words offered at least a bit of salve.

In that meeting, we were all asking the big question of "how?" How could we help bring this horror to a halt? Better organization, better communication, better local community action, better leadership, more money, more global engagement? After all, our organization's mission is to save lives by closing the gap between knowledge and action in global public health. But with Ebola, we were all staring hard at that yawning gap. We didn't know enough, so we didn't know what actions to take. As experts, we were doing everything in our combined experience that we knew how to do to treat the sick and prevent the spread of disease, but the challenge was like trying to swim in a tsunami.

After that meeting, I also kept asking myself another big question: Why? Why had it taken months for the World Health Organization (WHO) to declare a global public-health emergency? Why was there still no Ebola vaccine after more than 20 outbreaks of the disease since it was discovered in 1976? Why had the director of the Centers for Disease Control and Prevention (CDC) and the governor of Texas insisted the public was safe from this terrible disease, only to find days later that two nurses had contracted it at a Texas hospital from an infected man who had apparently come in from West Africa under the radar, potentially spreading the disease to an entire American city?

I began to reflect on what I had experienced firsthand or learned through colleagues about AIDS, avian influenza, severe acute respiratory syndrome (SARS), and other infectious-disease outbreaks. I also studied credible scenarios of the magnitude and impact of future epidemics. And I became more and more frightened.

What frightened me? Certainly the prediction by Bill Gates and his team that an epidemic like the 1918 influenza pandemic that killed 50 million people could happen again today—and that in the first 200 days it could kill 33 million people.[1] That's almost as many people as AIDS has killed over four decades. Even scarier was the Bank of America/Merrill Lynch assessment that the threat of a global pandemic is "arguably higher than at any time in human history" and that a severe pandemic could claim more than 300 million lives and cost the global economy as much as $3.5 trillion.[2]

We already know how to stop local outbreaks before they spread. But time and time again, our human failings—various mixtures of fear, pride, complacency, hubris, denial, and financial self-interest—have created, worsened, or delayed the response to past epidemics. I asked myself, why does this keep happening?

Yet I've also seen how, at our smartest, we have overcome our human failings.

I know of myriad inspiring examples of intelligent, compassionate people—from presidents to paupers—who, throughout history, did the right thing. I have worked closely with colleagues and studied the success stories of those who eradicated smallpox, transformed AIDS from a death sentence into a treatable disease, contained the avian influenza outbreak in the late 2000s—and, of course, handled the nearly two dozen Ebola outbreaks in Africa that preceded the West Africa epidemic of 2014–15. Based on my observations and experience, I firmly believe that achieving the impossible is possible.

I was a little kid in May 1961 when President John F. Kennedy committed the U.S. to "achieving the goal, before the decade is out, of landing a man on the moon and returning him safely to the earth." Over the next eight years, along with millions of other kids, I became more and more enthralled with all things astronaut. Like everyone else, I was awestruck on July 20, 1969, when *Apollo 11* astronaut Neil Armstrong became the first person to put a foot onto the lunar surface and radio back to earth his famous line, "That's one small step for man, one giant leap for mankind."

When Kennedy set his famous goal in 1961, the technology that would take the three *Apollo 11* astronauts to the moon did not exist. Neil Armstrong once observed that during the years of strategizing, innovating, and testing that led up to his landing, NASA engineers and scientists repeatedly ran into ferocious, unscalable walls. They often thought they would have to halt the mission. Nevertheless, each time the moon shot looked like a certain failure, they were firmly told: "We are going to the moon." They went back, reimagined the impossible, and made it happen.

By contrast, when leaders shrug their shoulders in resignation, nothing happens. World Health Organization director-general Dr. Marcolino Candau spent most of his career in public health believing that smallpox eradication was impossible. After all, smallpox had been around for at least 3,000 years and was fatal in 30 percent of cases. That's probably one of the reasons why, when WHO finally committed to smallpox eradication in 1966, Dr. Candau's home country of Brazil was the only one in the Western Hemisphere that hadn't yet dedicated itself to joining WHO's mission. It had taken global health leaders fifteen years to decide to rid the world of smallpox for good. But once they did so, it took just over ten years to eradicate the scourge.[3]

In late April 2003, at the height of an epidemic of the new respiratory disease known as SARS, reporters asked then–CDC director Dr. Jeffrey Koplan whether SARS could be eliminated in Hong Kong. He said he would be shocked if it was. "To be realistic, what we can hope for is the suppression and a minimization of the disease and viral spread," he told them.[4] A mere two months later, Hong Kong was declared SARS-free—ahead of Toronto, Beijing, and Taiwan. The virus has never returned. The impossible had again happened.

In this book, through examples and evidence, I will establish the seven fundamental sets of actions needed for preventing epidemics: (1) ensuring bold leadership at all levels; (2) building resilient health systems; (3) fortifying three lines of defense against disease (prevention, detection, and response); (4) ensuring timely and accurate communication; (5) investing in smart, new innovation; (6) spending wisely to prevent disease before an epidemic strikes; and (7) mobilizing citizen activism. I'm convinced that a combination of these actions could be achieved within a decade. Working together, The Power of Seven would put us well on the path to an epidemic-free world.

Dangerous microbes will always be out there, and small outbreaks that kill tens or hundreds of people will continue to occur. But if we can send people to the moon, if we can eradicate smallpox, if we can mount the largest public-health treatment effort in history as we did for AIDS, surely we *can* end epidemics.

In response to skepticism about sending a man to the moon, John F. Kennedy said, "We choose to go to the moon. We choose to go to the moon in this decade and do the other things, not because they are easy, but because they are hard." Pursuing the vision of making the world's last epidemic the very last one will be hard. To the skeptics who believe we cannot end epidemics, I say, "Let's imagine the impossible—then make it happen." Humanity simply cannot afford not to do this.

My sense of hope springs from my four-decade journey in global health. As a third-year medical student, I traveled to Latin America, Africa, Asia, and the Western Pacific to document pioneering efforts to bring modern medicines to the world's poor and underserved. As a family physician at the U.S. Public Health Service hospital in Talihina, Oklahoma, I delivered babies, treated snakebites, and healed gunshot wounds. I lived in Pakistan and Kenya, where I helped to strengthen local primary health care. As a director at WHO headquarters in Geneva, I worked to expand access to quality essential medicines, including AIDS treatment. And as former president and CEO and now senior fellow at Management Sciences for Health, I have worked with inspiring local leaders around the world to build strong health systems.

Throughout my journey, I have witnessed intense suffering, but I have also seen the stunning results of concerted effort in turning around public-health catastrophes. My experience as a family physician has put me face-to-face with the profound human pain experienced by families who lose a child, a beloved parent, or a sibling. Yet I have also observed the remarkable impact on entire countries when government officials, public-health leaders, activists, and average citizens galvanize action against a global health threat like AIDS, maternal mortality, or a preventable childhood illness. This book is driven by my personal response to the human anguish caused by missed opportunities to help, and by the intense joy I feel when our work saves lives. In it, I'll describe what happens when disease takes hold and spreads due to all-too-human failings, and how the heroic actions of others help to slow or stop viruses. I'll suggest how forward thinking could save us from global threats like Ebola, Zika, and pandemic influenza.

At the end of that MSH global staff videoconference, Ian Sliney spoke again from his hotel room in Liberia. His fatigued but stalwart voice was the last one we heard. "Wish us the very best of luck," he said. "Pray that we get this right."

With this book, I hope that we can all work to get this right.

PART I

THE PANDEMIC THREAT

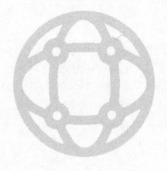

CHAPTER 1

STOP EPIDEMICS WITH THE POWER OF SEVEN

We can end epidemics with seven sets of concrete actions proven over a century of epidemic response.

The enormous health and financial impacts of epidemics are made worse through human foibles like fear, denial, panic, complacency, hubris, and self-interest. But we can end epidemics by facing up to them and applying concrete actions I call "The Power of Seven": (1) ensuring bold leadership at all levels; (2) building resilient health systems; (3) fortifying three lines of defense against disease (prevention, detection, and response); (4) ensuring timely and accurate communication; (5) investing in smart innovation; (6) spending wisely to prevent disease before an epidemic strikes; and (7) mobilizing citizen activism.

I had my first lesson in epidemic forecasting back in 1975, when I was 24 years old. As a second-year medical student at the University of Rochester in upstate New York, I was fascinated by the stories one of my young professors, Dr. Steve Kunitz, told of his search for predictors of the bubonic plague outbreaks, which occurred every few years in the American Southwest. "Six hundred years after the Black Death killed half the population of Europe and swept through Asia and Africa to claim roughly 50 million lives worldwide,

Native Americans and others in the Southwest endured sporadic outbreaks of this ghastly disease," Kunitz said. "They suffered abdominal pain, bleeding, blackening of the extremities, and other awful but classic symptoms. The question is: How were these Native Americans getting infected with plague?"

"Fleas on rats," somebody said.

"You're half right," Kunitz replied. "The disease came from fleas, but not rat fleas."

"Dog fleas?" another student suggested.

"Close," the professor said. "Prairie dog fleas hitchhiking on dogs. Native American families kept as many as ten domesticated dogs. These dogs often would hunt prairie dogs, picking up prairie dog fleas along the way."

We were perplexed. So where did the human plague come from?

Kunitz was a clever investigator. When he and a colleague visited the Navajo Reservation at Tuba City, Arizona, to discover how nature might signal when the next outbreak would occur, they began interviewing the locals. They suggested that clusters of dead prairie dogs ("die-offs") might carry a clue.

In class, we students learned that plague is caused by the *Yersinia pestis* bacteria, which is transmitted by the bite of an infected flea from a rat or other small rodent, like the prairie dog of the Southwest. The fleas that infested the prairie dogs came from rats that migrated on steamships from China, which suffered a plague epidemic in the 1860s. Over generations, the infected fleas migrated from ship rats to San Francisco squirrels, and the insects then made their way to the American Southwest. Kunitz and his colleague found that local domestic dogs regularly came in contact with prairie dogs and their fleas but rarely became visibly sick themselves.

Kunitz wondered whether the dogs might be getting a mild illness and developing antibodies to the disease. Could he measure that possibility by asking veterinarians to take blood samples when dogs came in for rabies shots? And what if the level of antibodies to plague among dogs meant that an outbreak of human plague was not far behind? "If both were true," he told us, "then regular testing of dogs could be used as an early warning alert for human plague."

Kunitz's research confirmed both of these hypotheses. Soon after, public-health officials began taking annual surveys of antibodies in dog populations. When dog antibody levels increased, community health representatives would spread the warning via local radio and TV and intensify education programs that teach people to protect themselves from fleas and recognize plague symptoms. The effort continues today, albeit with some modifications (such as sampling from coyotes instead of domestic dogs).

I was mightily impressed by this medical Sherlock Holmes. As a student, I had no idea how an epidemic disease could migrate around the world over centuries while occasionally jumping from its animal "host" to humans, inflicting death on tens, thousands, or millions of people. Nor did I have any inkling that, many years later, I would take on the challenge of preventing epidemics from starting.

Three Tales from Killer Diseases

The 1918 Spanish flu that sickened a third of the world's population almost a century ago still exists in weaker, seasonal strains today. For a tiny view of what could happen with a new pandemic, let's take a look at the moment when twentieth-century modernity was taking hold and World War I was winding down.

Based on clinical reports and genomic studies, scientists today believe that the influenza virus had been circulating within the armies of the World War for a long time—even years—before the pandemic of 1918–19.[1] Like all influenza viruses, the Spanish version mutated. In the western trenches, that flu likely took hold among those who had no immunity to it and were living in filthy, wet, cold conditions. It then erupted in far-flung port cities: Freetown, Sierra Leone; Brest, France; and Boston, Massachusetts.[2]

In the summer of 1918 in the U.S., the Spanish influenza first touched someone in Philadelphia. Americans were hoping for an end to the war and the return of their surviving fathers and sons. Many of the nearly 2 million citizens of Philadelphia flocked to theaters to see vaudeville, plays, and big events and concerts, exchanging occasional coughs. Nobody had paid attention to the fact that 8 million Spaniards were sick and dying from a strange new disease named the "Spanish influenza" or that people in Boston had come down with the same thing. The alarm bells were silent.

But by the time early autumn arrived, the coughing had spread the disease throughout the city. The coughed-upon developed fevers and pneumonia; the mortally ill suffocated because their lungs and organs collapsed, their bodies turning a hideous blue-black. By October 4, there were 636 new cases of the Spanish flu in Philadelphia; 139 people died. In less than a week, there were an astounding 5,531 new cases. In response, officials closed all the vaudeville and picture theaters, saloons, schools, and churches in the city. Most of the city's doctors had been sent to Europe to tend to soldiers while the flu was raging. Many remaining healthcare workers succumbed too. The most common treatment was whiskey, the stronger the better. But as whiskey ran out, frantic shoppers stripped pharmacy shelves bare. Medical care was in very short supply. Snake-oil salesmen advised patients to treat themselves with oil of balsam or to try "Munyon's Paw Paw" pills.

By mid-month, parents were so sick that they could not care for their children. Hospitals were so full that beds were set up in the armory. When volunteers showed up to hospitals to help, they could do little more than to carry away the dead. People died so fast that the coroner's office could not keep up with the demand for death certificates. Like some nightmare from plague-ridden fourteenth-century Europe, volunteers drove horse-drawn carts through the city streets, calling for people to "bring out the dead." Cemetery directors in Philadelphia raised prices for a plot by 50 percent and charged families an exorbitant $15 for the privilege of digging their loved ones' graves themselves.

In the streets, little girls jumped rope to a grim new rhyme:

> "I had a little bird / and its name was Enza / I opened the door / And in
>   flew Enza."[3]

Before it was over, the Spanish flu of 1918 wiped out 13,000 people in Philadelphia and between 50 and 100 million worldwide. It remains the most deadly flu outbreak in history.

*   *   *

Gaëtan Dugas was a handsome, charming Air Canada flight attendant who claimed to have had more than 2,500 sexual partners. For years, epidemiologists considered him "patient zero" in the AIDS epidemic. Early researchers believed he contracted AIDS while in Africa. In his iconic 1987 history of AIDS, *And the Band Played On*, Randy Shilts portrayed Dugas as recklessly spreading AIDS through unprotected sex even after he was diagnosed. Dugas died from his illness in 1984.[4]

As is the case with most epidemics, the first two decades of AIDS were rife with conspiracy theories about the origin of this other twentieth-century

A Century of Deadly Outbreaks

Influenza and HIV/AIDS have been among the most deadly of the viral pathogens of the last 100 years.

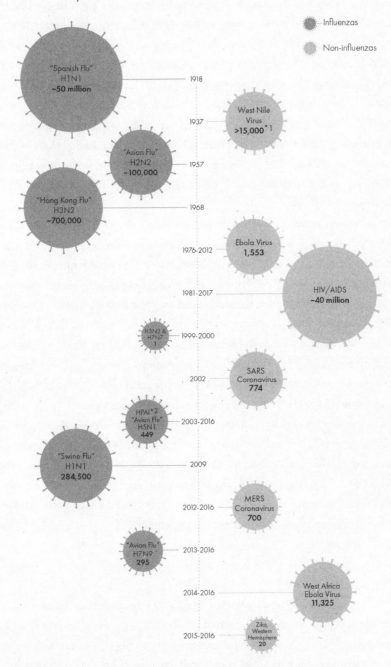

Influenzas

Non-influenzas

"Spanish Flu"
H1N1
~50 million

1918

1937

West Nile
Virus
>15,000*[1]

"Asian Flu"
H2N2
~100,000

1957

"Hong Kong Flu"
H3N2
~700,000

1968

1976-2012

Ebola Virus
1,553

1981-2017

HIV/AIDS
~40 million

H5N2 &
H7N7
1

1999-2000

2002

SARS
Coronavirus
774

HPAI*2
"Avian Flu"
H5N1
449

2003-2016

"Swine Flu"
H1N1
284,500

2009

2012-2016

MERS
Coronavirus
700

"Avian Flu"
H7N9
295

2013-2016

2014-2016

West Africa
Ebola Virus
11,325

2015-2016

Zika,
Western
Hemisphere
20

SOURCE: Bean A, Baker M, Stewart C et al. Studying immunity to zoonotic diseases in the natural host—keeping it real. *Nature Reviews: Immunology* 2013; 13:851–61.

Black Death. Some people blamed smallpox immunization; others blamed a polio vaccine grown in chimpanzee cells; still others claimed that AIDS was a government-sponsored genocide weapon used against the black or gay communities. Over the last decade, however, gene sleuths have unraveled the mystery. Scientists have now found proof that five successful "species jumps" of the simian immunodeficiency virus (SIV) from primates to humans occurred in Africa during the last century. "Successful" means that the SIV virus adapted, through rapid mutation, to a form of human immunodeficiency virus (HIV) that would thrive and multiply in humans. The first species jump happened around 1910 in southeastern Cameroon. The biology of the HIV virus subtype tells us that it came from a chimpanzee, which a human probably killed to eat or barter as "bushmeat," ultimately igniting the AIDS pandemic.

From the first human infections in Cameroon, the HIV virus spread down the Sangha River—probably through sexual contact among those living near and traveling along the river—to the bustling city of Leopoldville (modern-day Kinshasa in the Democratic Republic of Congo). Leopoldville became the cauldron in which the pandemic slowly cooked over the next decades.[5] In the early 1960s, following the end of the Belgian colonial government, the HIV virus was carried from the Congo to Haiti—most likely via Haitians returning from Africa after working for the colonial government. Around 1970, a single infected person or a container from a plasma-donation clinic brought the AIDS virus from Haiti to the U.S. and from the States to Europe.

Gaëtan Dugas certainly contributed to the spread of AIDS. But he was not patient zero. The HIV virus was already in North America when he contracted AIDS. AIDS had smoldered virtually unnoticed for more than 50 years in Africa before one strain passed into Western countries via Haiti, while other strains were carried from Africa to Asia and beyond. By 2014, the HIV virus had infected almost 78 million people.[6]

*   *   *

The recent Ebola epidemic in West Africa also began with an animal. In late December 2013, a two-year-old named Emile Ouamouno had been playing in a hollow tree, grabbing and poking insect-eating bats. Shortly afterward, he grew seriously ill and died in a small Guinean village near the great rainforest where Guinea, Liberia, and Sierra Leone come together. His family mourned the little one with all the appropriate traditional rites, including holding and kissing his corpse.[7]

There had been 22 previous Ebola outbreaks in Africa, all of which had been contained. In none did the caseload exceed 425, and there were rarely more than 50 deaths. Just months before the West Africa outbreak, experts had even declared Ebola to be a "dead-end event" because it burned out too quickly to spread very far.

But within weeks of little Emile's death, the Ebola virus that killed him had exploded into a three-country epidemic. By late 2015, it had infected nearly 30,000 people, killed more than 11,000, and touched people in Africa, Britain, France, Germany, Italy, the Netherlands, Norway, Spain, Switzerland, and the U.S.[8] The conventional wisdom about Ebola had proven fatally wrong.

*   *   *

These three stories of devastating sickness—and others that I draw into this book—illustrate how murderous diseases erupt when a microbe jumps species from animals to humans, as in the cases of plague, AIDS, influenza, and Ebola, and then spread from human to human. The majority of new infectious diseases with pandemic potential actually result from these animal-to-human species jumps. Infectious-disease outbreaks also happen whenever humans are exposed to a virus, bacteria, or other microbe against which they have little or no immunity—just as Europeans, who had long endured smallpox, introduced the disease to the indigenous populations of the New World, very nearly exterminating them. Outbreaks also occur when a microbe to which humans have developed immunity mutates, as often happens with influenza.

A Gigantic Threat

Somewhere out there a dangerous virus is boiling up in the bloodstream of a bird, bat, monkey, or pig, preparing to jump to a human being. It's hard to comprehend the scope of such a threat, for it has the potential to wipe out millions of us, including my family and yours, over a matter of weeks or months. The risk makes the threat posed by ISIS (Islamic State in Iraq and Syria), a ground war, a massive climate event, or even the dropping of a nuclear bomb on a major city pale by comparison.

A new epidemic could turn into a pandemic without warning. (For definitional purposes, an "outbreak" refers to a localized epidemic—something that affects hundreds, sometimes thousands; an "epidemic" refers to an illness or infection that is in excess of normal; and a "pandemic" is an epidemic that occurs over a very wide area, crosses international boundaries, and touches thousands or millions.) It could be born in a factory farm in Minnesota, a poultry farm in China, or the bat-inhabited elephant caves of Kenya—any place where infected animals are in contact with humans. It could be a variation of the 1918 Spanish flu, one of hundreds of other known microbial threats, or something entirely new, like the 2003 SARS virus that spread globally from China. Once transmitted to a human, an airborne virus could pass from that one infected individual to 25,000 others within a week, and to more than 700,000 within the first month. Within three months it could spread to every major urban center in the world. And by six months, it could infect more than 300 million people and kill more than 30 million.

This is not alarmist science fiction or tabloid fearmongering. It is one of several highly plausible scenarios—and far from the worst—developed by infectious-disease specialists working with disease-modeling experts. Just ask Bill Gates, who funds a group that uses computer simulations to predict the spread of diseases. In an interview with *Vox*, Gates said, "The Ebola epidemic showed me that we are not ready for a serious epidemic, an epidemic that would be more infectious and would spread faster than Ebola did. This is the greatest risk of a huge tragedy. This is the most likely thing by far to kill over 10 million people in a year." He put the likelihood of a catastrophic epidemic at "well over 50 percent" in his lifetime. Gates's model estimates that a perilous virus, carried via cars, planes, ships, and trains, and spreading quickly in packed cities, could kill up to 33 million people in just over 200 days.[9] Some experts put the potential first-year death rate at over 300 million people. To imagine what such a catastrophe would look like, imagine what happened in Philadelphia in 1918 occurring again, on a much larger scale, throughout the world. We would be in a world where scrappy, ravaged survivors struggle for life in a zombie-movie wasteland.

In the last century alone, smallpox killed 300 to 500 million people. The 1918 Spanish flu killed 50 to 100 million in a two-year period, and AIDS has taken 40 million lives since it was first recognized in 1981. The annual influenza outbreak still claims half a million people a year worldwide. The West African Ebola crisis took more than 11,000 lives—seven times the total of the 22 Ebola epidemics that preceded it. But widespread death isn't the only threat. For those who survive the initial infection, an epidemic leaves its own particular trail of disfigurement and disability. People who contracted small-pox suffered characteristic, sometimes horrific, scars along with blindness, limb deformities, and other disabilities. As a lifelong condition, AIDS and the side effects of treatment can affect nearly every body system from brain to bone.

In the early stages of a new epidemic—before it has been recognized or how it spreads has been determined, and before appropriate protection measures are in place—health workers die in high numbers. This was certainly true in the early phases of Spanish flu, AIDS, SARS, and Ebola. As with war, where common illness can take more lives than war injuries, epidemics sometimes take more lives from disruption of primary health care than from the epidemic itself. Because health workers are diverted to emergency response centers and health facilities are sometimes closed, epidemics can also disrupt routine public healthcare needs such as immunization, treatment of acute illness, and facility-based births.

Finally, there is the stunning financial and economic cost of epidemics to households, communities, businesses, and entire countries. As I show in chapter 5, such a pandemic could cause a global stock market crash that obliterates the livelihoods and savings of millions of survivors. "A severe and prolonged global pandemic could ... hit global GDP by as much as 5-10 percent in the first year," noted the authors of the Bank of America/Merrill Lynch 2014 Global Pandemics Primer report.[10] The World Travel & Tourism Council/ Oxford Economics has suggested that the cost of a global pandemic scenario, including spillover across industry sectors, could be as great as $3.5 trillion—an impact far greater than the magnitude of the great financial crisis of 2008.[11]

Every year, the world spends more than $50 billion controlling epidemics like avian influenza, HIV/AIDS, malaria, and polio, and responding to new threats like Ebola. In addition to the direct cost of preparedness, immunization, and emergency response, there's the indirect cost of disruption in travel, transportation of goods, tourism, financial markets, and other areas of economic activity. Wherever it has been measured, this indirect economic impact is at least equal to and usually greater than the direct cost, bringing the total cost of infectious-disease epidemics close to $100 billion per year. In short: even in the absence of Bill Gates's imagined pandemic, we can expect to spend $1 trillion on epidemics over the next decade unless we fundamentally change course.

Scientists don't know which microbe it will be, where it will come from, or whether it will be transmitted through the air, by touch, through body fluids, or through a combination of routes, but they do know that epidemics behave a bit like earthquakes. Scientists know that a "big one" is coming because scores of new, smaller earthquakes pop up around the globe every year. Some say the next pandemic is overdue. Thankfully, most epidemics are stopped in their tracks by public-health rapid-response teams.

*   *   *

I write this book not just because I'm scared. I'm also furious. Many leaders, economists, and scientists believe that the risk of potentially devastating epidemics could be prevented for a fraction of the cost of battling an out-of-control global pandemic. Despite tremendous advances in science and public health, and our success fighting many epidemics, we have been unable to keep small outbreaks from erupting into something much more devastating. The obvious question is this: *Why aren't we deploying absolutely everything we have to make sure that the next disease outbreak doesn't turn into a global catastrophe?*

The answer is depressingly simple. Rather than grappling with the threat directly, we hide behind our biases. Small infectious-disease outbreaks explode into global pandemics through human action or inaction. We human beings are too often victims of our own psychological, political, and sociological failures. Since the earliest times, the human failings that have stopped or delayed effective prevention and response include:

> **Fear:** We are all afraid of death. We respond to the fear of epidemic
> disease by wanting to blame someone else. Anytime a threat
> arises, we want to blame the "other," those not like "us." At the
> outbreak of the 1918 Spanish flu, Americans blamed "the Hun."
> AIDS was blamed on gay men. We want to punish those with
> the disease, pretending that whatever makes them other has
> cursed them. The most contagious behavioral reaction that af-
> fects political leaders, businesspeople, and the public is panic
> that disproportionately exceeds the actual event. Scared people
> overpersonalize the news, and their worries increase. Fear is a

warning system intended to alert us to impending danger, just as it is in animals. When we let it override our rationality, we make things much worse.

Denial, complacency, and hubris: We humans are fantastically arrogant. When we can't believe the evidence before our eyes, we dodge into all kinds of coping behaviors that support our personal worldviews. We choose to believe—or at least pretend—that a problem staring us in the face either isn't happening or will never happen here or to us. (Denial has a more specific psychological name: "normalcy bias.") Just as the people of Europe stood frozen during the Nazi takeover and the people of Philadelphia ignored warning signals of flu from Europe and Boston in 1918, many of us never take preventive action even as the worst is unfurling. Denial often starts at the top, with political leaders or public-health officials who reject the reality before them. Ironically, denial undermines the very trust needed to combat an epidemic. And complacency sets in when the last epidemic passes. We think, "Whew, that one missed me!" Related to complacency, hubris (the ancient Greek word for "pride") is the arrogant belief that we know how to handle a disease when we don't; that we'll have the silver-bullet vaccine in time; that technology will save us, so we don't need to spend time and money on basic prevention.

Financial self-interest: How many vaccines never get developed because poor people can't pay for the drugs that pharmaceutical companies could develop? How many times do governments and leaders plead that there is no budget for preparedness? How many disease-fostering agribusiness companies line the pockets of politicians who conveniently overlook the threats bubbling up from factory farm sewage? Greed is the bottom line, and when it comes to exchanging dollars for human lives, greed is unforgivable.

Unless we understand how we can respond more intelligently to disease outbreaks and do everything we can to rally scientists, healthcare workers, leaders of all stripes, and the general public, human beings everywhere are just sitting ducks. Failing to recognize our human failings—and to do everything we can in spite of them to prevent a potentially staggering loss of life and livelihood—would be not just irresponsible, but criminal.

Hope from The Power of Seven

How can we end epidemics? In this book, I ask you to join me in understanding the story of smallpox eradication, the continuing risk of pandemic influenza, the human and economic catastrophe of AIDS, the rapid containment of SARS, and the disastrous, perfect storm of the initial response to Ebola in West Africa. Some stories have very happy endings; others don't. What emerges is a picture of, yes, microbial villains that have inflicted on humans disfigurement, blindness, lasting misery, and death. But I also show how heroic men and women have overcome both microbial killers and human failure to succeed against overwhelming odds.

Specifically, I reveal how The Power of Seven—seven essential sets of actions—can end epidemics forever. You will learn about important acts of courage that demonstrate The Power of Seven, proving that we actually *can* prevent major epidemics. You will learn how, for less than $1 per year for every person on the planet (spent on the right things), we could prevent the next local disease outbreak from turning into Bill Gates's feared global pandemic. That's less than half of what Americans alone spend on video games each year and a small fraction of Bill Gates's net worth. It's far less than the current annual cost of dealing with AIDS, an epidemic the world allowed to spin out of control by people who slept in denial through its first decade. And it's nothing compared to what a pandemic would cost the world in emergency response and economic disruption. Those investment funds would support innovation for prevention, strengthen developing countries' health systems for epidemic control, and support emergency response to ensure that microbial invaders never arrive at the gates.

The Power of Seven emerged from a three-step process. First, I conducted in-depth analyses of five epidemics: smallpox, influenza, AIDS, SARS, and Ebola. I chose these five diseases because together they killed more than half a billion people in the last 100 years and because they reflect different types of epidemics. (An online appendix at www.endofepidemics.com describes the major outbreaks, characteristics, clinical illness, prevention, and treatment for each disease.)

Second, through interviews, lectures, and publications, I mined the expertise of scores of policymakers, political leaders, public-health experts, research scientists, field epidemiologists, and frontline workers. In the process of researching this book, I've asked everyone from African village chiefs to the head of the World Health Organization (WHO): How can we work together individually and together to prevent the next epidemic from ever happening? In short, how can we make the last epidemic the world's *very last* epidemic?

Finally, I put all this information together into The Power of Seven, a big call to action on seven levels:

1. *Lead Like the House Is on Fire.* In the face of an epidemic, what does public-health leadership look like? Just as firefighters race into the burning building, those responsible for protecting public health need to act rapidly, decisively, and on the basis of scientific evidence, not political interests. Leaders at the highest level must put the public good above parochial interests. If we are to end epidemics, presidents, prime ministers, and community leaders around the globe must pledge themselves and their countries to achieving this goal.

2. *Resilient Systems, Global Security.* Strong national public-health systems are the foundations for prevention and preparedness. National governments, the private sector, communities, and faith-based organizations have been enormously successful when they work in concert to fight disease. Robust international agencies and nongovernmental organizations are essential to support even the poorest countries in mounting successful defenses.

3. *Active Prevention, Constant Readiness.* Major epidemics can be stopped by active prevention through healthy self-care habits, immunization, and fighting mosquitoes; early detection of disease through surveillance at all levels; and rapid response to treat the sick, prevent the spread, and maintain routine health services.

4. *Fatal Fictions, Timely Truths.* In the face of an epidemic, terror, blame, rumors and conspiracy theories, distrust of authorities, and panic can take hold simultaneously. This is why establishing and maintaining trust through honest, clear communication at the local level is paramount. History continues to show us that health communication lies at the heart of epidemic control. Fighting rumor with truth is a job for professional communication teams working with local and national governments, international agencies, communities, print and broadcast media, and social media.

5. *Disruptive Innovation, Collaborative Transformation.* We also need to do everything we can to support the work of scientists who are applying breakthrough techniques to identify new viruses and prevent them from jumping to people, and we must help those who are working to nip outbreaks in the bud. We can't keep doing the same old things. We need to do better research and development to diagnose illness quickly and treat it immediately. We must discover new vaccines, make more of them, and figure out better distribution strategies.

6. *Invest Wisely, Save Lives.* A severe worldwide pandemic could cost the global economy up to $2.5 trillion alone in disruptions to travel, tourism, trade, financial institutions, employment, and entire supply chains. But an ounce of prevention, in terms of dollars, is truly worth a pound of cure when it comes to stopping epidemics. By investing an average of just $7.5 billion more annually for the next 20 years ($1 per person per year for every person on the planet) in the right preventive and response measures at the right times, we can substantially reduce the chance of epidemics and more than repay ourselves in savings.

7. *Ring the Alarm, Rouse the Leaders* with local, national, and international voices that track capacity, performance, and resources. This is a job for citizens and concerned stakeholders. We achieve progress through a combination of good science, strong leadership, and committed advocacy to keep the bell ringing and the spotlight on.

The Power of Seven

Catastrophic epidemics can be stopped with seven sets of concrete actions.

	Lead Like the House Is on Fire	When leaders work with urgency, decisiveness, and courage, they can defeat the deadliest viral enemies.
	Resilient Systems, Global Security	Strong national public health systems and robust international agencies can ensure health security for all.
	Active Prevention, Constant Readiness	Vaccines, mosquito control, and other measures will stop killer diseases before they spread, and constant readiness will save lives.
	Fatal Fictions, Timely Truths	Trustworthy communications, close listening, and local engagement are the best weapons for fighting disease and quelling rumors, blame, distrust, and panic.
	Disruptive Innovation, Collaborative Transformation	Breakthrough innovations bring new tools for preventing, controlling, and eliminating infectious-disease threats.
	Invest Wisely, Save Lives	Just $1 per year for every person on the planet will save lives and pay for itself in lower emergency costs and reduced economic disruption.
	Ring the Alarm, Rouse the Leaders	Citizen activists and social movements must mobilize the public and hold leaders' feet to the fire.

SOURCE: Authors.

Imagine the Impossible: Then Make It Happen

"Plagues are as certain as death and taxes." That was the shrugging assertion of the prestigious *British Medical Journal* in a March 2003 editorial about the SARS epidemic when the outbreak was at its peak. Even Louis Pasteur once noted, "The microbes always have the last word."

The prospect of a new global epidemic is extraordinarily frightening. However, this book is ultimately about hope. It contains the stories of many heroes, past and present, who have succeeded in their fights to stop the spread of illness and death. And it shows exactly how, by taking seven sets of decisive actions, we *can* prevent and end epidemics in the future.

I have no doubt that we can achieve this seemingly impossible goal. Why am I so convinced? Because I have seen what happens when visionary leaders imagine the impossible and then make it happen. Consider AIDS: in 2000, the epidemic was fast becoming a manageable chronic disease in the Northern Hemisphere, with dramatically reduced mortality rates and rapidly increasing life expectancy for HIV-positive people. Yet AIDS remained a death sentence in Africa, as in most low-income regions. Within a decade, however, large-scale, widespread prevention efforts stemmed the tide of new infections, and the number of people in Africa on treatment increased 100-fold, from fewer than 50,000 in 2000 to more than 5 million by 2010.

If in January 2000 you had described to the global health community the progress that occurred over the next decade, many would also have said, "Impossible. Not in the world I know." One of the nonbelievers was Andrew Natsios, then head of the U.S. Agency for International Development. He opposed U.S. support for treatment scale-up, actually arguing that the treatment regimens were too complex for people in Africa living with AIDS because they weren't familiar with clocks, and therefore they would not remember when to take their medicine.[12] The barriers to AIDS treatment included the exorbitant price (more than $10,000 per person per year for medicines alone), woefully inadequate funding, scarce diagnostics facilities, and lack of systems for large-scale treatment.

I vividly remember the debates we had among global health professionals about AIDS treatment in the year 2000 and the sense of achievement we felt in 2010. During that decade, the unthinkable became reality before our eyes. A determined group of activists, people living with HIV/AIDS, health officials, and political leaders, built a global movement that proved Natsios and the other naysayers wrong by successfully overcoming each barrier to build the largest public-health treatment program in history. That experience transformed my understanding of the word "impossible" and what we can do to stop epidemics.

In short, I refuse to accept that the inevitable local disease outbreaks will continue to explode into epidemics that kill thousands or millions. If we can eradicate smallpox, mount the largest public-health treatment effort in history as we did for AIDS, stop SARS in its tracks, and stop hundreds of outbreaks every year, then surely we can use The Power of Seven to end devastating epidemics.

This book is mostly about the helpful actions we can take. But like Dante's Virgil, I first have to lead you through the inferno of sickness before we can arrive at those happier gates. To understand what we're up against, let's take a good, hard look at who the real viral and human enemies are in the following three chapters.

CHAPTER 2

THE BUSH—LESSONS FROM EBOLA, AIDS, AND ZIKA

How deforestation, climate change, and population movement are turning wildlife into pandemic incubators.

We humans like to think that we're special, but to a killer virus we are just the same as a bat or a baboon. A virus such as AIDS that once hid in the bloodstream of a jungle beast can swiftly explode into an unconquerable pandemic, killing millions around the world. When a human eats or is bitten by a disease-carrying creature, a virus like SARS, Ebola, or Zika gains a foothold. Our own selfish behavior raises the risk at every turn. The Brazilian farmer who burns a forest to make way for cattle invites disease closer. And all of us who greedily warm the planet through our consumption of fossil fuels make it easier for disease-carrying creatures like mosquitoes to thrive.

My wife, three daughters, and I have snacked on eel in Indonesia and roasted gazelle, crocodile stew, barbequed ostrich, and crunchy, dried mopane worms in Africa. That's only the stuff I can name. In our journeys around the world, we've probably consumed plenty of other unidentified creatures as well. I shudder to think about it. Without the help of immunizations against cholera, hepatitis, rabies, typhoid, yellow fever, and meningitis, our immune systems probably wouldn't have fought off disease. Any or all of us might have grown very sick or even died from eating strange stuff.

If you live in one of the poorer locations on the planet, your risk of picking up a viral disease is much higher than it is in the U.S. or Europe, not only because of lack of access to good health care but also because desperately poor people need to consume whatever animal protein they can find. When a wild animal is killed, the creature's infected blood or feces can pass to a human with devastating effects. And no wonder: blood is a hospitable home for a new virus, and human blood is the same wonderful, nourishing bath as that flowing in the veins of a bat or a baboon.

Mammals of all kinds are a happy host for zoonotic pathogens. Since the year 2000, 75 percent of new human infectious diseases have originated in animals, the majority of these from wildlife. Bacteria such as bubonic plague can hide out for a century or more in the fleas that infest the prairie dogs in New Mexico. Lyme disease flourishes within a mouse or a deer waiting to be transported by ticks to humans. The Ebola and Zika viruses float around in the bloodstream of monkeys. These viruses often kill animals, but people don't pay much attention until the bug jumps to humans through infected animal meat or biting vectors like fleas, ticks, or mosquitoes. Eventually, if enough people sicken and die, we begin to pay attention, but typically too late.

The Ebola, AIDS, and Zika epidemics have much to teach us about the ways viruses from the African jungle—combined with human lassitude, denial, and ignorance—can unleash hell on an unprepared world.

The Bat Plague: Ebola

In the poor villages of the steamy, massive West African rainforest, you can't sit down in a restaurant and order a juicy, USDA-inspected filet mignon. You're lucky to get chicken or goat stew. But there isn't much of that kind of meat to go around, so the next-best source of animal protein is bushmeat. If you're lucky, you can occasionally bag monkeys or squirrels; otherwise, you can hunt down a colony of bats that have migrated from deep parts of the jungle. You can chop up the bat meat, mix it with some root vegetables, and stir it into a spicy stew. Otherwise, you can pick up bat meat from a market vendor who roasts the animal over an open fire, the smell of the meat mingling with that of burnt fur.[1]

Like most remote African jungle outposts, the tiny village of Meliandou in the forest region of southern Guinea is a good place for hunting bushmeat, including free-tailed bats nearly as big as crows. The camel-colored creatures group in a gigantic tree close to the river where the women of the village wash clothes. Children love to play in the massively curved roots of the tree that forms a generous, hollowed-out cave.

When two-year-old Emile Ouamouno grabbed or poked a dead bat from the tree, a few particles of blood or guano probably landed on his hands, and, as toddlers do, he put his fingers in his mouth.[2] Soon afterward, the little boy grew agonizingly ill. He developed a very high fever and a sore throat. He couldn't stop vomiting; his stool was black and runny. His pregnant mother took him to his grandmother's house, where Emile grew sicker. His sweat, vomit, blood, and feces distributed his germs to his caretakers. Within a few days, he bled internally and went into septic shock. His internal organs shut down. Then he died.[3] Emile's family followed the sacred burial custom of washing, touching, and kissing the child's corpse. An improper burial, they believed, would cause Emile's spirit to bring harm and illness to the family.[4]

But harm and illness visited them anyway. Emile's body was full of the killer Ebola virus, and a corpse carries an even more massive viral load than does a living person.[5] Emile's three-year-old sister, his pregnant mother, and his grandmother died within a matter of days. More dominoes began to fall. The virus's incubation period of a few weeks, in which symptoms lie dormant, was long enough to allow it to spread to anyone who'd touched Emile's family members. Within a month, hospitals in the area began reporting clusters of a disease that looked a lot like cholera, malaria, or Lassa fever, although the Ebola virus was no stranger to West Africa. Unaware that the virus was present in their region, local doctors and health workers missed the diagnosis. It wasn't until mid-March, three months into the outbreak, that medical investigators at the Geneva offices of Médecins Sans Frontières (MSF or, in English, Doctors Without Borders) realized that they were looking at a deadly strain of Ebola.

As the disease spread from Guinea to Liberia and Sierra Leone, health authorities were completely unprepared to deal with the onslaught. This was hardly surprising: after years of civil war, health systems in West Africa were decimated. Even on good days, keeping up with comparatively routine work such as treating malaria victims or helping birthing mothers was a challenge. The number of those sick with Ebola quickly overwhelmed brave healthcare workers from around the world. The work was wearying and endless. There was no treatment for the suffering other than to isolate and hydrate patients in the hope that their immune systems were strong enough to fight the disease. To the health workers, it must have felt like working in hell. Caregivers had to wear hot, plastic hazmat suits in the burning African sun, in which they themselves could quickly become dehydrated, making them more vulnerable to disease. It was worse than being in a war, some said.[6] One worker called it "a scene out of Dante."[7]

Joanne Liu, the passionate, French-Canadian pediatrician and international president of MSF, sent an urgent warning to WHO in April 2014. "When I had my first encounter with [WHO head] Margaret Chan, I said, 'Something needs to happen! We're very worried!' But she told us she was not that pessimistic." Throughout April and May, a lull in cases occurred because sick people were in hiding.[8] By June, MSF was overwhelmed. A Belgian newspaper published a story about the mayhem; social media picked it up.

It took another four months before WHO declared an international health emergency—a full eight months after Emile died.[9] Meanwhile, the World Bank made early, large financial commitments to the Ebola response, but its own systems proved too cumbersome to move the funds quickly and effectively.[10] Donor countries—the U.S., the U.K., and France—only sent their financial and scientific resources to help the individual countries, fragmenting a bigger, broader response.

By mid-June 2014, MSF doctors declared that the disease was totally out of control. So many health workers perished that in some places there was nobody to care for the infected. Every day, MSF doctors and volunteers drove into the villages in an effort to try to collect the sick people and bring them to the isolation centers, strange-looking places surrounded by waist-high orange plastic fencing and housed under white tarpaulins. But the villagers feared going to the hospital in the belief that they might catch the disease there or that MSF doctors were stealing their blood and harvesting their organs.[11] The healthcare workers in their frightening, head-to-toe plastic suits could issue reassuring sounds to their patients, but, with only their eyes visible, they looked as frightening and threatening as space aliens. No wonder that villagers hid from them. More rumors flew: people calling in to a hotline believed the outbreak had been fomented by Guinea's president in an effort to delay elections. One spiritual guide said the epidemic was due to the death of a white snake.[12]

*   *   *

The U.S., too, was unprepared, but it was only when the disease came to the country that the rest of the world woke up to the crisis. In August 2014, two American health workers returned to the U.S. and were treated at Emory University.[13]

A month later, Thomas Duncan, a 45-year-old personal driver from Liberia, boarded a plane for Brussels en route to Dallas, Texas, to visit his partner and their five children. Within ten days, Duncan began running a 100-plus-degree fever. He had a runny nose and some sharp abdominal pain. He didn't have a doctor or health insurance, so he did what most everyone in his situation does— he checked into the emergency room at the closest hospital, where he spent five long hours as a "Dallas resident," according to the intake information.[14]

Other than the fever, Duncan's vital signs were "unremarkable." He was given a diagnosis of sinusitis, acetaminophen to lower the fever, a prescription for antibiotics, and shown the door. When he came back a few days later, some observant health worker brought up a previously unnoted item about his travel history: Duncan had come from Monrovia, Liberia, a place where a particularly gruesome, deadly disease was raging. Finally, he was tested for Ebola.[15]

Within hours of the test, Duncan was vomiting explosively. His virus-laden blood and diarrhea-covered garments and medical materials were handled via the regular hospital system. Soon after his diagnosis was confirmed, two of the nurses who had cared for him contracted the virus. After word got out, the head of the Centers for Disease Control and Prevention, the chief executive at Texas Health Presbyterian Hospital in Dallas, and Rick Perry, the governor of Texas, each reassured the public there was no need to worry about the spread of Ebola. "Our system is working as it should," Perry crowed.[16]

But obviously, it wasn't.

Thomas Duncan's subsequent death and its aftermath unleashed considerable vitriol toward these public figures. "I thought America had this!" ranted the comedian and commentator Bill Maher. "One guy comes here from Liberia. One guy! And we couldn't keep [the disease] contained because those morons in that f—ing hospital in Dallas. . . . What could go wrong? This!"[17]

As shocking as the situation was to Bill Maher, it was entirely and sadly predictable. The West African epidemic proved to be a perfect storm of failure in preparedness and response. The conventional wisdom about Ebola had proven fatally wrong. The rapid spread through several countries in West Africa and the unfortunate events at Texas Health Presbyterian Hospital in Dallas showed how this outbreak was different.

The AIDS Explosion

In the opening scene of the 1993 movie *And the Band Played On*, a convoy of muddy trucks rolls through a monsoon rain. The mud on the jungle road is several inches deep. The drivers can barely see out the filthy windows. The first truck, emblazoned with the laurel-leaf blue seal of the World Health Organization, pulls up to a field hospital, a long building with a corrugated tin roof. Before exiting the truck, two doctors in blue hospital gowns and gloves strap on gas masks. They walk into the building and look around. The place is deserted and everything looks awry, as if the building has been robbed.

A young boy appears in the doorway. The doctors take off their masks and smile at him. "Where's the doctor in charge?" they ask in a friendly way.

"Doctor," says the boy. "Yes. I take you."

They follow the boy from the building. The boy points to a row of corpses lying on the ground.

"Doctor," the boy says, pointing to the dead white man.

One of the visitors hears the sound of groaning and follows it into a hut where a woman lies dying on the floor. When he comes closer, she grabs his arm, babbling, and vomits blood onto his hand.

Later, the two doctors burn all the corpses. As one of them stares at the flames, words appear on the screen: *"The Ebola fever outbreak was contained before it could reach the outside world. It was not AIDS. But it was a warning of things to come."*

And the Band Played On was based on a book of the same name by *San Francisco Chronicle* reporter Randy Shilts. The irony in the opening scene is deep from a contemporary perspective—the warning on the screen pertained not just to AIDS but to the future Ebola epidemic that would devastate West Africa in 2014. Both the book and the film offer brutal portraits of confusion, fear, denial, and indifference in the face of the catastrophic AIDS epidemic that resulted in millions of needless deaths. The book was published in 1987, seven years after AIDS began decimating gay communities in the United States. The movie came out a decade before Ebola's next terrible version reached the outside world.

Like Ebola, HIV also sprang from intimate contact with a jungle animal. Scientists think it jumped from chimpanzees to humans in the early part of the twentieth century, most likely when a hunter in Cameroon slaughtered a chimp for food.[18] While the hunter was wielding his knife, he probably cut his own skin and the animal's blood got into the hunter's bloodstream.[19] The hunter infected his wife and family. The virus he contracted was not just the most deadly new virus of the twentieth century, it was also the first new human pandemic pathogen to appear in at least a thousand years. It ranks with a small number of diseases that are so virulent that, left untreated, they are 100 percent fatal. By 2015, AIDS had infected nearly 80 million people worldwide and killed nearly 40 million of them, leaving waves of survivors and orphans in its wake.

Was the AIDS epidemic inevitable? Some AIDS experts (and a number of my colleagues) would say yes, because the HIV virus, all by itself, is one of the most awesome viral geniuses ever observed. It's highly adept at evading the body's immune system, a secretive characteristic that has completely stymied development of an AIDS vaccine for more than 30 years. Unlike smallpox or Ebola, whose symptoms become clear in pretty short order, HIV takes a long time to turn into AIDS. Symptoms typically begin with a mild fever and sore throat that start within weeks of becoming infected and quickly pass. The virus hides out in the bloodstream, doing its dirty work, for more than a decade before clinical signs of AIDS appear. Throughout this period, the infected individual can transmit the virus through unprotected sex, dirty needles, and via blood from a pregnant mother to a fetus. When it turns into full-blown AIDS, it destroys the body's immune system, rendering virtually every part of the body vulnerable to opportunistic cancers or infections.

In the 1970s, many years after the first human infection in Africa, AIDS first began sickening San Francisco's gay men. The virus wasn't discovered until the early 1980s, when a cluster of men in San Francisco suddenly came down with a variety of strange symptoms including swollen lymph nodes, rashes, sores, skin cancer, pneumonia, and wasting fevers; the disease was initially called GRID (Gay Related Immune Deficiency). By 1981, it was clear that one of the most mysterious and awful diseases the international medical community had ever known had been unleashed, and it had rolled a gravestone over what had been a rainbow-happy celebration of sexual freedom.

The story of AIDS is long, complex, and unutterably tragic. AIDS spread because of three tenaciously intractable human behaviors: sex, injectable drugs, and especially the politics and ideology that took precedence over public health (a topic I will explore in more depth in a later chapter). For public-health professionals, AIDS has been a long war on both the individual and collective fronts. As Michael Hobbes of the *New Republic* observed, "Just as the AIDS virus seems almost designed to perfectly exploit the weaknesses of the human immune system, treating it seems designed to exploit the weaknesses of our national health systems."[20]

From the earliest days of the epidemic, conservatives in the U.S. demonized and stigmatized those with AIDS, resisting preventive measures such as condom use and clean-needle programs. Even today, needle exchanges are banned in almost every state in the southern U.S., where the AIDS epidemic is now concentrated and HIV infection rates are ten times higher than in other parts of the country.[21] At the same time, in the early years of the epidemic, liberals and gays also fueled the epidemic by opposing proven public-health practices such as testing, case finding, and telling public-health authorities the identities of their partners.[22] In contrast to the U.S. dynamics, Australia's conservative government put science first and quickly enacted sound public-health practices.

AIDS and the Blood Curse

But AIDS, which is passed through bodily fluids including blood, semen, vaginal fluids, and breast milk, didn't just attack gay men and heroin addicts. Soon after President Ronald Reagan was elected, scientists noted that the so-called GRID also attacked women, babies, and hemophiliacs. The hemophilia story offers a particularly tragic case study of human culpability.

Hemophiliacs (nearly all of whom are male) can quickly die of blood loss; a razor nick can kill them because their blood doesn't clot. To survive, hemophiliacs need to receive blood proteins called "clotting factors" that control bleeding through blood transfusions. Making the clotting factor requires taking blood plasma from thousands of people and combining it to extract the material.

Blood is a big business, despite its lifesaving, feel-good aspect. Blood banks made (and still make) a lot of money from generous plasma donors. The banks sell the blood to hospitals, and the patient's insurance (or the patient) pays for it. Blood is also a source of income for poor donors who sell it to the banks. Back in 1981, a pint of blood could buy a sexually active junkie a decent meal and maybe even a flea-ridden room in San Francisco's Tenderloin district. (Dr. Jacques Pépin, an infectious-disease specialist at the University of Sherbrooke in Quebec, also hypothesizes that AIDS might have been unwittingly spread by Haitians who were hired by the UN to teach Africans in the Congo. Pépin thinks that in 1966, a Haitian with AIDS gave or received blood through a Haitian plasma center with poor hygiene standards. That center exported 1,600 gallons of plasma to the U.S. every month.[23])

Among the victims was a teenager named Ryan White, one of the first hemophiliacs to be diagnosed with HIV following a blood transfusion. He quickly became a scapegoat for frightened, ignorant people. Ryan endured terrible discrimination before he died at the age of 18 in 1990. "People were really cruel," his mother wrote. "People said that he had to be gay, that he had to have done something bad or wrong, or he wouldn't have had it. It was God's punishment. . . . That somehow, some way he had done something he shouldn't have done or he wouldn't have gotten AIDS."[24]

The real-life protagonist of *And the Band Played On* (played by the actor Matthew Modine in the movie) is a sandy-haired, compassionate yet angry 74-year-old named Dr. Don Francis. Francis is the founder of a San Francisco–based organization called Global Solutions for Infectious Diseases (GSID), which works to develop vaccines. A former pediatrician and epidemiologist who spent 21 years working at the U.S. Centers for Disease Control and Prevention (CDC), he was in fact a member of the WHO team that investigated an African outbreak of Ebola in the 1970s. Francis was among a group of CDC doctors and scientists who attempted to draw attention to the tainted blood problem.

Since time immemorial, killer diseases have always been signifiers of an "otherness" and cultural curse. This cultural bias has played out starkly in the age of AIDS. In the Reagan era, the "just-say-no" political establishment saw gays and IV drug users as "icky" and unworthy of discussion, let alone treatment.[25]

Francis recalls that despite the CDC's pleas, the Reagan administration directed its health policy people *not* to ask about where blood came from. This immoral and inhumane refusal to face scientific facts filtered down to the blood banks. Since blood donors weren't screened for their sexual or drug history before 1985, the HIV virus infected the clotting factor. "A better way to transmit an infectious agent than that would be difficult—that is, you take thousands of people, put them into a bottle, and then send that out and inject it into other people with a needle," Francis told PBS's *Frontline*.[26]

As a result, thousands of hemophiliacs and transfusion recipients around the world—in Japan, the Middle East, Europe, Canada, and the U.S.—received infected blood. In January 1983, Francis's group presented their data to the blood banks and described how the banks could avoid infecting patients. The blood bankers "obstructed it from the get-go," Francis recalled. "It was as frustrating a [meeting] as I've ever been in." He pounded on the table and yelled at them, asking how many people they wanted to kill. "If it's five now, instead of having another meeting of this kind, I just said: 'Just tell us the number. You want 10 dead? You want 20 dead? You want 100 dead? Then we'll make these [recommendations]. We can make the recommendations today, and then you can just count the cases.' That didn't go down very well."[27]

Francis was, and remains, furious with the Reagan administration's failures to respond to the national and international AIDS crisis. In his view, their political nearsightedness cost millions around the world their lives, millions of others their health, and millions of children their parents. The dead include well-known people such as the science fiction writer Isaac Asimov; the actor Rock Hudson; tennis pro Arthur Ashe; dancer Rudolph Nureyev; the French philosopher Michel Foucault; musicians Tom Fogerty and Liberace; and Randy Shilts, the author of *And the Band Played On*.

Zika: Mosquitoes Crossing Continents

When Guilherme Amorim was born in Ipojuca, Brazil, his parents, Germana Soares and her husband Glecion, were elated. The little boy appeared to be very healthy, and friends and relatives in the waiting room celebrated with dancing. But then a nurse measured Guilherme's head. It was 32 centimeters—much smaller than it should have been.[28] He was diagnosed with a condition called microcephaly, which manifests as an abnormally small head size and cognitive disorders in infants.

As I was beginning to write this book, a virus first identified in African rhesus monkeys was cursing mothers and children in the Western Hemisphere, in the urban slums of equatorial Brazil. Zika is spread by the bite of the *Aedes aegypti* mosquito, which also carries yellow fever, West Nile virus, and dengue fever. The first human cases of the infection were discovered in 1952 in Uganda and Tanzania.[29] Though Zika was common in Africa and Asia, it only reached the Western Hemisphere in May 2015, probably by way of Polynesia.[30]

While not as deadly as Ebola or AIDS—the vast majority of people who have it experience no symptoms—Zika is alarming nonetheless because it leads to a neurologic condition in the infected person called Guillain-Barré syndrome and microcephaly in developing fetuses. Because people in the Western Hemisphere aren't generally immune to Zika, the pregnant women of the Western tropics were in special danger of having babies with microcephaly.[31] By April 2017, there were more than 3,000 confirmed cases of Zika-induced microcephaly and related birth defects, including 2,650 in Brazil and nearly 100 in the U.S. and Puerto Rico.[32] There is no treatment to prevent microcephaly, and a potential vaccine against Zika is many years away.[33] Many countries in Central and South America, including Brazil, don't allow pregnant women whose babies may have the condition to abort.

The Zika threat is yet another frustrating example where researchers and health professionals have been caught flat-footed in the face of a disease, but it's not as if the medical community knew nothing about it. In fact, we've been around this particular block before. In the 1940s and 1950s, women infected with rubella (German measles) in their first trimester of pregnancy were having babies with birth defects including blindness, deafness, and, yes, microcephaly.[34] Had we been paying attention to this fact, we might have been more aware of the danger of Zika-like infections. And because most people who have Zika are asymptomatic, scientists dismissed it as trivial when it was first discovered. It was occurring in places far from Europe and America, so there wasn't a lot of research done on it. "This really goes back to funding priorities," Ken Stuart, founder and director for the Seattle-based Center for Infectious Disease Research, told National Public Radio. "Much of the funding devoted to infectious disease today is in reaction to outbreaks. Therefore, we're not generally prepared to respond quickly."[35]

If there is one thing we know for sure about epidemics, it's that the poor get hit first and hardest. Nearly 10 percent of Brazil's people live on less than two dollars a day.[36] More than half of those poor live in hot, dense, garbage-strewn urban slums. In such places, it's hard to get access to running water, so people store water in containers that attract mosquitoes. Rainwater also stagnates in potholes, tires, and trash. It's hard enough to be poor, but if you are pregnant and have little access to decent health care and you are already struggling to put food in your mouth and a roof over your head, then caring for a baby with severe cognitive problems is going to be close to impossible.[37]

Little Guilherme's parents are among those who are struggling. Glecion lost a welding job that paid well and the private insurance that went along with it. He now averages a little over $625 a month giving dune buggy rides to beachgoers. Guilherme's parents fear getting evicted from their house. Germana can't work because caring for Guilherme is a full-time job. He has muscle spasms that presage convulsions; he is likely to develop speech and hearing problems and to have difficulty learning.[38]

Unfortunately, Zika is rapidly on the move. It's spreading fast because the *Aedes aegypti* mosquito that carries it is very common and because it can be sexually transmitted. By mid-2017, the CDC reported risk of Zika in Africa, India, Central and South America, and the Caribbean.[39] By early 2017, the U.S. had experienced more than 5,200 symptomatic cases and Puerto Rico more than 35,000 cases. Every state in the U.S. from Maine to Hawaii had reported cases, with the largest numbers coming from Florida, New York, California, and Texas, reflecting travel patterns between these states and high-prevalence countries.[40]

In addition, Zika has turned into a catastrophic epidemic because the Brazilian government failed to control the mosquito population, despite the fact that the country had the world's biggest problem with dengue fever. Instead of investing in public health, Brazil's well-off decision-makers chose to pour money into infrastructure for the 2016 Summer Olympics—ironically an event that many people, including some athletes, were afraid to attend due to Zika. The failure to invest in public health is particularly tragic in the case of Zika, because the expense of caring for thousands of disabled children will be much greater than it would have cost to keep up with mosquito control. And since Brazil's oil revenues have dried up, the country is undergoing a terrible economic downturn, making the government even less able to care for Zika victims.

Bushmeat and Poverty

Dr. Nathan Wolfe is a brilliant scientist with close-cropped black hair and an intense gaze. An energetic and charismatic Harvard-educated immunologist, Wolfe is a polysyllabic academic who slaps people with facts at machine-gun speed. Wolfe speaks with the directness and velocity of an entrepreneur comfortable with giving elevator pitches to Silicon Valley venture capitalists. In his orb, you feel as if this is the last chance we all have to heed his warning before some viral bomb goes off. "If you don't get this," he's basically saying, "you, I, our kids, and everyone we know could die."

Wolfe is no conspiracy freak. He just wants to stop epidemics before they start. He does this by tracking killer diseases to their bushmeat sources in viral hotspots like Central Africa. (I'll describe his innovative work in more detail in chapter 10.) He gets the bushmeat connection and communicates its dangers brilliantly.

In 2009, Wolfe gave an impassioned speech at the TED Conference, where he showed the audience some gripping slides and film clips of jungle treks with Cameroonian bushmeat hunters. In one film clip, the TED audience sees Wolfe slashing through the jungle like Indiana Jones, tagging along with bushmeat hunters in an effort to locate an animal virus that could spark an epidemic. CNN's Anderson Cooper follows behind, asking questions as Wolfe and his African partner look for animals in set traps. Then Wolfe shows the audience a picture of a man carrying a haul of three colorful, dead monkeys on his back. "One of the things I want you to note from [the picture] is blood—you see a tremendous amount of blood contact," he says. The picture illustrates what he calls "a very intimate form of connection" from one species to another.[41]

Like mosquitoes, monkeys, and people, viruses want to stay alive. Viruses have a much better chance of survival in places where there is profound instability and intense poverty. And poverty, Wolfe insists, lies at the very root of the viral threat. In many African nations, decades of war, clear-cutting, and mining have stripped natural resources, leaving millions of people to live in extreme poverty. Women lack access to basic health care and birth control. The more babies a woman has, the poorer she is. In Africa, one in six children dies before the age of five from malnutrition and sickness. Millions of children have been orphaned by AIDS. A third of the people are underweight.[42]

At TED, Wolfe put up another slide of the same man carrying the dead monkeys, this time dressed in shredded purple rags, his hands folded as if in supplication. "Bushmeat," Wolfe told the TED audience, "is one of the central crises which is occurring in our population right now, in humanity, on this planet. But it's not the fault of the man in rags hunting bushmeat to stay alive. It's all our faults. And if we neglect this problem," Wolfe said, "we do it at our own peril."

Hot, Flat, and Crowded

Pandemics don't just happen. All kinds of complex and interconnected social, economic, and environmental risk factors contribute to the emergence and spread of disease.

Consider how just one risk factor, population growth, leads to a whole set of others. The *New York Times* columnist and author Thomas Friedman was right: the world is hot, flat, and crowded,[43] and it's getting more so. The world's human population is now more than 7.5 billion. It's projected to increase by more than two billion people by mid-century, exploding to 8.1 billion by 2025 and 9.6 billion by 2050.[44] More than half of that number will be born in Africa, and most of them will be packed into dense urban areas where an epidemic can spread like wildfire.[45]

The more people there are, the greater the demand for shelter, food, and water. Imagine that you are a poor person living in a remote part of Guinea or the Amazon jungle, and you want to do the thing that is most instinctive for all of us: to stay alive. If you are lucky enough to procure cows, goats, or chickens, you need room for a pasture. And if you need wood for fires or to build a house, you chop down the trees. But your own personal needs are nothing in comparison to the demands of agribusiness and industry, which obliterates millions of acres of forestland each year. Between 2000 and 2010, these industries annually consumed some 13 million hectares (500,000 square miles)[46]— an area roughly the size of Alaska, South Africa, or Peru.

Clear-cutting brings people in closer contact with primates, rodents, and bats that carry dangerous pathogens. Some researchers believe that ravaged tropical forests and increased human activity in countries like Liberia and Guinea presented an ideal opportunity for the Ebola virus to jump from its natural reservoir to humans.[47] Deforestation also leads to flooding, which of course attracts mosquitoes. The hotter the jungle (and the planet) becomes as a result of all this deforestation, the happier mosquitoes are. If you're living near a forest in Africa and have the leisure to be focused on more than your survival, you may have begun to notice that some amphibians and birds that hunted mosquitoes have disappeared because they are in fact extinct. Those that are not extinct may have migrated to more northerly realms that are rapidly becoming more hospitable, thanks to global climate change.[48]

Viruses such as Ebola, AIDS, and Zika aren't like fastidious plants that stay rooted in only one place. On any given day, millions of people around the world are moving around on planes, trains, boats, trucks, and automobiles, some of them from places where as-yet-undiscovered viruses are festering in the bloodstreams of wild beasts and fowls. An average of 10 million people per day take to the skies; there are 3.5 billion passenger flights each year.[49] All this creates huge opportunities for the transcontinental spread of pathogens like SARS, Ebola, or Zika. A person who has been infected in a hot zone somewhere won't feel ill for days or weeks until after the fact, not until they land in Dallas, Singapore, London, or New York. And the duration of the longest intercontinental flights is now greater than the incubation period of several common pathogens. A person may be asymptomatic when they get on a jumbo jet in Hong Kong, but by the time they land in New York, they will have spread the virus to the crew and passengers on the plane.

Of course, people can carry diseases by train, car, truck, boat, and foot, too. In the case of AIDS, the virus spread slowly at first. Then, as Africa became more urbanized and roads connected remote regions to cities, men went to the cities to look for work. Those men hooked up with infected prostitutes who spread the virus to clients.

Disease travels especially fast in West Africa, where the population is seven times more mobile than it is in other areas in the world.[50] People move around a lot to look for work or food or go to visit extended family members across borders. Also, sick people will travel to countries that have the resources to treat them when their own countries do not. One sick individual crossing a border to seek a cure could start a wave of new infections across a country that has all but succeeded in controlling an outbreak. The problem is compounded by the illegal trade of goods, animals, and people; there is often no record of who or what may have entered a country, or when or where that person or animal carrying a deadly virus might have done so, making the prevention and treatment of the disease very difficult.

Finally, we can't overlook the role of human behavior in the spread of disease. Like the proverbial butterfly whose beating wings can set off a hurricane somewhere far away, any single human being can do something that sets off catastrophic consequences. People need to have sex; before AIDS broke out, thousands spread the disease through unprotected sex, and a few irresponsible ones continued this behavior even after discovering they had contracted HIV. Human beings need to hug and kiss their friends and relatives: during the Ebola crisis, containing the disease was made far more difficult not just because of an ancient tradition of kissing dead bodies but because people insisted on touching each other. And human beings need to eat: given a choice between starvation and risking disease, most people would prefer to roast a monkey or a bat.

A Web of Risk Factors Drives the Increase in Epidemics

A combination of social, economic, and environmental factors is accelerating the emergence and spread of novel viruses and new epidemics.

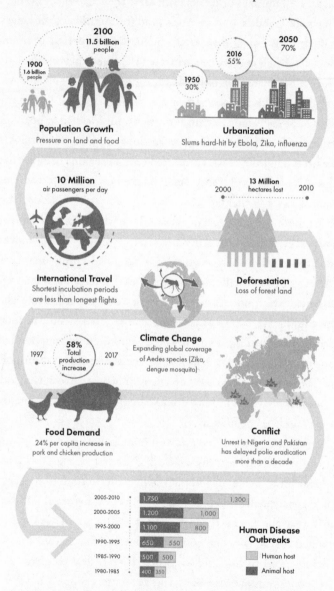

1900
1.6 billion people

2100
11.5 billion people

Population Growth
Pressure on land and food

1950
30%

2016
55%

2050
70%

Urbanization
Slums hard-hit by Ebola, Zika, influenza

10 Million
air passengers per day

International Travel
Shortest incubation periods are less than longest flights

2000 **13 Million** 2010
hectares lost

Deforestation
Loss of forest land

1997 **58%** 2017
Total production increase

Climate Change
Expanding global coverage of Aedes species (Zika, dengue mosquito)

Food Demand
24% per capita increase in pork and chicken production

Conflict
Unrest in Nigeria and Pakistan has delayed polio eradication more than a decade

Period	Animal host	Human host
2005-2010	1,750	1,300
2000-2005	1,200	1,000
1995-2000	1,100	800
1990-1995	650	550
1985-1990	500	500
1980-1985	400	350

Human Disease Outbreaks

Human host
Animal host

SOURCE: Adapted from World Health Organization. *Research priorities for the environment, agriculture and infectious diseases of poverty.* Geneva, Switzerland: World Health Organization; 2013. https://www.mcmasterhealthforum.org/docs/default-source/Product-Documents/stakeholder-dialogue-summary/capacity-to-respond-to-future-pandemics-sds.pdf?sfvrsn=4 (accessed 18 November 2016). Smith K, Goldberg M, Rosenthal S et al. Global rise in human infectious disease outbreaks. *Journal of Royal Society Interface* 2014; 11: 20140950–20140950. DOI: 10.1098/rsif.2014.0950.

Are We Entering the Century of Pandemics?

Ebola, AIDS, and Zika each arose in the first half of the twentieth century and spent their first several decades in the African bush, largely unnoticed by the rest of the world. But they are three very different examples of emerging infectious diseases. And they are just three of nearly 400 new infectious diseases that have been identified in the last 75 years. Since 1971, scientists have discovered at least 25 new pathogens for which we have no vaccine and no treatment. Even more worrisome is the rate at which emerging infectious diseases are appearing: the number of new ones has been increasing each decade, more than tripling between 1940 and 2000. During the 1980s, the number of new infectious diseases spiked to nearly 100, reflecting an association with the AIDS pandemic.[51] In 2014, WHO recorded more than 100 disease outbreaks with exotic names like MERS and Zika, most of which attracted international attention.

Given the rate at which population, deforestation, global warming, urbanization, climate change, international travel, and emergence of new pathogens are accelerating the risk of pandemics, it's reasonable to ask: Are we entering the century of pandemics? It's certainly possible. As if this thought is not frightening enough, let's take a closer look at the risks from even more contagious germs that live in the domesticated creatures that many more of us eat: chickens, pigs, and cows.

CHAPTER 3

THE BARN

Our global animal food industry and the renegade
influenza viruses it spawns could one day annihilate
the people it feeds.

Our addiction to chicken, steak, and bacon could easily kill us, and not just
from eating too much of it. At any given point in the year, there are 19 billion chickens, 1.5 billion cows, and 1 billion sheep on the planet—more than
three times the number of people. Most of these animals are raised for meat
in factory farms, where they are packed together by the millions in fetid disease incubators before slaughter. Factory farms present the greatest animal-
borne potential for catastrophic disease because they are the source of
influenza—the most mercurial, hardest-to-control, and fastest-spreading
potential killer there is.

In late 1989, my wife, our two preschool daughters, and I arrived in Peshawar,
Pakistan, our first overseas assignment with the World Health Organization.
Conflicts between the "freedom-fighter" mujahidin and the Russian-installed
Afghan government in Kabul were tapering off, but Pakistan remained a very
scary environment for my family. Aside from worrying about car bombs, flying bullets, and trying to stay cool and hydrated in the hellish heat, our greatest daily concern was food safety. We steered clear of the roadside shops, with

their still-bleeding beef and mutton carcasses drawing clouds of flies. One potential relief for the children—ice cream made from unpasteurized milk—was off the menu because it posed a risk of tuberculosis.

Some years later, after a stint in Kenya that posed more dangers from car bandits, bullets, bugs, and bellyaches, we eventually moved to Geneva. In this Swiss Eden of mountains, lakes, and pastures full of happy cows, I thought we would be safe on the street and at the dining table. But soon after our arrival in Europe, mad cow disease had the public in a panic, thanks to a killer virus that turned cow-eating people's brains into sponges. Like millions of others, my family and I stopped eating beef entirely. Mad cow was never to become the next Ebola—it wasn't that kind of pathogen, and the number of cases was small. But it was a vivid lesson in the risk that the animal food industry posed to human health, and in the serious infectious diseases that can be created or accelerated by it.

In the previous chapter, I warned you about the risk of the next catastrophic disease springing from the African jungle. In the following pages, you'll learn about the much higher risk of pandemic disease from animals raised for meat.

The Spanish Flu

Like HIV, influenza is sneaky. It lies hidden; it's easy to underestimate; it's devilishly mercurial; it's uncontrollable; and it's impossible to eliminate. The flu virus changes so fast that it outraces scientists' ability to develop potent vaccines against it, which is why we're all encouraged to get a new shot each year.

From an everyday human standpoint, it's hard to believe that the sniffles, fever, or a cough could signal the onset of something that could actually kill you. To most of us, the seasonal flu is just a nuisance, like a noisy neighbor. We get it when an infected person nearby us sneezes, coughs, or touches things we touch. The germ works silently within us for a few days before it grasps our throats and limbs, laying us flat with fatigue, sore throat, and fever. We develop a cold and a cough, spend some miserable days in bed, drink a lot of fluids, eat chicken soup, and generally recover nicely because our immune systems have enough *oomph* to help us return to health. If things get really bad, we can go to a doctor who can prescribe a drug called Tamiflu, which usually does the trick.

Normally, the annoying seasonal flu kills a very tiny percentage of people who come down with it—a minuscule fraction of 1 percent. If you caught the flu last winter, there is a chance that it was a descendant of the 1918 version.[1] Nevertheless, millions of people around the world contract a severe form of seasonal flu and end up in the hospital; between a quarter and a half million people die of it.[2]

*   *   *

Imagine surviving the horrors of one of the deadliest wars in human history, only to come home to another, even more terrible and personal experience of death.

In 1917, Dr. Ward J. MacNeal, a 36-year-old professor at New York Graduate Medical School and leading researcher, bid farewell to his wife Mabel and three sons and headed off to the trenches of World War I, where he served in France as one of the Great War's first medical officers. MacNeal's job was to help control infectious diseases among the American forces. His lab tested thousands of solders for syphilis, tuberculosis, and typhoid; processed hundreds of thousands of laboratory tests; autopsied the deceased; and investigated military and civilian outbreaks throughout France.

In April 1918, the final year of the savage trench fighting of World War I, MacNeal noticed that something besides bullets and bombs was killing the soldiers. He received reports of patients in southern France, Italy, and Spain who were seized with the flu, though MacNeal reported that "complications were so rare as to be non-existent." By late August, however, the condition of patients grew more dire. Something had changed. The outbreak had become "distinctly more malignant," MacNeal observed. The sick suffered from high temperatures, sore throats, exhaustion, headache, aching limbs, bloodshot eyes, coughs, and sometimes violent nosebleeds. The mortally ill soldiers developed a bluish-gray skin. Many died less than 48 hours after their symptoms appeared. When doctors at autopsy opened the chests of the dead, they found that the normally light, elastic lungs were clogged with heavy, bloody fluid.[3] The patients basically suffocated to death.

Three months after an armistice was declared in November 1918, Dr. MacNeal returned to New York, anticipating a joyful homecoming to a world far away from disease and war. Instead, he found that the same illness killing the Europeans had gripped New York and threatened his own family. Two of his three sons, Perry and Edward, were terribly sick. He and Mabel took turns comforting the two boys around the clock, trying to quell their fever. Perry recovered, but just five days after his father's return, Eddie, a previously healthy 12-year-old, died. MacNeal expressed his grief in this epitaph: "Now come the sad days when death has broken through / The circle of our loved ones / And taken him for whom we dreamed so much."[4]

Experts say that something as awful as the Spanish flu pandemic could very easily happen today. To understand how such a disaster might unfold, I recommend watching the 2011 movie *Contagion*. In the film, a woman goes on a business trip to Hong Kong, picks up an airborne virus from a restaurant chef on a visit to a casino, and returns home to Chicago. On the way she develops a fever and a cough; her illness looks like the everyday flu that so many of us pick up while traveling, but it's not. Every time she or the chef touches a surface—her son, a wineglass, the standing bar in a bus—the virus delivers a tiny knife-thrust into the mouth, nose, or eye of a new victim. Within hours, the woman has a seizure and dies in the hospital; within another few days, her son dies, too. Meanwhile, the virus spreads with geometric internet speed from hand to lung and from city to city. Days pass before anyone understands the gravity of the situation; some suspect a bioterror attack. Society begins to break down. Kids can't go to school; nobody goes to work; streets and airports are empty. Supermarket shelves are stripped bare; chaos ensues as people fight over resources and a snake-oil salesman's useless herbal remedy.

Contagion's chilling scenario isn't just a disaster-film fantasy dreamed up by Hollywood scaremongers. Experts including the American epidemiologist Larry Brilliant and Pulitzer Prize–winning author Laurie Garrett acted as consultants on the film, and it received high kudos from other epidemiologists for its accuracy.[5] Scientists agree that if a highly contagious strain of flu one day combines with a highly pathogenic one and is spread from human to human, the *Contagion* scenario could easily play out in real life.

Beware of the Birds

Human influenza—seasonal and pandemic alike—usually starts with wild aquatic birds because avian flu is very common in waterfowl. Once in a while, a wild bird virus gets friendly with another strain inside another bird, or even a pig. When that combination of viruses from birds and beasts finds its way into a human, it can kill us because we have zero immunity to it.[6] And because birds are free to fly anywhere they please, they can drop their viruses everywhere.

Poyang Lake, the biggest freshwater lake in China, has scientists worried. The lake attracts enormous numbers of migratory birds that hunt for food in and around the many poultry farms in the area. The Chinese eat a lot of chicken, ducks, and geese; they prefer to buy live poultry because they (understandably) tend to distrust the quality of meat from factory farms. At the small farms around the lake and in the live poultry markets of the city of Nanchang, thousands of birds intermingle, trading their genetic material in droppings ingested by other fowls. This makes the Poyang Lake area an ideal breeding ground for deadly strains of bird flu.[7]

Epidemiologists fear that avian flu from the wild birds will fall into a viral mixing bowl of genes from people, domestic fowl, and animals around the lake, mutate, and jump to humans. China has required poultry farmers to vaccinate their flocks, but there isn't much enforcement, and quarantining poultry is a big challenge for small farmers.[8]

The most frightening flu virus scientists know of today killed its first human victim in May 1997. A three-year-old boy named Lam Hoi-Ka died a few days after being admitted to a Hong Kong hospital. The child's autopsy showed that he died of acute respiratory, liver, and kidney failure as well as "disseminated intravascular coagulopathy," meaning that the child's blood had effectively curdled.[9]

While his death was terrible for his family, death from influenza in Hong Kong was not so unique in itself; after all, the Hong Kong flu of 1968 killed a million around the world.[10] But the death of Lam Hoi-Ka was different because the virus that killed him, H5N1, was completely unheard of. Scientists believed that humans were only susceptible to H1, H2, and H3 viruses. When Keiji Fukuda, an epidemiology expert at WHO, was asked what his first thought had been upon hearing the news that a brand-new flu virus had killed a child, Fukuda replied that he remembered thinking, "This is how it begins."[11]

The Influenza Alphabet:
The Most Notable Human Influenza Viruses[12]

Three types of influenza virus infect humans: A, B, and C. Influenza type A is divided into subtypes based on two surface proteins: hemagglutinin (H) and neuraminidase (N).

Seasonal influenza vaccines target the most common causes of worldwide annual flu epidemics: influenza A (subtypes H1N1 and H3N2) and influenza B. Influenza C infections are mild and are not known to cause epidemics.

In order of known pandemic deaths, the influenza A subtypes of greatest concern are:

- **H1N1 caused "Spanish flu" and the 2009 swine flu outbreak.** It is one of the most common strains affecting humans today. A virulent and contagious mutual of this virus caused the 1918 Spanish flu (50 million deaths) and the 2009 swine flu (575,400 deaths).

- **H2N2 caused "Asian flu" in 1957** (also called "avian influenza" or "bird flu"). It led to about 2 million deaths and is still a threat.

- **H3N2 caused the "Hong Kong flu" in 1968,** which led to 1 million deaths. It is also one of the most common strains affecting humans today.

- **H5N1, "highly pathogenic avian influenza (HPAI),"** caused several hundred deaths between 2003 and 2016. It kills 50 percent of the humans it infects, which makes it a global influenza pandemic threat.

- **H7N9, another avian flu, first detected in 2013,** has killed 295 people as of 2016. It has the potential to become a pandemic.

- **H5N6 is an avian influenza first identified in China in 2013.** It has caused 14 laboratory-confirmed cases of human infection with six deaths. It also has the potential for an outbreak.

Where did this new killer come from? Two months before the little boy died, thousands of Hong Kong chickens asphyxiated from H5N1. The birds' bodies shook; their faces turned dark green and black; they strangled on big blood clots stuck in their windpipes. Laboratory samples of the virus showed it to be a thousand times more infectious than typical human strains.[13] H5N1 probably jumped to a human through contact with the blood and organs of a diseased bird slaughtered on a poultry farm or in one of Hong Kong's poultry markets.[14]

Lam Hoi-Ka's death immediately alarmed scientists because the 1918 Spanish flu epidemic likely started the same way.[15] In short order, 17 other people in Hong Kong who exhibited the same symptoms as the child were admitted to hospitals; six, including the boy, died. Had H5N1 spread beyond Hong Kong in 1997, Lam Hoi-Ka would have been patient zero for a global pandemic. Understanding the danger, officials lost no time in killing every last chicken in Hong Kong. The tactic appeared to have worked; there were no more human victims. "We felt we had dodged a bullet," Fukuda recalled.[16] (Of course, chicken farmers, their families, and others whose livelihood and dinners depended on fresh chicken doubtless wished that the bullet of H5N1 had never been fired.)

But unlike the satisfying ending of a movie where the bad guy is finally shot and killed, H5N1 didn't just disappear. It escaped from Hong Kong, went underground for a while, and started working on a sequel, distilling itself into something more lethal before erupting in a more virulent way and in a different place. Sometime later, a stronger version of the virus swept rapidly to Southeast Asia. In 2003, a Vietnamese 18-year-old was admitted to a hospital that specialized in treating infectious disease. An X-ray showed a small cloud at the base of her lungs. Four days later, her lungs were completely filled with fluid, and she later died. Eight other patients admitted to the hospital with H5N1 also died. By August 2004, the new virus killed 40 people in Vietnam, 12 in Thailand, 4 in Cambodia, and at least one in Indonesia.[17] Then, in 2005, a 10-year-old named Ngoan picked up H5N1 from the chickens that died on her family's farm in Vietnam's Mekong Delta. She died, along with 50 others in Southeast Asia. Since then, H5N1 has shown up in birds in 16 countries.[18]

"But wait a minute," you might say. "What's the big deal? Why are scientists so scared? After all, not that many people have died from H5N1." Certainly, from a sheer numbers perspective, you're correct. But the story changes when you look at the *percentage* of people who died from that strain of flu. By the end of 1997, 6 out of 18 infected people in Hong Kong died of H5N1—that's a 33 percent death rate. When H5N1 showed up again in Thailand in 2003, it killed 346 out of 587 people reported to have been infected—that's 60 percent.[19] From 2003 through January 20, 2016, there were 846 laboratory-confirmed human cases of H5N1 virus infection from 16 countries, according to WHO. Of these, more than half died.[20] And those are only *the officially reported* numbers. The percentage is probably a lot higher because a lot of people don't make it to the hospital. By comparison, the Spanish flu epidemic of 1918 was no big deal; it had a mortality rate of between just 2 and 3 percent.

This makes H5N1 one of the most contagious and pathogenic—i.e., deadliest—viruses scientists have ever come across. And it's still very much out there.

The CAFO Threat

Mitchell Weiner, an assistant principal at an intermediate school in Queens, New York, was a beloved dad and adored teacher who knew every kid's name. "The heart and soul of the school," Weiner was also a Little League coach and a rabid baseball fan.[21] He had only one health problem: a form of inflammatory arthritis.

In 2009, Weiner went to the hospital with a flu that looked a lot like the humdrum seasonal one, but then he was suddenly overwhelmed by the illness and died.[22] Meanwhile, on the other side of the U.S., Nancy Pinnella, a 47-year-old sales manager at a Sacramento, California, news affiliate, left work saying that she felt unwell. She went into the hospital the next day, where they sedated her and put her on a ventilator and dialysis because her kidneys and lungs were failing. She died three days later. Family members said that Pinnella, who did not get a flu shot, was in great health before she died.[23]

Weiner's and Pinnella's deaths were shocking because they didn't catch the flu directly from other people or directly from birds. This time, the disease that killed them came from pigs—more specifically, from a strain of flu born of massive pig farming. Before the version of H1N1 "swine flu" that started killing people in 2009 was over, an estimated 575,400 people worldwide died of it, though estimates vary.[24]

Swine flu sprang from what one might call "animal kitchen chemistry." Pigs eat almost everything, so their guts are the perfect mixing bowls for flu. When pigs eat the droppings of sick wild birds or the chickens living near them, their digestive systems become creative microbial chefs that recombine the variety of genetic material to create new pathogens. Pig guts can flavor the viral soup with multiple human germs, too. (In the movie *Contagion*, one of the last, quick scenes is that of a wild bird dropping something into a pig feeding trough.)

To find out where the murderous 2009 flu strain that killed Mitchell Weiner and Nancy Pinnella started, scientists traced the viral gene to pig farms.

They found that the virus first appeared in 1998 at a big pig-breeding facility in Fayetteville, North Carolina, where 2,400 of the facility's sows came down with a familiar, flu-like cough, and pregnant sows spontaneously aborted their litters. An animal disease laboratory discovered that the virus killing the litters had three human flu genes; within a few months, the virus had acquired two bird flu gene segments as well. The sows in the Fayetteville operation turned out to be a wonderful viral stirring pot. When infected sows and their offspring were transported to other places, more hogs all over the United States fell ill and died. Although the virus was circulating in North American swine, it did not develop into a virus capable of infecting humans until it mixed with strains from European swine, likely via the livestock trade, just before 2009.

Just as the H5N1 virus laid low for a while in birds and transformed itself before hitting humans with a mighty blow, the swine flu didn't begin to attack humans until a more dangerous version broke out in a 60,000-sow factory farm operation in Mexico run by Smithfield Foods, a North American meat conglomerate. CAFOs (short for "Concentrated Animal Feeding Operations") like Smithfield's are mostly owned or subsidized by large agribusiness companies such as Tyson Foods, Perdue, and Cargill that supply meat to fast-food chains as well as supermarkets.[25] These factory farms are enormously profitable; a reported 50 percent of Americans' meat comes from their feedlots.[26] The United Nations Food and Agriculture Organization (FAO) estimates that 80 percent of all growth in livestock production around the world takes place within "industrial" CAFO-type systems; in the United States, CAFOs remain the heart and soul of poultry, egg, pork, and dairy production. The animals live in fetid conditions until they are slaughtered, stripped, and rendered; their meat is then shipped all over the globe. CAFOs have spread quickly and their numbers are increasing around the world—particularly to places like China—because they are so profitable and because consumer demand for the meat and dairy they produce is rising.[27, 28]

If you've ever taken a drive through central California or the American Midwest where CAFOs are common, you can't possibly miss them. You can recognize them from a distance by their enormous green silos, but what really stamps them is their awful stench. The feedlots are packed with thousands or tens of thousands of beef and dairy cows, hogs, chickens, and turkeys, all squished together in concentration camp conditions as they're fattened up for milking or slaughter. Meanwhile their waste and attendant genetic material is stored and mixed into a viral soup in gigantic, reeking lagoons.[29] With issues of infectious disease, antimicrobial resistance, environmental health, and animal welfare at stake, regulatory oversight remains woefully inadequate.[30, 31]

CAFOs were the birthplace of swine flu, and they could very likely be the birthplace of the next killer pandemic. Here's how one can imagine the outbreak scenario that occurred in 2008: A poor Mexican man working in a Smithfield slaughterhouse catches a pig- or chicken-borne flu. He begins to feel sick, develops a fever and a cough. He has no choice but to work despite his illness; he's poorly paid and if he doesn't work, his family doesn't eat. He tends to the pigs, whose feedlots may not be far from those of chickens or from lagoons where the waste of other animals is stored. Some chicken, wild goose, or duck poop gets into the feedlot, which a pig eats; the sick Mexican man coughs on his hands while he handles the pig; the sick pig sprays the combined bird/pig/human virus on other pigs and handlers, who pass it on in a vicious cycle.

In 2009, H1N1 moved from the Mexican Smithfield operation to local workers and their vulnerable relatives—the very young or the very old, or people who had a history of medical problems. Despite efforts to close public and private facilities in Mexico City in an attempt to contain the spread of the virus, swine flu continued to spread globally; some clinics were overwhelmed by infected people.[32]

This same scenario could happen virtually anywhere, at any time.

Mad Cow: The First Man-Made Epidemic

Andrew Black was a bright, good-looking, fit, funny fellow who worked as a freelance radio producer in England. One day in 2004, he stopped acting like himself. He didn't want to work any longer. At first, doctors diagnosed depression, but things got progressively worse. He found that he could no longer open a can of soup; when his sister opened it for him, he couldn't pour it into a pan. He began losing his eyesight and balance; he eventually became paralyzed. After writhing for days in his mother's arms, he died. "Find out who did this to me," he begged his mother, Christine.[33]

Andrew lost his mind to Creutzfeldt–Jakob disease (vCJD), known in the vernacular as "mad cow." This incurable disease steadily kills off brain cells, causing progressive dementia, memory loss, personality changes, hallucinations, seizures, and a host of other neurological problems. It is invariably fatal. Mad cow derives its nickname from a phenomenon that British cattle ranchers first noticed in their herds back in the 1980s. The ranchers observed that their cows became aggressive and eventually stopped being able to walk. The culprit was a strange protein called bovine spongiform encephalopathy (BSE for short) that had basically turned their brains into porous sponges; in its human form, it turned Andrew's brain into a pore-pocked sponge, too.

BSE is the first man-made epidemic. It's what I might call a "Frankenstein" disease, a pathogen that some agricultural scientist inadvertently made when he cobbled together the meat and bone meal (so-called MBM) of dead cattle, sheep, and goats to provide a source of protein.[34] Feeding MBM to herbivorous cattle effectively turned them into carnivores, to horrific and unforeseeable effect.[35] That change in cattle feeding habits allowed an age-old animal pathogen to enter the human food chain. After cattle started dying off from BSE in the 1980s, the British government killed between 3 and 4 million of them; thereafter, Kenneth Calman, the government's chief medical officer, insisted that British beef was safe to eat. But it wasn't, because the MBM material that made them sick in the first place was still in circulation.[36] (The British government eventually banned the use of MBM in ruminant feed, but the animal feed trade was given a grace period of five weeks to clear its stock—leading to the infection of thousands of additional animals.[37])

Among other things, the story of mad cow is a cautionary tale of official denial, politics, and greed trumping sound public-health science. It wasn't until 12 years after the first identified case of BSE that the British government finally admitted that there might be a serious risk to human health.[38] Unfortunately, BSE has a very slow incubation period. It didn't begin to show up in cattle for four to five years after infection, and vCJD took even longer to show up in humans. It first appeared in humans in 1996, long after infected meat products had entered the food supply. A single hamburger could contain meat from more than 100 animals. BSE-infected material found its way into school lunches, soup, and even vaccines. Even though Andrew's mother decided not to serve beef when her son was just a little boy, he still managed to contract vCJD, and she still doesn't know how.

Mad cow became a political football and a blame game. An official U.K. report noted that the danger to the public was not identified quickly enough, and found fault with scientists, government officials, and bureaucrats. But ultimately, British politicians fought to protect the agribusiness industry, siding with it over public health. (The report's "mistakes were made" tone offered a lot of outs to the culpable: in answer to a question at the press conference launching the report, the government's point person, Lord Phillips, said the meat industry had come out of the crisis "relatively unscathed."[39])

Meanwhile, the disease had spread not just throughout Britain but also to several European countries and even into Canada. The epidemic was enormously costly to the British and European beef industries; in France alone, some suppliers noted that demand for beef dropped by half.[40] The European Union mandated a beef labeling system[41] and banned beef from Britain for ten years, from 1996 to 2006.[42] The cost to the U.S. beef industry was an estimated $6 billion,[43] and the overall economic loss to the beef industry (as well as to restaurants and other businesses in its supply chain) dwarfed whatever profits came from BSE-fed growth of individual food animals. The human blood supply was hurt too: anyone who had lived in, visited, worked, or stayed in the U.K. for more than six months between 1980 and the end of 1996 could not be a blood donor anywhere else in the world because they were seen as "at risk" of carrying mad cow. Even today, the disease continues to menace the British blood supply.[44] Like all devastating pathogens, mad cow snuck under the radar. With Darwinian adaptation, it could come back again in a much more virulent form.

Fortunately, Andrew's case turned out to be pretty rare. There were only 177 cases of vCJD in Britain since 1980, and just a few in other countries. That's cold comfort for Andrew's mother, who remains dedicated to holding the British government responsible.[45] Like so many germs that show up when people aren't paying attention to their own destructive practices and behaviors, mad cow is another canary in the proverbial coal mine. At the very least, Andrew's tragedy demonstrates how sloppy animal husbandry practices, greed, and political arrogance lead to the spread of killer diseases from the barn.

When Antibiotics Don't Work

David Kirby is the kind of writer any journalism major—or any deeply curious person, for that matter—would love to share a few long beers with. Blessed with a full head of curly brown hair, smart eyeglasses, and strict, Bob Woodward–style earnestness, the 57-year-old is a gumshoe investigative journalist of the great old school. He's determined to get to the bottom of a story, pick out the heroes and villains, and follow them regardless of where the story leads or what it might cost him personally to peer too deeply into the cracks and folds of evil.

About a decade ago, Kirby wandered into an investigative wilderness. He was looking into mysterious diseases that were killing river fish and affecting the health of people in rural agricultural areas. He was shocked by what he found. The fish were dying of poison connected to CAFOs. "I had no idea that we feed chicken feces to cattle," he says. "I didn't know that we feed cattle to cattle."[46] His investigation led him to factory farms in the area, places he studied so closely that he himself came down with so-called "manure flu" (also known as "olfactory fatigue") from merely breathing the air in and around them.

Manure flu happens when your nose is so burned out from prolonged exposure to the stench from CAFOs that you can't smell them anymore. It brings on headaches as well as muscle and tendon pains. In Randolph County, Indiana, where more than 40 CAFOs are in operation, manure flu is legion and the stench is so overwhelming that people can't distinguish many smells any longer. Many have to use inhalers to breathe.[47] In his gripping 2010 book about factory farming called *Animal Factory: The Looming Threat of Industrial Pig, Dairy, and Poultry Farms to Humans and the Environment*,[48] Kirby clearly showed that when poultry, pig, and cattle factories are placed in proximity to each other, as they are in places like Iowa, Idaho, or California's Central Valley, the chances for interspecies mingling of influenza virus skyrocket. But beyond that, the CAFO feedlots, buried ankle deep in urine and feces, introduce even more viral killers that scientists have not yet figured out how to prevent.

Other issues such as animal cruelty aside—which is not at all a trivial matter—just think about the volume of waste from CAFOs and the viral risk it represents. A single cow produces hundreds of times more waste than a human being.[49] As the fecal matter from thousands of animals evaporates, the wind carries it throughout the area, which is one of the reasons why CAFOs make horrible neighbors and why Kirby caught manure flu. The wind from CAFOs carries more than unneighborly stink. Kirby learned that on CAFOs, livestock are given low doses of antibiotics to prevent the spread of bacteria (a big hazard in their living conditions) and to make the animals grow faster and bigger. In 2010, 80 percent of antibiotics sold each year in the U.S. were used to grow beef cattle, hogs, and poultry.[50] In an experiment, Texas researchers who placed air samplers near beef and dairy feedlots found that all the samples tested positive for two antibiotics used to treat people: monenisin and tetracycline. They also found high concentrations of antibiotic-resistant bacteria in the air.[51]

According to a CDC report, *Antibiotic Resistance Threats in the United States, 2013*, world health leaders have described antibiotic-resistant micro-organisms as "nightmare bacteria" that "pose a catastrophic threat" to people in every country in the world. Antibiotic resistance is a worldwide problem crossing international boundaries and spreads between continents with ease.

If you're not depressed and alarmed enough, there's more.

Let's say you live near a CAFO and get an infection that lands you in the hospital. The doctors and nurses tuck you in, take your blood pressure and pulse, and stick an IV tube into your arm. Because the hospital staff might not have been as diligent as they need to be when they stuck the needle, another germ called MRSA, prevalent in the ward, could find its way into you. Short for "Methicillin-resistant *Staphylococcus aureus*," MRSA is a bacterial infection resistant to antibiotics, thanks to all the stuff floating around in the air that CAFOs have exhaled. MRSA can spread like wildfire in hospitals and health-care settings, especially among patients with open wounds, catheters, and immune-deficiency problems. And MRSA makes it much harder for doctors to treat infections. In 2005, in the U.S. alone, 278,000 people were infected with MRSA; of those, 18,650 died.[52] In fact, more people died from MRSA infections that year than from HIV/AIDS.[53] And if you live near a CAFO, particularly one that feeds pigs, your risk of getting MRSA is three times higher than it is if you don't.[54]

Recently, scientists have been raising the alarms about "superbugs"—diseases that are resistant to *all* antibiotics.[55] "One day," Kirby predicts, "influenza from birds and swine will combine into a superbug. It's not a matter of if, but when." Bill Gates agrees. "We've created, in terms of spread," he told *Vox*, "the most dangerous environment that we've ever had in the history of mankind."[56] Kirby lays the blame not only on the corporations that own the CAFOs but on the failure of regulators and politicians at the state and federal levels to do anything to restrict CAFO operations. "Without proper regulations," he warns, "the diseases will keep coming."[57]

"Not Whether, but When"

Eddie MacNeal, Lam Hoi-Ka, the 18-year-old in Vietnam, Ngoan, Mitchell Weiner, Nancy Pinnella, and millions of others all died from diseases that originated in wild birds and then spread to humans and domesticated animals.

These diseases still lurk. H5N1 continues to stir in the blood soup of chickens and ducks. Swine flu still replicates in the blood of pigs and remains a threat to humans. Meanwhile, mad cow remains a threat as MBM is fed to cattle in the third world,[58] and antibiotic-resistant bacteria continue to threaten people in hospitals and in the community.

An overriding fear among scientists is that some highly pathogenic marriage of viral genes will produce a bug that becomes airborne and leaps fast, as in the movie *Contagion*, from human to human. Such a thing may have already happened. A girl dying of H5N1 flu in Thailand passed it to her mother and aunt, who nursed her; it jumped from a man who ate pudding made of raw duck to his brother, a cement trader, who cared for him.[59, 60] If a highly contagious, airborne strain of H5N1 or some as-yet-unidentified virus hitchhiked with an unwitting passenger onto a cruise ship or an airplane and landed in a crowded place like Hong Kong, London, Mexico City, Nairobi, Manila, or New York, the pandemic situation would look very much like the one in the movie.

Infectious-disease experts agree that under present conditions the question is not whether a superbug will occur and create a global pandemic. The question is when. Experts also agree that the most likely superbug candidate will be an influenza virus mutation. For those of us who want to keep ourselves, our children, and their children alive, there is nothing more important than fighting these incipient viruses that fly through the air, lurk in animals, and live on the ground.

CHAPTER 4

THE TRIPLE THREAT: BIOTERROR, BIO-ERROR, AND DR. FRANKENSTEIN

The threat of an epidemic unleashed by terrorists,
lab errors, or irresponsible scientists
has never been greater.

A deadly virus, all by itself, is positively benign compared to what an evil human being can do with it. Right now, microscopic killers like smallpox and anthrax sit stewing in labs around the world. People who study bioterrorism believe that it's not a matter of whether, but where and when a maniac from ISIS or anywhere else gets hold of some deadly spores and releases a cloud of disease in a big city. Nobody, but nobody, is fully prepared for such a catastrophe.

Imagine the following scenario occurring toward the end of the year that you are reading this book.

October 29: A scruffy terrorist with an advanced degree in microbiology has inoculated himself against smallpox. He custom-designs a small aerosol sprayer disguised as an air freshener. Then he develops smallpox culture in his home laboratory in London.

December 9: The terrorist inserts the weaponized virus into the sprayer.

The spray is so light and small that not even a mosquito would immediately notice it. Disguised as a security guard, he smuggles it into an enclosed sports arena where a world-famous rock band is giving a concert. The arena is dark, the lights are flashing, and it's full of happy, fist-pumping fans, all of whom are riveted upon the band's lead singer. Nobody notices as the man discreetly attaches the sprayer to an air vent close to the stage. He sets it off, then leaves the arena. The stuff coming out of the sprayer, completely invisible and odorless, enters the noses, eyes, and mouths of the rock stars and then the audience.

December 16: The band members, crew, and some who were closest to the stage develop fevers and coughs. The band's lead singer feels quite ill, so they cancel the next night's scheduled concert in Paris. In areas around London, some audience members commute to work or school though they feel a little unwell, spreading contagion everywhere they go. Those who do visit their doctors are told the same-old, same-old flu recommendation: "Take Tylenol for the fever. Drink lots of water. Go to bed. And if it doesn't get better, come back in a few days."

December 17: The band members and others show up at emergency rooms, their faces covered with blisters that look like chicken pox. The patients are put into isolation.

December 24: The band's lead singer dies. The other members are extremely ill.

December 25: By the time a quarantine and vaccine campaign is fully mounted, many of those who were at the arena, along with their initial contacts in London and elsewhere, will have sickened and died, and global panic will have taken hold.

Such a scenario is not the stuff of science fiction.[1] A laboratory-engineered pandemic following a scenario like the one above has been identified as one of the top "global catastrophic risks"—that is, a risk that could lead to the deaths of approximately one-tenth of the world's population—by the U.K.-based Global Challenges Foundation (the other two giant risks are a natural pandemic and a nuclear war).[2] Short of a nuclear bomb, which is much more difficult to unleash, the tool of destruction for terrorists would be a cupful of either naturally occurring or bioengineered pathogens that could be relatively easily produced and dispensed. An anthrax attack alone would devastate a city.[3]

It would not be terribly daunting for someone with sufficient know-how to get hold of dangerous material. A European Parliament report noted that today, anyone with college-level chemistry and biology can now produce a crude but effective terrorist weapon.[4] It's also getting easier, quicker, and cheaper for scientists to experiment with potentially dangerous material in the lab, thanks in part to a gene-splicing technology called CRISPR-Cas9 that has taken the scientific world by storm. (CRISPR stands for "clustered regularly interspaced short palindromic repeats," and Cas9 refers to "CRISPR-associated protein number nine.")

A Short History of Biological Attacks[5]

Disease has been used as a weapon of war since time immemorial. According to the memoir of Gabriele de' Mussi, a main source chronicling the origin of the Black Death, the Mongol army attacked the walled city of Caffa in Crimea by catapulting corpses infected with plague into the city. Those who survived fled to the Mediterranean Basin, taking the disease with them and spreading it in their wake.[6] In World War II, Japan dumped cholera into wells used by the Chinese populace. Fleas were carefully collected, infected with plague, and then dropped in aerial bombs over Chinese cities.[7]

Time	Event
1155	Emperor Barbarossa spreads cholera by poisoning water wells with human bodies in Tortona, Italy
1346	Mongol forces use catapults to throw bodies of plague victims over the city walls of Caffa, Crimean Peninsula (now Feodosia, Ukraine)
1495	In Naples, Italy, Spanish forces take blood from leprosy patients and mix it with wine to sell to their French foes
1710	Russian troops hurl human bodies of plague victims into Swedish cities
1763	British distribute blankets infected with smallpox to Native Americans
1797	Napoleon floods the plains around Mantua, Italy, to spread malaria
1863	During the U.S. Civil War, Confederates sell clothing infected with yellow fever and smallpox to Union troops
World War I	German and French agents rumored to use glanders and anthrax
World War II	Japan uses plague, anthrax, and other diseases; several other countries work to create biological weapons programs
2001	Anthrax-laced letters sent through Washington, D.C., post office

The Threat of Bioterror

Back in 2011, a bunch of harmless-looking, grizzled, gray-haired, gun-loving Vietnam veterans, ranging in age from their late fifties to close to 80, liked to drink and "talk bull" in Gainesville, Georgia. A common theme of the conversation was their hatred for the U.S. federal government. They tossed around ideas for killing all the judges employed by the U.S. Justice Department, as well as the federal employees at the IRS and the U.S. Bureau of Alcohol, Tobacco, Firearms, and Explosives in downtown Atlanta. (They appeared to have at least a drop of moral compunction, because they drew the line at killing kids.)

Following a sting operation, two of the group, Frederick Thomas and Dan Roberts, were arrested, tried, and sentenced to prison for plotting to blow up federal buildings.[8] That might have been the end of it, but the crazy talk turned out to be a lot more serious than just "bull." A few years later, two other men from the same group, Ray Adamas and Samuel Crump, were found guilty of plotting to make ricin, a biological toxin, which they hoped to use in a terrorist attack.[9] "These guys were incredibly stupid," said Mark Potok of the Southern Poverty Law Center, which tracks the rising number of hate groups, many espousing similar beliefs, in the U.S. "They were going to throw the ricin out the window of a car, which would have blown back in their faces."[10]

In fact, you don't need to be a rocket scientist to make ricin, a poison that can cause respiratory failure and other maladies. It's made from castor beans, the same raw material as castor oil. The beans grow wild and abundantly along some U.S. highways, and there are recipes aplenty to be found on the internet. In 2013, an Elvis impersonator sent several ricin-laced letters to President Obama, a judge, and a U.S. senator.[11]

The U.S. CDC defines a bioterrorism attack as "a deliberate release of viruses, bacteria, or other germs that are typically found in nature and are used to cause illness or death in people, animals, or plants." These can be spread through the air, through water, or in food. An aerosol sprayer would be a preferred method for airborne delivery. Biological agents are hard to detect and don't cause illness for up to several days. Some bioterrorism agents, like the smallpox virus, can be spread from person to person, and some, like anthrax, cannot.[12] Organisms that are easily spread (e.g., anthrax) or transmitted from person to person (e.g., smallpox) are especially dangerous and would produce high death rates, public panic, and social disruption.[13]

A Matrix of Terrorist Weapons

Infectious-disease bioterror threats rank second only to nuclear devices in their potential to inflict mass casualties.

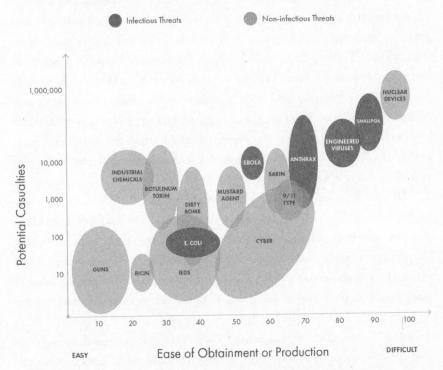

SOURCE: Adapted from Coleman K, Ishisoko N, Trounce M, Bernard K. Hitting a moving target: A strategic tool for analyzing terrorist threats. *Health Security* 2016. DOI:10.1089/hs.2016.0062.

Biological weapons may be more difficult to obtain or produce than attacks with assault rifles or improvised explosive devices (IEDs), but they have the potential to cause far more mass casualties (see chart).[14]

Far from the southern U.S., terrorists have been busy hatching different plots involving various microbial agents and spreading them proudly. In 2009, an animated, smiling, white-bearded professor from Kuwait named Abdallah Al-Nafisi appeared on Al Jazeera television. He described in detail how one person armed with four pounds of anthrax—"in a suitcase this big—carried by a fighter through tunnels from Mexico into the U.S.," could "kill 330,000 Americans within a single hour, if it is properly spread in population centers there." The 9/11 attacks would be "small change" in comparison. "There is no need for airplanes, conspiracies, timings, and so on," Al-Nafisi continued, noting that the anthrax could be made in laboratories run by Al Qaeda or

Hezbollah. "One person, with the courage to carry four pounds of anthrax, will go to the White House lawn, and will spread this 'confetti' all over them, and then will do these cries of joy. It will turn into a real 'celebration.'"[15]

Consider, too, the blood-chilling material that Abu Ali, the leader of a group of Syrian rebels, discovered back in 2014. In a bombed-out building on the border of Turkey and Syria, Ali found a Dell laptop. He had no idea what it contained, so he gave it to reporters from *Foreign Affairs* for a look. The reporters opened the laptop and found nothing on its hard drive—its owner, one Muhammed S., had the presence of mind to erase everything, perhaps just before Ali and his men burst into the building. But then the reporters discovered all the "hidden files," which they copied onto a thumb drive and took along with them for deeper inspection.

They found plans that sounded almost like a Third Reich–style blueprint for the mass extermination of so-called "unbelievers." The hidden files included a 26-page document that was a fatwa, or Islamic ruling, on the "rules" for using bioterror, written by an imprisoned Saudi jihadi cleric. "If Muslims cannot defeat the unbelievers in a different way, it is permissible to use weapons of mass destruction . . . even if it kills all of them and wipes them and their descendants off the face of the Earth."

One 19-page document detailed how to safely test weaponized bubonic plague before using it in a terrorist attack. Muhammed S. understood that, delivered through an aerosol sprayer and then transmitted person to person, the plague would be almost impossible to control. Without early treatment, those exposed to it would die.[16] "When the microbe is injected in small mice, the symptoms of the disease should start to appear within 24 hours," the document noted. "Use small grenades with the virus,[17] and throw them in closed areas like metros, soccer stadiums, or entertainment centers. . . . Best to do it next to the air-conditioning. It also can be used during suicide operations."[18]

*   *   *

It doesn't seem to matter to those who hope to unleash such horrors that they would likely die themselves, along with their enemies. Before suicide bombers came along, experts argued that bioterrorism simply would not work. Releasing anthrax, smallpox, plague, botulinum toxin, tularemia, Ebola, or some other ghastly disease upon innocents would delegitimize the terrorists' cause, generate defectors, and bring the full force of government prosecution on their heads. But suicidal bio-bombers' willingness to act on their beliefs changed the game, as the events of September 11, 2001, proved. The bombers care about only two things: destroying the perceived enemy and perhaps being richly rewarded in an afterlife.

Like a venomous viper released from the dark hole of the misbegotten Iraq war, ISIS has already deployed chemical weapons such as mustard and chlorine gases in Iraq and Syria. A European Parliament briefing published in December 2015 reported that the radical Islamic group has everything it needs—money, scientists, innocent suicide-bombing children,[19] and an abundance of deadly toxins stockpiled by the tyrants of Syria, Iraq, and Libya, in addition to the ones its scientists can make—to unleash the dogs of hell on victims.[20, 21]

When will someone get hold of deadly spores and release a cloud of disease in a big city? Fortunately, "weaponizing" dangerous microbes is still difficult. But it's probably just a matter of time until someone figures out how to do it, says Randall Larsen, an amiable, talkative Texan and retired air force pilot who is one of the top bioterrorism experts in the U.S.[22]

Larsen observes that "a non-state actor can make a pretty deadly weapon for a couple of thousand dollars. They don't need sophisticated labs and engineers." He quotes, with much respect, the microbiologist and Nobel laureate Joshua Lederberg: "'Today, one man can make war. A lucky bio-buffoon could kill 400,000 people.'"[23]

Larsen already takes it for granted that a lucky-buffoon attack would be frighteningly simple to pull off. He himself has proved the point at least a dozen times. In 1998, a friend at the CIA gave him a vial of weaponized *Bacillus globigii*, a germ closely related to anthrax.[24] Larsen's vial of powder has since been carried into high-security areas of Congress, the CIA, and the Pentagon, as well as past every single TSA agent he's ever encountered. "If the TSA people ask me what it is, I just say sweetly, 'It's my powdah.'" After scrutinizing him (Larsen is getting up in years), one TSA agent teased him: "Honey, it'll nevah work."[25]

A few days after 9/11, Larsen was called to the Eisenhower Executive Office Building near the White House for a meeting with a few top national security people, another biodefense expert named Tara O'Toole,[26] and Vice President Dick Cheney. The meeting had been called to discuss what might occur in the event of a smallpox attack. Prior to the meeting, Larsen went through security screening, including a pat-down. When security guards pulled out a gas mask from Larsen's briefcase, he explained that it was for demonstration use in the meeting. (He had forgotten that the tube containing the powder was also in the briefcase; radiation-sniffing machines and inspectors failed to find it.)

In the middle of a what-if scenario presentation, Cheney asked an obvious question: "What does a biological weapon look like?"

Suddenly remembering, Larsen pulled the powder-filled tube out of his briefcase. "It looks like this. And by the way, I just carried it into your office."[27] Recalling the incident, Larsen laughs. "The Secret Service didn't like me for several years after that, but the truth is that this stuff is undetectable and anyone can make it with a recipe they can find online. Today, Americans are asked to remove their shoes in airports years after a 2001 attempt to blow up an airplane by a man who put a bomb in his shoe. We started flying jets in the fifties," Larsen points out, "but it took four decades for someone to figure out that planes could be used as a weapon. Now terrorists want to be more inventive."

I asked Larsen another obvious question. Can't we prevent a bioterrorist attack?

His curt reply: "No, you can't."

Where Have All the Scientists Gone?

In the fall of 1992, a dark-haired, heavy-set, bespectacled Russian microbiologist with a Cupid's-bow mouth left the crumbling former Soviet Union for the U.S. with a wife and three children in tow. Kanatjan ("Ken") Alibekov also brought with him harrowingly detailed descriptions of the work he and at least 30,000 other scientists did for Biopreparat, the Soviets' secret biological weapons program, under the assumption that the U.S. was doing the same, despite a 1972 international ban.

Four years after Alibekov set foot in the U.S., the investigative journalist Laurie Garrett went to Russia to check out the remainders of the Biopreparat program for herself. She described a gigantic but seedy biological research facility outside the largest city in Asian Russia, Novosibirsk. It was an "enormous complex of a hundred large concrete and steel buildings, surrounded by an 8-foot concrete wall, topped by three rows of electric wires," she wrote. Then she described what lay inside the walls:

Scattered about, dressed in tattered uniforms, Russian soldiers idled away the long, cold, boring hours, guarding microscopic charges. In Building Number 1, for example, row upon row of industrial freezers housed Ebola, Lassa, smallpox, monkeypox, tick-borne encephalitis, killer influenza strains, Marburg, HIV, hepatitis A, B, C, and E, Japanese encephalitis, and dozens of other human killer viruses. And there were dozens of different strains of smallpox viruses—140 of them were natural, wild strains. Some were hand-crafted by the bioengineers . . . giving them greater powers of infectivity, virulence, transmissibility.

The Russian Army guards didn't fully understand what was in Building Number 1. They called them "superbugs."[28]

She wondered what would happen if, under such terrible conditions, the germs were to escape their frozen test tubes. And then she thought about all the people who once worked in the Soviet Union's massive biological weapons program, composed of 47 institutes, 40,000 employees, 9,000 scientists, and 11 full-scale research institutes employing 2,000 people with special expertise in pathogens. "By 1997," she noted, "most [of the scientists and technicians] were no longer to be found toiling in the laboratories, bioweapons factories or test sites. Where did they go?" she asked.[29] U.S. officials wondered the same thing. By way of an answer, Alibekov informed them that several of the specialists from Biopreparat had found work in other countries, including North Korea[30] and Iraq.

Following the 9/11 terrorist attacks on New York and Washington, Alibekov insisted to a U.S. congressional subcommittee that there was "no doubt" that Saddam Hussein had procured weapons of mass destruction.[31] Of course, no biological weapon of mass destruction was ever found in Iraq, and some experts have since questioned Alibekov's characterizations of the threats. (The Russian subsequently emerged as one of the most persuasive voices in favor of "Project Bioshield," a multibillion-dollar U.S. program designed to counter anthrax, smallpox, and other potential bioterrorism agents.[32] He has also profited quite handsomely from government contracts.[33])

But one thing is certain: even if Alibekov was wrong about Iraq, he certainly raised awareness about the bona fide threat of biological terrorism—a dark threat that, with the growth of fanatical groups like ISIS, has grown even darker. In 2010, Al Qaeda in the Arabian Peninsula made a call for "brothers with degrees in microbiology or chemistry to develop a weapon of mass destruction."[34]

The Threat of Bio-Error

At the time of Garrett's reporting for her 2000 book *Betrayal of Trust*, there were 453 known research labs with repositories in the U.S. and Europe, but also in China, Russia, Bulgaria, Iran, Turkey, Argentina, and 60 other nations. Of those labs, 54 sold or shipped anthrax; 64 sold the organism that caused typhoid fever; 34 offered the bacteria that produced botulism toxin; 18 repositories in 15 countries traded in plague bacteria. "Some of these repositories did business over the Internet, offering overnight shipment of microbes for nothing more than a credit card number," Garrett noted.[35]

Eighteen years have passed since Garrett did her count. Since then, the number of biolabs has exploded. In the United States alone, there were 1,371 high-security bioweapons labs in 2009. By 2013, according to *Newsweek*, the U.S. Government Accountability Office (GAO) reported that due to a lack of counting and registration standards, it could no longer provide an accurate estimate.[36] And the risk of bio-error is serious. Even if all the people who work in all these labs turned out to be responsible people doing legitimate work, what are the chances of a mistake happening and someone getting exposed to deadly viruses?

The scientists who work in the highest-level (BSL-4) biolabs take their own lives into their hands. Like the health workers in Ebola-ridden West Africa, they have to wear what look like spacesuits to protect themselves. To develop vaccines that stop the spread of disease, these scientists try to reverse-engineer a pathogen until they decipher its lethality, and then figure out how to defeat it. In addition to working with known disease agents like smallpox and anthrax, they try to develop drugs that could counteract a weaponized virus.

Lab Safety Levels

- *A Biosafety Level 1* (BSL-1) lab is suitable for work with well-characterized agents that do not cause disease in healthy humans. In general, these agents should pose minimal potential hazard to laboratory personnel and the environment. At this level, precautions are limited relative to other levels. Lab work is done on open benches.

- *A Biosafety Level 2* (BSL-2) lab involves work with agents of moderate potential hazard, including hepatitis A, B, and C; HIV; salmonella; and staphylococcus. In both BSL-1 and BSL-2 labs, laboratory personnel have specific training in handling pathogenic agents and are directed by scientists with advanced training. Access to the laboratory is limited when work is being conducted, but in BSL-2 labs, some procedures involving infectious aerosols or splashes are conducted in enclosed, protected workspaces called biological safety cabinets.

- A *Biosafety Level 3* (BSL-3) lab involves working with potentially deadly microbes—including tuberculosis, SARS, yellow fever, West Nile, and certain forms of encephalitis—that could be inhaled. In addition to the precautions taken in BSL-1 and BSL-2 labs, personnel wear protective clothing, and they are offered immunizations and receive medical surveillance. The facilities must have a series of safety features to prevent accidents, including special ventilation systems.

- A *Biosafety Level 4* (BSL-4) lab requires the highest levels of precaution. Personnel work with agents that could cause severe to fatal disease in humans for which there are no available vaccines or treatments, including Ebola. At this level, precautions may include airflow systems, multiple containment rooms, sealed containers, special pressurized suits, and established protocols for all procedures, including decontamination of materials, extensive personnel training, and high levels of security to control access to the facility.[37]

Unfortunately, even the highest-level biosafety labs aren't foolproof. One would assume that labs at the CDC in Atlanta, just one of two facilities in the world that officially holds smallpox, would be about as secure as it's possible to get. But even in such places, frightening accidents can happen. In February 2009, four CDC scientists in hazmat suits entered a decontamination chamber where they were to be showered in virus-killing chemicals before changing into their clothes. The shower didn't start. The gasket around the exit door deflated. When the scientists started an emergency chemical shower, the door back into the infectious-disease lab wouldn't shut either. Air pressure alarms blinked. Monitors went red. One biosafety expert called the incident "like a screenplay for a disaster movie."[38]

Consider some of the other accidents that occurred in the U.S. during 2014 alone:

- The army's Dugway Proving Ground lab in Utah accidentally sent specimens of live anthrax—which had been labeled as killed—to several labs across the country and around the world.[39]

+ Someone found 60-year-old vials of smallpox in a storage facility in a Bethesda, Maryland, lab. Even after three generations, the virus was still alive.[40]

+ Scientists at the U.S. Department of Agriculture asked the CDC for samples of an ordinary flu virus for some experiments. But when the USDA scientists noticed the virus wasn't behaving as they expected, they realized that it was deadly H5N1.[41]

+ 86 CDC workers were potentially exposed to live anthrax at the CDC's lab.[42, 43]

In October 2015, the White House issued directives to improve safety at federal labs. In response, the U.S. Department of Agriculture and the CDC published a report about the findings of the "Federal Select Agent Program," the purpose of which is to "regulate the possession, use and transfer of biological select agents and toxins so that important work with potentially dangerous and deadly pathogens is conducted as safely and securely as possible." The report noted that there were more than 230 safety incidents with bioterror viruses and bacteria in 2014 alone. Hundreds of employees had to be screened for potential exposures. Some labs had their permits suspended because of violations that raised "significant concerns for imminent danger."[44]

Following up on these alarming findings, the U.S. Government Accountability Office tried to find out exactly how often such incidents occur. The investigators found it was "impossible to determine" how often this kind of problem occurs in public and private labs in the U.S., mostly because the reporting forms that regulators use aren't designed to capture and track such incidents. In summarizing the GAO findings, USA Today reported that "neither the Federal Select Agent Program nor the National Institutes of Health, which separately oversee work with certain genetically altered pathogens, could provide the GAO's investigators with an accurate count of inactivation incidents from 2003 through 2015."[45] The report also noted that the U.S. still lacks a national strategy to identify the risks associated with the expansion in this kind of research.[46]

Laboratory mistakes can also happen anywhere in the world.[47] A scientist in Germany pricked herself with a needle contaminated with a strain of Ebola. At one laboratory in Austria, deadly H5N1 bird flu virus samples were mixed with seasonal flu samples.[48] In England, scientists meant to send dead anthrax samples to other labs in England and Ireland, but the tubes got mixed up, and the live stuff was sent out instead of the dead material. (The *Guardian* newspaper reported in 2014 that there had been more than 100 safety breaches in U.K. labs, the latter one being the most egregious.[49]) Such mistakes happen all over the world.[50]

And then there's the stuff going on in the countries with more limited resources. To find out what the labs looked like in Africa, U.S. senator Richard Lugar and a team of Pentagon arms-control experts visited Burundi, Uganda, and Kenya in 2010. Their findings made them shudder. One Kenyan research lab housing anthrax, Ebola, and Marburg viruses had low walls that could be easily scaled; the lab backed onto a slum. The African researchers had to use large samples of the viruses because their equipment was old.[51]

A pathogen can even escape a lab without anyone knowing how. At Tulane University in Louisiana, a couple of rhesus monkeys came down with *Burkholderia pseudomallei*, a deadly disease that lives in soil and water and that's found in Southeast Asia. Nobody could figure out how the monkeys were infected, but there was significant worry that the bacterium had spread to the facility's grounds.[52]

And of course, we need to ask: Who exactly works in all these labs? And does anyone do any sleuthing if a colleague routinely works late? "No one is doing due diligence on any of the labs [in the U.S.] so we don't really know if they're well run," Edward Hammond, a policy researcher and cofounder of the now-defunct Sunshine Project, told *Newsweek*.[53] (According to the report on the Federal Select Agent Program, the FBI also stopped 16 people who posed security risks—including six convicted felons, two fugitives, and a person found to be a "mental defective"—from working in the labs.[54])

When Scientists Play God

In September 2011, on the island of Malta, a friendly, blue-eyed, silver-haired Dutchman named Ron Fouchier gave a presentation to fellow researchers from the European Scientific Working Group on Influenza. Fouchier, of Erasmus University, announced that he and his colleagues had "mutated the hell out of H5N1 [highly pathogenic avian influenza]" and spread the highly contagious new germ around to ferrets in the lab. A dangerous life form that had previously existed only in nature had had its genetic sequence altered by serious scientists working in a respected lab.

Fouchier is not a bad guy by any stretch of the imagination; he's one of the good guys. In order to protect the public from the next naturally occurring pandemic, scientists like Fouchier have to understand how the microbes work.

"What is the difference between an ordinary zoonotic virus and a pandemic one?" he asks. "If we can understand that, then we can monitor those viruses in nature and know which ones we should keep an eye on."[55] But the kind of research he was doing sparked frightening stories in the media and a vigorous debate in the scientific community.[56, 57] Critics say the specific kind of work he is doing, called "gain of function," in which a germ gets stronger through gene manipulation, is just too dangerous.[58] Some worry that a lab-altered virus might escape through errors, like those I just cited, or else fall into the wrong hands.[59]

Fouchier insists that his high-security lab has so many redundant safety and security levels that the risk of a virus escaping, while not utterly impossible, is infinitesimally small. "This work is highly regulated and we are under continuous inspection," he says. "The animals with the genetically engineered viruses [ferrets] are kept in air-tight steel cages. If there would be a small leak, the virus still couldn't escape because the area that the cages are in is under low air pressure. My people go in wearing full protective gear, and they are vaccinated against the viruses we work with. The lab and equipment are always electronically monitored for pressure drops and leakages. In the many years we have done this work we have not had a single incident."[60] Personnel are also carefully screened.

But Marc Lipsitch, an epidemiologist at the Harvard School of Public Health who has been carrying on a fierce debate with Fouchier in various scientific journals, remains unconvinced, saying that an official in the Netherlands responsible for biosafety noted his own country's relatively poor record. "No matter how careful the lab is, failures can happen," Lipsitch says. "The scenario of a lab technician breathing in something from a ferret in one of the highly secure labs doing this research may be unlikely, but the empirical record shows that multiple times a year, there are cases of someone taking what should be treated at a high biosafety level and confusing it with something else. Even if you made the high-level labs completely impregnable, you still have the human problem. Humans tend to make a series of assumptions that are best case when the evidence goes in the opposite direction."

And while it may be awful yet "acceptable" for one person to die from an exposure accident, the consequence of hundreds of millions of deaths is very different, Lipsitch argues. "If even a small outbreak occurred as a result of this kind of research, it would set all scientific work back for decades. Besides, there are lots of ways to study flu. There are many experiments that have demonstrated many of the same things that the gain of function research shows, conducted in a safer way."[61]

Noting that scientists keep publishing more studies that involve genetically altered flu viruses, Dr. David Relman, a microbiologist at Stanford University, has observed that "every time that one of these experiments comes up, it just ups the ante a bit. It creates additional levels of risk that force the question: Do we accept all of this?" The Cambridge Working Group of scientists, concerned about the number of accidents and errors occurring in labs, believes that researchers should put a stop to experiments that would lead to risky new pathogens until there's a better assessment of the dangers and benefits. Another group called "Scientists for Science" thinks that limiting experiments is the wrong way to go; focusing on lab safety, they say, is the best defense. Each of these two groups boasts more than 100 supporters, including Nobel Prize winners. (The March 2016 National Academy of Sciences Second Symposium on Gain-of-Function Research added new evidence and insights to the debate, as well as an important international perspective.[62] But it's unclear how much closer it took us to an optional balance of benefits and risks for this type of research.)

The question is: What kind of research jumps over the line of acceptability? It's a stop-and-think question, and an old one. In Mary Shelley's classic novel *Frankenstein*, the scientist who creates the monster sees himself on a pure mission: to discover the source of life and prove his knowledge by creating a living human being. In his search for pure knowledge, Victor Frankenstein doesn't think about the consequences of his work: "One man's life or death were but a small price to pay for the acquirement of the knowledge which I sought, for the dominion I should acquire and transmit over the elemental foes of our race," he writes.[63] What would Mary Shelley have made of the fact that messing around with genetic sequences is all the rage now in the scientific world, thanks to a technology that allows scientists not only to mutate genetic material but even to create life?

That technology—CRISPR—was developed by two researchers, Jennifer Doudna of UC Berkeley and Emmannuelle Charpentier of Berlin's Max

Planck Institute. Genome engineering has been around since the 1970s, but CRISPR-Cas9 allows scientists to make changes to the DNA in cells. It's a system that bacteria have used since the beginning of time to shed their DNA genomes of little viruses called phages, and scientists everywhere are going wild over it. The bacteria-based CRISPR technology is cheap, elegant, accurate, and promising. Many see it as the end to the many blights humankind has suffered. Scientists are already using it to genetically modify mosquitoes to fight the Zika virus, to look for cures for HIV/AIDS, cystic fibrosis, cancer, Parkinson's and Alzheimer's diseases, and more.

The tool has incited a patent war, and now scientists all over the world are racing to win all kinds of pharmaceutical gold medals with CRISPR's help. Research teams from many countries are now playing with genes to discover ways to make pig organs safe to use in people, prevent inherited blindness, develop new medicines, and even bring back extinct animals like the mastodon.[64]

The CRISPR technology has even allowed scientists to create artificial microorganisms. In 2010, Craig Venter, head of the J. Craig Venter Institute (JCVI), a genomic research organization in La Jolla, California, announced that his team had used CRISPR-Cas9 to create a truly synthetic new life-form called JCVI-syn1.0. JCVI-syn1.0 is based on an existing bacterium that causes mastitis in goats, but it's constructed from chemicals made by 20 scientists who spent more than 10 years and an estimated $40 million on the project. JCVI-syn1.0 can reproduce itself and double its population size every three hours, passing on its genes through a novel form of evolution. As Venter claims in his speaker's bio, JCVI-syn1.0 "heralds the dawn of a new era in which new life is made to benefit humanity,"[65] starting with bacteria that can create biofuels and more.[66]

There are many obvious ethical issues surrounding the use of CRISPR-Cas9, not least of which are worries about "designer babies"[67] and gene manipulation in humans (the "human germline"). Also worrisome is the possibility of an accident. It's not beyond the pale to imagine that some biolabs around the world are using CRISPR to develop more virulent pathogenic viruses. As Garrett has pointed out, no country has yet adopted CRISPR-specific regulations, and what if a giant, uncontrolled DNA experiment, or some version of smallpox, gets loose?[68] As Dr. Gigi Kwik Gronvall, a senior associate at the Center for Health Security, has noted, "With gene synthesis technology accessible to people all over the world, and most genetic sequences for viruses including smallpox available on the Internet, there is now the potential that smallpox could return."[69] And diseases that have been extinct for many years could be brought back to life by bioterrorists using mail-order DNA kits and openly published sequence data.[70]

Like most technologies, CRISPR-Cas9 can be used for good or ill, but in this case the dividing line is particularly murky. What if a scientist, in pursuing a cure for HIV/AIDS or bubonic plague, accidentally produces a much more dangerous bacteria virus, with catastrophic results? Gene editing could result in an accident that could make humans more susceptible to diseases. The Future of Humanity Institute at the University of Oxford has issued recommendations regarding such risks, arguing that scientists doing the kind of research in which Fouchier is involved should "acknowledge that some of these experiments may pose unacceptable risks and should not be pursued in the absence of adequate mitigation measures." The Oxford authors also call for mandatory liability insurance for such research, to ensure that researchers have incentives to maintain high levels of laboratory biosafety.[71] Others advocate a systematic licensing protocol to prevent synthesis of dangerous DNA sequences.[72] Some think governments should put a curb on the publication of research that "could lead to adverse outcomes."[73]

Or what if a scientist working for a terrorist organization uses the technology to unleash a new form of bubonic plague? According to the *Guardian*, geneticist Robin Lovell-Badge of the Francis Crick Institute is "very, very concerned about this whole notion of there being rogue clinics doing these things." "It really scares me; it's bad for the field," he told reporters at the American Association for the Advancement of Science conference in Washington, D.C.[74] Daniel Gerstein, a former undersecretary at the Department of Homeland Security, said, "It's interesting that we have something that is clearly a technology that was designed for legitimate biotechnology research which has been associated in this way with weapons of mass destruction."[75]

Could strong international agreements and security checks on the use of genetic engineering technology help? Perhaps, but given the time differential between the frantic speed of genome development and the tortoise-like plodding of national and international agreements, the odds of winning the experimental race are heavily with the biolabs. Currently, most countries have forbidden the use of the technology for improving human genes to make designer babies, and so on, but not all. Although legislation and guidelines exist in 39 countries, and 29 have rules that could be interpreted as restricting genome editing for clinical use, the bans in several of these countries—including Japan, China, and India—are not legally binding, and the rules in nine other countries—among them Russia and Argentina—are ambiguous.[76] Moreover, guidelines and ambiguous rules are difficult to enforce.[77, 78]

And if you are a rogue scientist intent on helping a terrorist organization kill a lot of people, you really don't care. Indeed, Dr. Kenneth Bernard, a biosecurity expert who has worked with WHO and in the Bill Clinton and George W. Bush White Houses, thinks the idea of international compliance is close to laughable. "Russia made three tons of smallpox after they signed the Biological Weapons Convention," he told me. "The idea that people's behavior will be changed as a result of such an agreement is like taking your shoes off for a metal detector at the security line at the airport because it is easy. They never make you take your underwear off, although there was also an underwear bomber. Whether it is an international treaty or removing items of clothing at the airport, everyone wants to take action and do something, even if it may not be making us appreciably safer."[79]

What Can Be Done?

Every two years, the British government assesses the risks of civil emergencies facing people in the U.K., including events or situations that threaten human welfare. They lay out the seriousness of a risk based on the likelihood of something awful happening over the next five years. In response to smaller-scale biological attacks, the British government recommends that

- emergency responders receive specialized training for dealing with biological incidents, and have protective equipment to allow them to operate in hazardous environments and to rescue and treat casualties;

- ambulance and fire rescue services have the capability to decontaminate people;

- local authorities have plans in place to open centers for those forced out of their homes or otherwise caught up in the incident;

+ nonspecialist emergency responders are trained to perform life-saving activities;

+ regular testing is in place for effective and integrated response;

+ national stocks of medical vaccines, supplies, and other counter-measures are maintained and their distribution is arranged;

+ evacuation locations and shelters are planned for and built;

+ communications are improved so that the public knows what they can do to minimize risk.[80]

Since the terror attacks of 9/11, much has been done to put the U.S., too, on a more defensive footing. For example, the government has stockpiled enough smallpox vaccine to immunize every citizen, and a program called Bio-Watch set up a network of sensors in major American cities to detect harmful chemicals and biological agents. An agency called the Biomedical Advanced Research and Development Authority (BARDA) within the U.S. Department of Health and Human Services was set up to oversee the development and purchasing of vaccines, drugs, therapies, and diagnostic tools for public-health medical emergencies. BARDA is stockpiling vaccines against a variety of germs and is working to make sure that enough vaccine will be available should an epidemic occur.

Despite these and other precautions, biodefense in the U.S., regardless of all its capabilities and wealth, has been surprisingly rudderless with respect to unified command. Part of the problem is a culture clash between the militaristic biodefense world that deals with terrorism and the public-health world that doesn't want to, says Bernard. "It's like the difference between a pediatrician and a neurosurgeon—they can't switch positions for all kinds of reasons. If you go to a four-star general, he would say, 'I can't be concerned about bioterror,' he says, 'you are the health person, you do it.' You can't raise the profile of health in the realm of national security."[81]

This is very different from the preparedness stance of a country like Israel, which is accustomed to facing down terrorist threats. For example, Israel conducts a bioterror drill every two years in each of its hospitals. At the end of the drill, responders and hospital management have to take an exam. An American member of the U.S. National Biodefense Science Board who witnessed the exercise noted that "[w]e in the U.S. don't do this at all on a systemic basis, and certainly not at the regional scale," adding that the Israeli healthcare system is "remarkably well-coordinated."[82]

Preparation Is All[83]

In October 2015, a blue-ribbon, bipartisan panel of biodefense experts published a report that assessed the U.S.'s readiness for a biological attack. Above all, the report cried out for much more focused and coordinated leadership from the White House—including putting the vice president in charge of national biodefense—all the way down to local communities. "Simply put, the nation does not afford the biological threat the same level of attention that it does other threats," the report noted; "there is no centralized leader for biodefense. There is no comprehensive national strategic plan for biodefense. There is no all-inclusive dedicated budget for biodefense."

The U.S. Blue Ribbon report recommended a 33-point list of improvements to programs, legislation, and policies that, it urged, should be implemented "with the utmost haste, for lives are in the balance."

The report recommended the following actions, which it urged the U.S. government to complete in five years or less:

- Increase the development and availability of medical countermeasures, including drugs, vaccines, equipment, point-of-care technologies, and laboratory capacities.

- Establish a plan for coordinated decontamination and remediation in the event that disease-causing agents end up harming air, water, and soil.

- Ensure that emergency responders have what they and their families need to feel protected (if they don't, the report pointed out, "they will likely protect themselves and their families, not you and yours"). For example, only 20 percent of paramedics in one survey said they would remain on duty without a vaccine and protective gear—a number that rose to 91 percent if these protections were provided.[84]

- Increase hospital preparedness. During the Ebola outbreak of 2014, it became clear that hospital preparedness varied widely. A few hospitals were well prepared to serve as treatment centers for infected patients, but the vast majority of others were completely unprepared and struggled to catch up.[85]

- Improve intelligence collection and sharing. "A National Intelligence Manager for Biological Threats should manage biological intelligence," the report noted. "They, rather than the CIA, would be responsible for distributing funds for biological intelligence activities."

- Ensure full coordination among animal health and environmental health agencies, recognizing that every bioterror threat faced is zoonotic, except for smallpox. "This should include developing a nationally notifiable animal disease list and a reporting system which is accessible to agencies engaged in biodefense."

- Secure databases that contain genetic sequences of pathogens (including those of the most serious threat agents) against hacking.

- Mandate (by Congress) military-civilian collaboration on biodefense.

- Develop an environmental detection system for known and unknown biological threats.

The report also called for better biodefense budget analyses; multiyear funding for biodefense programs; enhancements to community intelligence; surveillance and emergency preparedness efforts; better apportionment of risk; making sure there is sufficient vaccine and medical emergency kits to safeguard citizens; improving logistics and innovation (especially for rapid point-of-care diagnostics); allowing research and security agencies to share needed data; overhauling the Federal Select Agent Program; and much more.

But ultimately, "it's all about leadership," insist Kenneth Bernard and Randall Larsen in duet, both of whom participated in the study. "If there were a deliberate attack, whom do you go to?" says Bernard. "Right now there is nobody at the White House or U.N. to be the point source for the national or international community. This is a national and international security issue; it's also a personal issue and community security issue. These are all very different, based on the population you are talking about." For his part, Larsen thinks things won't change until there is an attack.

*   *   *

In this chapter I have focused on bioterror, bio-error, and the Frankensteinian risks of engineered pathogens. If what I have said in this chapter and the previous two frightens you, it should. I wish the facts were different, but they aren't. Nevertheless, these warnings, dire as they are, impel all of us to think about intelligent responses to biological threats.

CHAPTER 5

THE COSTS OF COMPLACENCY

In addition to millions of deaths worldwide,
we could face global recession and massive
social upheaval.

It's a dystopian nightmare, and it could happen tomorrow. An uncontroll-able pandemic overwhelms public-health systems and wipes out millions of people in less than a year. Business and industry grind to a halt. Up to $3 trillion, a tenth of the country's global gross domestic product, evaporates as fear of infection stifles travel, tourism, trade, financial institutions, em-ployment, and entire supply chains. Children stop attending school. Rumors abound; neighbors scapegoat neighbors. Millions of unemployed poor, al-ways hit the hardest, resort to theft and violence in an effort to stay alive. People starve, even in the U.S. Those who do survive are left with their lives turned upside down.

Carlo Urbani's wife, Guiliani, was frantic. Why, she asked her husband and father of three, was he putting himself in such danger to treat desperately sick pa-tients in Vietnam?

"If I can't work in such situations, what am I here for? Answering emails, going to cocktail parties, and pushing paper?" he replied.

Urbani, a dogged protector of human life, was a hero in the fight against SARS (severe acute respiratory syndrome). In early 2003, the gentle, generous Italian doctor was working in Vietnam for Médecins Sans Frontières (MSF) when a troublesome case turned up in Hanoi. Local physicians were mystified. They called Urbani, a highly regarded expert clinical diagnostician, to see Johnny Chen, a 48-year-old Chinese-American businessman suffering from pneumonia, a high fever, and a dry cough.

Urbani first thought Chen had contracted bird flu, but the diagnosis didn't seem right. Urbani's clinical and epidemiological experience then led him to suspect Chen had something else, perhaps a new and highly contagious disease.

Between the time Dr. Urbani was summoned and the time he saw Chen, the microbe was already spreading rapidly among patients and workers at the hospital. Many would die within weeks.

Chen had picked up SARS during a stay at the Metropole Hotel in Hong Kong. His hotel room was across the hall from that of Liu Jianlun, a doctor who had recently treated patients with flu-like symptoms in Guangdong, China. Within days, both Jianlun and Chen became desperately ill. Another 15 hotel visitors would become infected too. But in the absence of any symptoms (yet) to warn of the danger they harbored, the tourists innocently boarded airplanes, unwittingly bringing the virus to Canada, Vietnam, Singapore, and Taiwan.

The first new and deadly infectious disease of the twenty-first century, SARS was an entirely unknown virus when Urbani saw Chen. Despite the fact that he had never encountered such an infection, Urbani immediately knew what to do. He instituted infection control procedures such as high-filter masks and double gowning, and he warned officials at the Vietnam Health Ministry that things looked bad. Then Urbani himself contracted SARS. Within weeks, he died in an isolation ward, hooked up to a ventilator. In one of his last conscious moments, he asked that his infected lung tissue be saved for science.[1, 2]

The Ricochet Effect: Scattered Risk and Amplified Costs

Killer diseases travel fast. After Carlo Urbani died, SARS quickly spread from South Asia to China to Canada and almost 20 other countries in 2003. In just four months, SARS infected around 8,000 people worldwide, killing nearly 10 percent of them.

Similarly, epidemiologists had predicted that Middle East Respiratory

Syndrome (MERS) would inevitably escape the Middle East to some distant place, but they had no idea where. MERS began its deadly path in May 2015 when a single traveler ("case zero") brought the "camel flu" home to South Korea from the Middle East. Within three weeks, a few dozen people were diagnosed with MERS and nine people died. By July, when the epidemic ended, 5,200 Koreans had been quarantined, 186 cases had been diagnosed, and 36 victims had died.[3]

The speed at which these diseases traveled demonstrates what I call the "ricochet effect." In today's world, a deadly virus that shows up in one place, carried by one patient who boards a plane, can rapidly ricochet around the globe to create an epidemic threat virtually everywhere. Zika, which first showed up in Uganda, blindsided Brazil in 2015. Ebola, which also broke out in Guinea, caught Dallas, Texas, unaware in 2014. H1N1 swine flu, which first appeared in Mexico, shocked southern California in 2009. If we think that such threats exist only "over there"—in Africa, in Asia—we're dangerously mistaken. This ricochet effect amplifies the risk and creates tremendous uncertainty for people, economies, and entire countries.

In addition to traveling fast, epidemics are unbelievably costly. SARS cost the global economy between $30 and $50 billion[4]; Toronto alone lost an estimated $1 billion in revenue.[5] In one holiday weekend, 250,000 fled Beijing; during the epidemic, the city received 1.5 million fewer visitors, a massive $2 billion hit to its tourist economy. Beijing closed schools and universities, movie theaters, internet cafes, and other leisure sites for a month. SARS also crippled hotel occupancy in Singapore by 20 percent, and even more in Hong Kong. Retail sales halved in both cities.

When MERS struck, the ensuing panic led the Bank of Korea, South Korea's central bank, to drop the prime interest rate to a record low—a move the bank's governor described as a preemptive action to reduce MERS's economic consequences. Despite the relatively low number of casualties in this case, MERS nevertheless caused a tremendous loss in revenue. Department store sales in affected countries dropped by 17 percent, and more than 100,000 foreign travelers canceled trips.

Why do epidemics cost so much? At least half of the price tag springs from disruptions to businesses local and global, small and large. An epidemic lands a gut-blow to virtually every sector of the economy, including manufacturing, trade, tourism, agriculture, financial institutions, employment, education, medicine, and more. The other half is spent by governments, charities, and

The Economic Impact of Recent Epidemics and Pandemics

Recent SARS, H5N1 avian influenza, and H1N1 swine flu pandemics have each cost the world $30 to $55 billion.

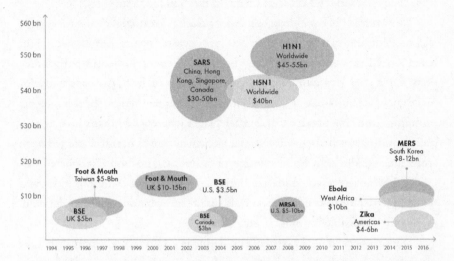

SOURCE: Adapted from Machalaba C, Daszak P, Berthe F, Karesh W. Added value of global health security. Consortium of Universities in Global Health 8th Annual CUGH Conference. 2017. Carroll D. The global virome project: A first step toward ending the pandemic era. Consortium of Universities in Global Health 8th Annual CUGH Conference. 2017.

nongovernmental organizations that try to keep disease from spreading. And those costs don't include losses from disruptions to social order or the cost of caring for survivors.

Aversion Behavior and the Epidemic Cascade

In a typical example of what psychologists and economists call "aversion behavior" (simply put, the human desire to stay away from scary events), the American TV personality Ali Fedotowsky canceled her big wedding in Mexico in 2016. "We were super excited," she told a reporter from *Sky News*. "We found the most amazing location and villa that would allow our entire family to stay with us. Then, all the news broke about the Zika virus and we had to cancel. It was such a huge disappointment." Since most of her friends were in "baby mode," she didn't think it was fair to ask guests to come to a place where Zika was active.[6]

For people with means like Fedotowsky—particularly those hoping to escape the bitter cold of a northern winter—the pearlescent beaches and turquoise water of Mexico's coasts, the Caribbean, and Florida are a magnetic draw. But in the event of an epidemic, anything associated with tourism (hotel rooms, food, and entertainment) gets wounded first.[7]

This aversion behavior can combine with the direct effects of an epidemic (sickness, disability, and death) to create a devastating "epidemic cascade" of health, social, economic, and business impacts in a country or entire region. Nobody wants to risk catching a disease or being quarantined. Aversion behavior makes people shun not only travel but also arts venues, malls, theaters, sports stadiums, amusement parks, and other places where we humans love to congregate. Our aversion behavior hurts anyone who works in travel and tourism, from tour guides and hotel owners to waitstaff and housekeepers. If an epidemic were severe, companies in the travel, tourism, arts, entertainment, and related sectors in these industries could lose 80 percent of consumer demand, making it impossible for most to stay afloat.[8]

The prospect of a catastrophic epidemic is a CEO's nightmare, whether the company is in the hotel, airline, towel-manufacturing, or any other sector in the global supply chain. Frighteningly, and despite the immense risks to business, experts note that most companies would be completely unable to protect their staff, profits, and reputation in the event of an epidemic. Three-quarters of companies have inadequate pandemic preparedness plans, and about one-quarter have no strategy at all. Only 22 percent are comfortable that they are prepared.[9]

Here are examples of economic threats to specific sectors:

Hospitals. The cost of individual patient treatment is astronomically high. If a severe epidemic were to strike, health systems would be quickly overwhelmed. During the Ebola epidemic, an article in the *Economist* noted, the estimated cost to build a 70-bed facility in Bong County, Liberia, would be $170,000. It would require a staff of 165 to treat patients and handle tasks like waste management and body disposal. It would go through 100 sets of overalls, gowns, sheets, and hoods every day. The monthly cost of running the unit would have been around $1 million, or roughly $15,000 a bed.[10]

In the U.S., treating just two Ebola patients cost the University of Nebraska's Medical Center $1 million.[11] According to the U.S. Department of Homeland Security, the direct cost to healthcare facilities, including new and temporary facilities in a severe epidemic, would be $80 billion in the U.S. alone. The U.S. healthcare system would be overwhelmed in seven to ten weeks, and it would be forced to turn away 3 to 4 million patients due to lack of resources.[12]

The Epidemic Cascade

The direct effect of epidemics, combined with aversion behavior, drives a cascade of sometimes devastating and lasting healthcare, social, economic, and business impacts.

Direct Impact

Severe pandemic could strike **2.5 billion** people, killing up to **400 million** worldwide

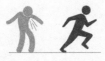

Aversion Behavior

Risk Avoidance, Fear of Contagion

Healthcare Impact

3-4 million patients could be turned away in a severe U.S. pandemic

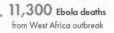

11,300 Ebola deaths from West Africa outbreak

10,600 additional deaths from AIDS, tuberculosis, malaria due to disrupted health services

Unexpected outbreaks hit health workers **513 died** from Ebola

Social Impact

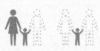

17,300 children lost one or both parents to Ebola

33 weeks of school closures due to Ebola

Business Impact

$5 billion in tourism losses from H1N1 in 2009

20-60% absenteeism with pandemic influenza

Up to **40% businesses closed** by a disaster, never to reopen

Economic Impact

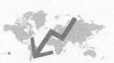

5% ($3.5 trillion) cost of severe pandemic to the global economy

Indirect Impact — Direct Health Impact

Two-thirds of the economic impact is losses in supply, demand, productivity, and jobs

SOURCES: Cost of the Ebola Epidemic, Centers for Disease Control and Prevention, 2016, https://www.cdc.gov /vhf/ebola/outbreaks/2014-west-africa/cost-of-ebola.html (accessed 6 July 2019); Machalaba C, Daszak P, Berthe F, Karesh W. Added value of global health security. Consortium of Universities in Global Health 8th Annual CUGH Conference. 2017.

Potential GDP Losses during a Severe Pandemic, by Industry, U.S.

The nonprofit Trust for America's Health analyzed the potential impact of a U.S. pandemic as severe as the 1918 influenza. Every U.S. state and every sector of the economy would be affected, with losses of $30 to $70 billion for manufacturing, transportation and warehousing, and accommodation and food services.

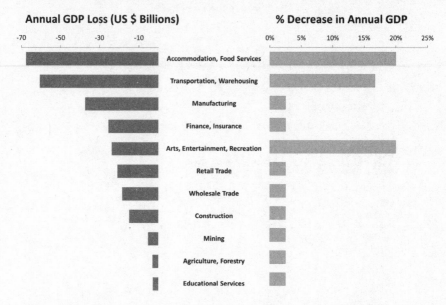

SOURCE: Pandemic flu and the potential for U.S. economic recession. Trust for America's Health. 2015. http://healthyamericans.org/reports/flurecession/FluRecession.pdf (accessed 24 June 2017).

If a health system shuts down, more people may die of disrupted health services than from the epidemic itself. Children go without immunizations, women go without maternal care, and those who suffer from chronic diseases like diabetes lack access to life-saving drugs. During the Ebola epidemic, with people scared to go to health facilities and healthcare workers themselves dying in large numbers, in addition to more than 11,000 deaths from Ebola, there were an estimated 10,600 deaths from AIDS, tuberculosis, and malaria due to disrupted health services.[13] Childhood immunization rates fell by 30 percent as resources were diverted to fight Ebola.[14]

Finance and Insurance. Stock markets and financial institutions are exquisitely sensitive to the effects of public fear, anxiety, and perceived risk. Anyone with investments in places where disease strikes would want to withdraw money to avoid the risk.[15] The Dow dropped 460 points during the Ebola epidemic, not because the disease directly affected financial personnel but because of its indirect impact on tourism.

Health, commercial property, casualty, and life insurance companies also worry about epidemics, because losses from mortality claims, absenteeism, and business disruptions could be catastrophic. One study predicted a loss of $40 billion for the U.S. insurance industry alone, assuming that 35 percent of the U.S. population would become ill and 200,000 would die.[16] For many insurers, disease is the number-one extreme mortality risk, and a severe pandemic could wipe out up to 20 percent of the value from insured losses alone.

Agriculture and Farming. In poor countries, an epidemic can also have a brutal impact on subsistence farming and local markets. Beyond the scares associated with beasts and fowl, as I showed in chapter 3, spreading illness can hurt agriculturally dependent businesses everywhere—not just because they may need to cull diseased poultry, pigs, and cows, but merely by virtue of their geographic location. For instance, the Ebola virus threatened the cocoa harvest in Ghana and Côte d'Ivoire, which supply 60 percent of the world's cocoa. By mid-October 2014, a drop in production caused international cocoa prices to jump by close to 20 percent.[17]

In Liberia, Sierra Leone, and Guinea, Ebola caused precipitous drops in agricultural production and income.[18] Farmers couldn't tend to their crops; at the same time, aversion behavior and travel bans kept people away from markets and thus their access to food.

A terrible snowball effect ensues. When farmers get sick, they can't work in the fields, resulting in lower wages and lack of available food. When health workers fall ill and die, health care becomes less available, leaving more people to get sick and die, too. And when parents get sick and die, children are left alone.[19, 20]

Mining, Manufacturing, and Infrastructure. Iron ore mining is a huge industry in West Africa, where Ebola hit with unmerciful force. ArcelorMittal, the world's largest steel company, was in the midst of a $1.7 billion expansion of its iron ore mine in Yekepa, Liberia, when the disease broke out. The company had been exporting 5 million tons of iron ore a year from the country and had employed scores of Liberians.[21]

When Ebola shut Liberia's borders, ArcelorMittal's management insisted it would not close up shop, and it made valiant efforts to protect the health of its employees, contractors, and the community in which it operated. But following an employee's death and the expanding horror of the epidemic, the challenges to the company's Liberia operations ballooned.

By the late summer of 2014, Liberia's civil service workers were told to stay home, which meant that ArcelorMittal had to find ways to move iron ore and supplies through its port, although no customs inspectors were on hand. When Liberia imposed a curfew that August, the company, which operated around the clock, had to obtain special permits for its vehicles so it could move ore at night. After Guinea shut its border, ArcelorMittal couldn't get the imported fruit, meat, and other goods it needed. Food supplies ran out in neighboring Monrovia, so ArcelorMittal had to charter planes to bring in fresh food. Meanwhile, 2,400 of the company's contractors fled the country. When airlines began canceling flights into and out of Liberia, ArcelorMittal evacuated 130 of its expatriates. Needless to say, morale among those who remained in the hot zone was abysmal.[22]

The Ebola virus interrupted infrastructure projects in West Africa too, including a road project linking Liberia and Guinea. The contractor, China Henan International Cooperation Group, pulled its workers from those countries, leaving more people desperate for employment in their wake.[23]

Social Costs: The Hit to Education

What if you or someone you loved were one of the millions who could die from a deadly disease? When confronted with numbers like those above, I know your eyes close. So do mine. Numbers numb us. But when we think about a single human being's suffering, we're much more interested. "If you are told that someone is drowning but you don't see or hear their cry," says behavioral economist Dan Ariely, "your emotional machinery is not engaged."[24] From afar, Ariely suggests, Earth is a pale blue dot. As you move closer, you can see the terrain of oceans and continents. It's a gorgeous thing. Zero in and you see all kinds of terror and horror, the scourge of epidemics, and the suffering of individuals.

Most of us never really stop to think about the secondary effects of epidemics. In fact, the victims aren't just those who get sick and die from the disease itself—they are also the children left with no one to care for them.

Delphia Akafumba Mwanagala, a teacher in Lusaka, Zambia, contracted AIDS from her husband, a retired soldier. After he died, his family took everything she had and left her with three sons. Her $50-per-month salary as an elementary school teacher was too small to pay for a doctor.[25]

Delphia grew deathly ill. The school where she taught, Kaplunga Girls High School, had a nickname: ABC, for "AIDS Breeding Center." Between

2000 and 2003, six of the school's beloved teachers had died of the disease. The deaths came so fast that the school stopped canceling classes for teacher funerals, and there weren't any more teachers left alive to take their places.

Epidemics can decimate school enrollment and attendance.[26] According to UNAIDS, more than a million African children lost a teacher to AIDS in 2001. AIDS traumatized whole communities where teachers were seen as leaders. The children where the schools closed often were forced to work to supplement family income or take care of sick siblings or relatives. Once that happened, older children often could not return to finish their education.[27]

For a moment, put yourself in the mind of an intelligent 11-year-old girl whose parents died of AIDS-related illnesses. Your mother never told you how she got the disease or how to avoid it. You spend the rest of your childhood looking after your three brothers and sisters and three other boys whose parents also died of AIDS-related illnesses. Someone from Save the Children comes along, and you say the following:

> When my mother died, we suffered so much. There was no food, and there was no one to look after us. We didn't even have money to buy soap and salt. We wanted to run away to our other grandparents, but we didn't have transport to go there. I tried to be positive, but it was difficult. Some neighbors say bad things about us: "Those children are so poor; they don't even have relatives. They don't belong." Some people also call us "AIDS orphans," and they say that maybe our parents infected us. We don't say anything.
>
> I don't go to school. I'd like to go, but my grandparents and neighbors told me to stay at home and look after the others. If I were educated I'd like to be a nurse. I want to treat other people and heal them from whatever they're suffering from. I want to do this because when my mother was sick, there was nobody to look after her because we had no money.[28]

Not only did this child lose her parents and her opportunity for an education, as is so often the case, but to make matters worse, her fearful community shunned her and her siblings.

Douda Fullah, 17 years old, lost his father, stepmother, brother, sister, and grandmother to Ebola when it struck Sierra Leone in 2014. Like so many in West Africa, the teenager was left to look after younger relatives. "Presently I am just left without my family," he tearfully told *Sky News*. "I have no one to take care of us. I am left with my younger ones. I want to follow my education.

I want to do a better thing in life to support my younger ones. I am begging. There's no hope for us. We need help."[29]

If Douda could safely go to school and contribute to the world beyond taking care of his relatives, how much would his life be worth? How much could he contribute to his country? How much could the siblings he was left to look after contribute?

The tragic result is that an epidemic ruins lives in multiple ways.[30] It's a vicious cycle that degrades a society year after year: besides killing and disabling a society's most productive adults (thus eroding the tax base needed to keep social structures like education and health care intact), it forces children to surrender their education. And less-educated children have less knowledge to pass on to their own offspring, affecting the next generation's health, productivity, and more.[31]

Survivors Are Costly Too

Liberian nurse Salome Karwah lost her parents, brother, aunts, uncles, cousins, and a niece to Ebola. Thanks to care from Médecins Sans Frontières, she herself recovered from the virus. Because she was now immune, she went to work caring for innumerable other victims. In 2014, *Time* magazine honored her with the title of "Person of the Year" for her tireless dedication in saving the lives of others. But when Nurse Karwah delivered a son by cesarean section in February 2017, she fell into seizures and died because none of the hospital staff would touch her, believing she was still contagious. She died in agony without treatment, a victim of stigma.[32]

Now fly far out into space, away from Douda and Salome—innocents whom psychologists call the "identifiable victim"—and multiply this story by millions. Does that exercise in imagination make us care any more than we did before? At what point do we become immune to his tragedy? At what point does his story fail to register? Mother Teresa once said, "If I look at the mass, I will never act. If I look at one, I will." How do we begin to care once they stream away into hundreds, millions, or billions?[33,34] What happens if something like pandemic flu sickens your neighbors, your employees, your loved ones? If a pandemic strikes, you or your children could be one of the millions of "identifiables" lost.

The fact is that if a deadly epidemic strikes, it can affect you or me or anyone we love in an instant. Ebola cost Douda his family and devastated the lives of thousands in West Africa, but the loss of life and so many children's futures was just one terrible effect of the epidemic. If you visualize an epidemic as an intricate spiderweb with the disease at its center, you can imagine the innumerable, sticky aftereffects spinning out from that center in all directions.

Liberia had only 117 doctors for a country of more than 4 million people. Imagine being Dr. Jefferson Sibley, director of Phebe Hospital in Liberia, who lost more than a dozen doctors and nurses to Ebola. When Ebola victims began streaming into Liberia's hospitals, staffers were overwhelmed. Doctors and nurses died. Other health workers, fearing for their lives, stayed home or fled the country. The crisis was so great that women needing prenatal and maternal care, or people needing treatment for malaria or measles or those who needed surgery, were sometimes left to fend for themselves.[35, 36] Outpatient care dropped by 61 percent from 2013. Care for newborns and their mothers shrank by 43 percent. And vaccinations for diphtheria, pertussis, and tetanus fell by more than half.[37]

The HIV/AIDS crisis in East and southern Africa decimated the most economically active segment of the population, those between the ages of 16 and 45.[38] If 35 percent of the people of a given country get sick, more than 70 percent of overall productivity is lost, which in turn drives down imports and exports. Add to such catastrophes the ongoing costs of treatment and care for those who survive an epidemic. According to the CDC, it costs more than $379,000, in 2010 dollars, to treat one HIV-positive person for a lifetime, and many people are uninsured.[39] In the case of Zika, caring for a single baby with microcephaly could run as much as $10 million for the life of the child.[40]

And people who contracted the SARS virus faced all kinds of chronic problems as a result. One study found that even after recovering from SARS, 88 percent of patients suffered ongoing problems like shortness of breath, muscle pain, and fatigue so debilitating that they could not return to work. In addition, many continue to suffer mental health issues like post-traumatic stress disorder.[41] Ebola survivors suffer many of the same kinds of symptoms as those who survived SARS.[42] Those who struggle with these problems often can't function as fully productive members of society like they once did.

We're Not Ready for the Big One[43]

In September 2014, Liberia's president and Nobel laureate Ellen Johnson Sirleaf wrote to President Obama begging for the U.S. to act against Ebola. "I am being honest with you," she wrote, "that at this rate . . . the virus will overwhelm us." She continued: "In a country that has barely emerged from a 30-year period of civil and political unrest, with the presence of a large youthful (mainly unemployed) population, some of whom were child soldiers, this health emergency threatens civil order."[44]

When an epidemic turns into a full-blown conflagration, civil society can reach a tipping point. Those who can flee, do. Soldiers, police, and healthcare workers leave their posts. Schools and financial institutions close. Basic services like food, water, and electricity might start to collapse. Looting increases. A severe pandemic would not only stop people like farmhands and truck drivers from working; there would also be too few people to man infrastructure systems like the electric grid and computer networks. Some experts posit that in a little over a year of a major pandemic like the 1918 Spanish flu, half the U.S. would be starving. Although starvation resulting from Ebola was widely predicted in West Africa, especially in quarantined rural areas, it was averted by aid agencies distributing food, according to Dr. Andrew G. Huff, a specialist in food supply protection. But in a worldwide pandemic, "There is no one to bail other countries out."[45]

*   *   *

As epidemics go, SARS was an amateur compared to the bubonic plague that killed about a quarter of Europe's population in the fourteenth century. And it was a mere blip on the radar compared to the 1918 Spanish flu, which sickened a third of the world's population and killed up to 50 million people.[46] If a Spanish flu–style pandemic were to strike North America or the rest of the world today, given the world's current lack of preparedness, the economic impact would dwarf that of the $30 to $50 billion lost to SARS.

The history and biology of the influenza virus tell us that we should expect another major global pandemic within the next 20 to 40 years. As I noted earlier, such a pandemic could kill 200 to 400 million people if it spread as readily and were as deadly as the 1918 flu, causing massive economic and social disruption. I believe this is the worst-case scenario on which our preparedness should be based. But is the projection of 400 million deaths realistic or alarmist rhetoric? Are we really at the same risk we were 100 years ago?

The good news is that medical care is vastly more advanced today. International communications, health regulations, and coordination mechanisms are light-years ahead of where they were in 1918. Nearly all high-income and a growing number of low- and middle-income countries have pandemic preparedness plans. Though far from perfect, communication methods for professionals and the public are vastly improved. And finally, we have better-nourished, healthier populations in many parts of the world.

The bad news is that, despite our medical advances, we still do not have highly effective vaccines to prevent, or effective medicines to treat, pandemic influenza viruses.[47] And the combination of international travel, global warming, food production, population growth, urbanization, and land encroachment together increases the likelihood of infectious-disease outbreaks.

In short, without the much more aggressive course of action that I am proposing in the seven areas described in part II, it's wishful thinking to believe that we are less vulnerable to a devastating pandemic than we were 100 years ago.

A Better Investment

The moral of the story is this: in both economics and epidemics, prevention always far surpasses even the best efforts at cure. If we proactively invest in prevention strategies to monitor and track outbreaks, develop vaccines, improve public-health systems, control disease-carrying mosquitoes, reduce deforestation, improve farm biosecurity, and so on, we can dramatically reduce the risk of catastrophic epidemics and global pandemics.

In chapter 11, I will show how, if you do the numbers, the cost of such investment would run roughly $7.5 billion per year over the next two decades—$1 per year for each person on the planet. That's a tiny fraction of the estimated $374 billion for a mild pandemic to $7.3 trillion for a severe pandemic.[48] It would save tens or hundreds of millions of lives and avert the social upheaval often created by pandemics. This is arguably the best investment we could ever make. The more we spend up front, the more lives and money we will save down the road.

One company that is making a serious investment in public health is

Unilever. "We believe in a three-pronged approach—prevention, relief, and rehabilitation," says Rebecca Marmot, who heads up advocacy and partnership for the multinational corporation. "The business case and social impact are linked. By ensuring we train and equip not only our employees but suppliers and distributors across our value chain, we help mitigate business risk but more importantly protect their livelihoods."[49]

The cost of inaction puts heads of state, leaders of national and international agencies, and corporate CEOs on special notice: given the risks, they should be doing whatever they can to step up their preparedness plans and invest in public-health systems. As citizens, we should be demanding such an investment with everything we have.

In the chapters that follow, you will learn more about the practical ways that we can defend ourselves against bioterror, bio-error, and threats that emerge from the bush and the barn. You will see what we can do in terms of personal, community, and national protection; you will also learn more about how better investment and innovation, strong leadership, timely risk communication, and on-the-ground activism can help us defend ourselves against disease. Indeed, if what I have told you so far has frightened you to the degree that you understand the threats that face us, then you will better understand the prescription for remedying them that I explain in the chapters that remain.

PART II

STOPPING PANDEMICS
BEFORE THEY START

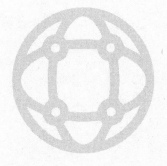

CHAPTER 6

LEAD LIKE THE HOUSE IS ON FIRE

When leaders work with urgency, decisiveness, and
courage, they can defeat the deadliest viral enemies.

Like firefighters racing to a burning building, the best leaders respond rapidly and decisively in the face of an epidemic. They put public well-being first, rising above complacency and political expediency. They encourage and support those at the front line. Most important, strong leaders learn from experience and are not afraid to change course or admit missteps in response to new information.

One of my first hands-on experiences as a medical student was assisting in an appendectomy. Dr. Bob Caldwell, the surgeon with whom I was working, called me into the emergency room to see Tom, a boy in his late teens with severe pain in his lower right side. The pain pattern and physical exam strongly indicated appendicitis. We also had to consider other possibilities such as the stomach flu or a bad case of constipation. While we awaited the results of the usual blood tests and X-ray, Dr. Caldwell looked at me and said, "These tests can be helpful, but there is no single test to confirm appendicitis."

This troubled me. When the X-rays came back, I didn't see anything but a bit more gas than usual in his intestines. Based on the strength of the clinical evidence, Dr. Caldwell had to make a judgment call. If we waited until we were 100 percent certain that Tom had appendicitis, the appendix could swell from inflammation and rupture, spilling a life-threatening infection through Tom's entire abdomen. If we operated, Dr. Caldwell noted, there was a 10 to 20 percent chance the appendix would turn out to be normal. For a few moments, he stared at the X-ray viewer on the wall. "We're going to the operating room," he concluded.

As it happened, Tom did have a red-hot appendix. The surgery was successful, and Tom made a speedy and complete recovery.

Despite phenomenal advances, medicine remains an imperfect science. Sometimes, as in the case of appendicitis, it can be a bit like predicting the path of a cyclone or a hurricane—a skill at which meteorologists have improved, but not to the point of 100 percent accuracy. In the case of a potentially dangerous weather event, presidents, governors, and mayors also face perplexing judgment calls: Do they order an evacuation of everyone in the storm's path, running the risk that the alarm might turn out to be false? Or do they take a less aggressive approach and risk widespread loss of life and property? Sometimes, you're damned if you do and damned if you don't.

*   *   *

The same is true for leaders in the face of a potential epidemic. Consider what happened when an outbreak of swine flu sickened a few people at Fort Dix, Virginia, in 1976. The flu looked like it had a lot in common with the 1918 flu strain. The head of the CDC, Dr. Dave Sencer, feared that the disease could affect up to 60 million Americans. With the blessing of the president and Congress, he ordered a mass inoculation to the tune of $137 million. More than 40 million Americans received the shot. The swine flu epidemic never materialized, but hundreds of people suffered a reaction called Guillain-Barré syndrome, the same paralytic condition brought on by the Zika virus. Twenty-five people died, and the government was forced to pay millions in damages.[1] Sencer lost his job and vaccine skeptics felt emboldened.[2]

"The principal players in the swine flu drama were people of immense goodwill, high ideals, technical competence and dedication to the public good. Yet the matter turned out in a way that was disappointing to all," wrote David A. Hamburg, president of the Carnegie Corporation and former president of the Institute of Medicine.[3] Sencer made an evidence-based judgment call that turned out to be wrong, but the harm done certainly was not intentional.

Unintentional mistakes are easier to accept when we know leaders make the best judgment calls that they can, based on careful consideration of the facts. But leaders truly err when they are presented with the evidence and refuse to take action. In *Shall We Wake the President?*, a history of disaster response by U.S. presidents, Tevi Troy cites U.S. president Woodrow Wilson as one of the five worst presidents at dealing with crises for his handling of the 1918 Spanish flu, because Wilson allowed the World War I effort to trump public health.[4]

Wilson was so focused on the war effort that he ignored repeated warnings about the spread of the flu, even from his personal physician and the admiral of the navy. More than 600,000 Americans died from influenza without a single word from Wilson. He refused to speak out about the epidemic publicly or privately. Nor did he mobilize nonmilitary government resources to help civilians. Worse, while influenza raged, and with Germany's allies rapidly abandoning the war, Wilson continued to send troops on ships from America across the Atlantic. Packed into dense quarters as they crossed the ocean, thousands of conscripts contracted the disease. Pandemic historian John M. Barry paints a horrific picture of overwhelmed sick bays, hemorrhaging patients lying on deck, and "waves of bodies" buried at sea.[5]

In the case of catastrophic epidemics, those at the highest levels of power are far more culpable when they deliberately avoid taking steps to prevent and contain outbreaks quickly. The toxic trio of denial, dithering, and distrust characterized the early phases of the AIDS epidemics in the U.S., SARS in China, Ebola in West Africa, and Zika in Brazil. In each case, failure to heed the alarms and to invest in preventive measures paved a road to disaster.

By contrast, the best leaders I know, including the ones I later describe, transcend denial, complacency, political expediency, and self-interest to prioritize the public's well-being. They rely on scientific evidence. They learn from experience and mistakes when things don't turn out as they expect or predict. With an unshakeable commitment to preventing unnecessary suffering and death, they create effective plans to prevent transmission and treat the ill. They tend to those most in danger. They defend civil liberties, even while they may have to temporarily restrict people from traveling or going out in public. They do what they can to prevent financial harm to people, cities, and companies.

They discourage scapegoating of the ill. And they inspire confidence, cooperation, and resilience. In short, they put humanity first.

Effective and focused leadership is the starting point for The Power of Seven, the essential steps that can end epidemics. Simply put, there is no chance of success without leaders who are wholly committed to putting humanity first. How do the best leaders, sometimes under threat to their reputations or even their own lives, do what they do? What are the essential qualities that they must possess?

D. A. Henderson and the End of Smallpox

In Charles Dickens's mid-nineteenth-century London, a compassionate maid named Charley drags her pretty mistress, Esther Summerson, to check on a sick homeless child in a godforsaken corner of the city. The young boy shakes with fever and emanates "a very peculiar smell" from a straw bed. Esther, a perennial do-gooder, insists that the boy be brought to the warm, safe house she shares with her adoptive guardian and others.

Infection and death then enter through the garden gate. The boy dies in the house. Within days, Charley's face is engulfed in blistering red pustules. She recovers, but Esther grows desperately ill. Bedridden for several weeks, Esther temporarily loses her eyesight and wavers between life and death. Finally recovering, Esther looks around her room and observes that her mirror is missing. Charley—now immune and able to safely nurse Esther—breaks into sobs, and Esther suddenly realizes why there is no mirror. Her face now looks like a minefield. "I called Charley back," Esther says. "I took her in my arms, and said, 'It matters very little, Charley. I hope I can do without my old face very well.'"[6]

Thus, in *Bleak House*, Dickens deftly explores the theme of smallpox infection. In this—one of Dickens's most acclaimed novels—no one is safe from the disease because everyone is connected. The author vividly captures the casualness of contact among classes, the uncertainty of survival, and the disfigurement experienced by the majority of survivors.

Caused by the *variola* virus, smallpox was a pain-wielding grim reaper with unremitting persistence. Nicknamed "the speckled monster," it ravaged humanity from the time of Egyptian pharaohs; mummies bear the signs of its deadly wrath. Throughout history, this microbial villain killed at least a third of its victims and disfigured most of the remainder. It was deadlier than the bubonic plague that obliterated a third of Europe in the thirteenth century. It wiped out huge segments of indigenous peoples. It's hard to believe, but smallpox buried and disfigured twice as many people in the twentieth century as all of that century's wars, from World War I and II to Vietnam and beyond.[7]

*   *   *

As early as 1796, long before Dickens described Esther's disfigurement, an English physician and scientist named Edward Jenner demonstrated the effectiveness of a vaccine. Like many innovators, Jenner stumbled on this discovery by the chance observation that women who milked cows seemed to be immune to smallpox.[8] Had a real-life Esther Summerson been vaccinated with cowpox vaccine at the time Dickens was conceiving *Bleak House*, she might have kept her milkmaid complexion.

Not long after Jenner's discovery, the wealthy of Europe and America began receiving immunizations. It would take another 170 years to eradicate the disease worldwide, because the poorest communities and countries had no access to the vaccine. The U.S. experienced its last case of indigenous smallpox in 1949. By 1966, only one country in the Americas was not yet smallpox-free, and by 1971 the entire Western Hemisphere was clear of the disease.

Many believed that eliminating smallpox for good in the rest of the world was impossible. But Donald Ainslie Henderson, a public-health physician known affectionately as "D.A.," begged to differ. D.A., who passed away in 2016 at the age of 87, was a man I knew personally and admired wholeheartedly. An avuncular, broad-shouldered, and compassionate doctor, D.A. cared deeply about smallpox victims. "Smallpox has been called one of the most loathsome diseases," he told the *Washington Post* in 1979. "No matter how many visits I made to smallpox wards filled with seriously ill and dying patients, I always came away shaken."[9]

During the eradication campaign, he worked closely with local people who were helping with the vaccinations. "He would go out into the field with the local workers, and he would put his hand on their shoulders and say, 'We couldn't do this work without you,'" recalled Dr. Sanjoy Bhattacharya of the London-based Wellcome Trust. "He had this wonderful way of making people feel they mattered."[10]

D.A. was the kind of doctor you would want as your own physician. He embodied a blend of caring, indefatigable determination, and the assuredness of a surgeon who is at home in his realm of scientific expertise. Those same qualities served him equally well as a leader. The American epidemiologist William Foege observed him as having "a sense of certainty on things . . . and people like to follow a leader that is quite certain about what they are doing."[11]

D.A. spoke with an authoritative, calming baritone as he described the drama of the international debates that led to smallpox eradication. When the proposal to eradicate smallpox from every country, which he helped to develop, was presented to the world's ministers and secretaries of health during the May 1966 World Health Assembly, it was put to a vote after three days of debate. "It came within two votes of being defeated," Henderson told me. "When the vote came, we had no idea how it would come out. We needed 56 votes. We got 58."[12]

As I describe in the prologue, one of the biggest eradication skeptics was the WHO director-general himself, the Brazilian malariologist Marcolino Candau. So he wanted an American to blame. "When it fails, I want it to be seen that there is an American there and the U.S. is really responsible for this dreadful thing that you have launched the World Health Organization into," Candau told the U.S. surgeon general. "And the person I want is Henderson."[13]

D.A. moved his family to Geneva and began his daunting task, armed with a tiny staff, telephones, mail, and airline tickets (there was no email, internet, or overnight delivery back then). Help and money were both in short supply. He took on a stack of challenges, not the least of which was the WHO director-general's skepticism. He battled with recalcitrant governments, a lack of sufficient vaccine, a strong antivaccine movement, and frightening geopolitical instability and civil disorder, including the ongoing Cold War between the U.S. and the Soviet Union. He confronted authorities in Moscow for shipping weak vaccines. When vaccination rates failed to rise enough in Ethiopia, he used his influence with the notorious emperor Haile Selassie's personal physician. Richard Preston, the author of *The Hot Zone* and *The Demon in the Freezer*, described D.A. as a "Sherman tank of a human being—he simply rolled over bureaucrats who got in his way."[14]

Despite his struggles with government officials, "It was surprisingly easy to get cooperation from the local people," D.A. told me. "For the whole program in West Africa, we had just 50 people. We were forced into doing things the most efficient way. We didn't have the people, the vehicles, the supervision—so we had to work it out."[15]

And work it out he did, in the cleverest manner. He relied on a "ring vaccination" strategy devised by Foege that was much more efficient and effective than vaccinating everyone. The idea was for the campaign workers to find smallpox patients, identifiable by their red blisters, and isolate them. The next step was to vaccinate anyone who'd been in contact with the infected patients—their inner circle. Workers would use an innovative two-pronged rod that made it easy for nonprofessionals to vaccinate people. The third step was to vaccinate the outer ring of people who'd had contact with those in the inner circle.

The strategy worked. The last wild case of smallpox was diagnosed on October 26, 1977, in Ali Maow Maalin, a hospital cook in Merca, Somalia. In 1979, after two years of intense verification efforts, WHO declared the disease eradicated. It was the single greatest achievement in the history of medicine. After suffering repeated epidemics over thousands of years, humankind was freed from this disease in about a decade.[16] Economists have calculated that by eliminating the need for routine immunization for smallpox in the U.S., the American investment continues to repay itself every 26 days to this day.[17] At a cost of just over $300 million, that makes a cumulative savings from smallpox eradication of $168 billion as of 2017.

D.A. hardly rested on his laurels. He went on to become the dean of Johns Hopkins School of Public Health in Baltimore and later founded a center for civilian biodefense. As director of President George W. Bush's Office of Public Health Preparedness, he had a mandate to combat bioterrorism. D.A. felt strongly that all traces of smallpox, even the last samples kept under lock and key in Biosafety Level 4 research facilities, should be destroyed, as humanity would have no immunity against the disease if it ever escaped. "I feel very—what should we say?—dispirited," he told the *New York Times* in 2002, when George W. Bush insisted on inoculating soldiers bound for Iraq against smallpox in the mistaken belief that Saddam Hussein was storing bioweapons. "Here we are, regressing to defend against something we thought was permanently defeated. We shouldn't have to be doing this."[18]

Ironically, D.A.'s final battle was with a problem all too common in the elderly—a hip fracture. He might have survived it had he not also been plagued by an antibiotic-resistant staphylococcus infection, the killer of so many in hospitals. It was a pathogen he himself had studied and worked to defeat.[19]

Peter Piot and the Battle Against AIDS

In 1976, a 27-year-old Belgian microbiologist named Peter Piot learned that many people in Zaire (now known as the Democratic Republic of the Congo) were falling ill with fever, diarrhea, vomiting, and bleeding. Then they died. Piot traveled to a remote part of Zaire to find out why so many people were succumbing to this terrifying, unknown disease. A Zairian doctor had sent a thermos containing blood from a dead nun to the lab where the young scientist worked. The blood contained a deadly unknown virus.

After experts around the world confirmed that the sample under the microscope wasn't Marburg, a disease found in African monkeys, the young scientist, along with his colleagues in Antwerp and at the CDC in Atlanta, got excited. "There was a feeling of being very privileged, that this was a moment of discovery," Piot would tell BBC News decades later, just as a new outbreak of the disease he'd discovered in 1976 was beginning to grip West Africa.

Not that it wasn't frightening. Piot and his colleagues flew to Kinshasa in a C-130 transport aircraft, arranged for them by the personal physician of President Mobutu, Zaire's leader. Then the team had to travel to the epicenter of the outbreak in the remote village of Yambuku. Sensing death in the vicinity, the pilots dropped the scientists off as fast as possible. Instead of bidding Piot and his colleagues "Au revoir" ("See you again"), they left them with "Adieu"— literally, "to God," which is something you would say to someone you will never see again.

When Piot and his colleagues arrived at an old Catholic mission, they found a sign on the doorbell that read, "Please stop, anybody who crosses here may die."

"The mission had already lost four nuns to the disease. They were praying and waiting for death," Piot told the BBC. The team needed to find out how the deadly virus was spreading and what the sources were. Who was being infected and by what means? They discovered that dirty syringe needles were one culprit; funerals, where people touched and kissed infected corpses, were another. Piot and his team insisted that nurses and doctors use soap and gloves. They isolated patients, ended the practice of reusing needles, and quarantined the contacts of those who were sick.

Piot and his colleagues decided to name the new virus after the nearest river—the Ebola.[20]

*   *   *

I met Peter Piot almost 20 years after he returned from Zaire. Back in 1996, I was working as director of essential medicines at WHO in Geneva. At the time, the world was already 15 years and 8 million deaths into the AIDS epidemic. Many national and international leaders were still in denial. The number of new cases was still rising. Deaths were accelerating, prevention efforts were patchy, and fewer than one in 20 people at risk of the disease knew their HIV status. In Africa, the core of the workforce—workers, business leaders, doctors, teachers— was being decimated. Hundreds of thousands of children were being orphaned.

Something had to be done. That something was the launch of an organization called UNAIDS. Its mission was to lead, strengthen, and support an expanded response to HIV/AIDS, a mission that included preventing HIV transmission, providing care and support to those already living with the virus, reducing the vulnerability of individuals and communities to HIV, and alleviating the impact of the epidemic. In a tightly contested selection process, Peter was chosen as the organization's founding executive director. He had been studying sexually transmitted infections for years, since people first began displaying HIV symptoms. "The dogma at the time," Peter recalled, "was that it was a gay disease. But I always thought that was a human judgment—from the perspective of a virus it's important to jump from one host to another; why would it care about your sexuality?"[21]

He certainly had his work cut out for him. For public-health professionals, AIDS was a long war on both individual and collective fronts. Once Peter was appointed, I was quickly impressed by his vision, personal credibility, and unrelenting sense of urgency. I marveled as he brought together eight UN agencies and built strong working alliances with national governments, corporations, media, religious organizations, community-based groups, regional and country networks of people living with HIV/AIDS, and other civil society organizations. Within five years, UNAIDS had launched a pioneering AIDS treatment program. World leaders were paying unprecedented attention to AIDS, and funding to fight the disease was on the verge of exploding into the largest financial commitment ever made to a single global health issue. The number of new cases started to decline in 1998, but it took another six years until the number of deaths began to decline.

*　　　*　　　*

Despite this progress, the battle against AIDS is far from over. According to UNAIDS, 36.7 million people globally were living with HIV in 2015.[22] In that year alone, 2.1 million people became newly infected with HIV and 1.1 million people died from AIDS-related illnesses. Since the start of the epidemic, 78 million people have become infected with HIV and 35 million people have died from AIDS-related illnesses. Although 17 million people accessed antiretroviral therapy in 2015, lack of money as well as ignorance continue to obstruct efforts to eradicate HIV to this day.

Gro Brundtland and the Containment of SARS

The twenty-first century's first major epidemic, SARS, was brought to heel by leaders who took strong action. One of those leaders was my former WHO boss: Dr. Gro Harlem Brundtland, the former prime minister of Norway. A straight-talking woman with a backbone of steel, Brundtland was the most effective leader and the best boss I've ever had the privilege to work with.

Her father, a career statesman, had taught her how to bring people together for common purpose. As a child, she fled Nazi-occupied Norway to Sweden with her parents, who had worked in the resistance. She was reared to take an equal place in a man's world. Of her childhood, she said that she was lucky to be "brought up in a family of strong convictions, deeply held values of solidarity, justice, and equality."[23] She describes her mother and father as "clearminded, deliberate parents who believed in social justice and equality between the sexes."[24] She might just as easily have been talking about herself.

Brundtland began her professional life as a general practitioner. But, given her activist upbringing and natural leadership qualities, she became increasingly drawn to politics and Norway's left-leaning Labour Party. She began writing articles about the need to protect the environment. When she was 35, the Norwegian prime minister called her to his office on the strength of some articles she had written and invited her to serve as Norway's environment minister. He wanted someone who wasn't an expert to bring in fresh ideas. In this new role, Brundtland quickly came to understand that environmental protection and public health are intertwined. "I realized environmental policies are public health policies," she said. "It's really the same thing." (Indeed, the sad history of pollution, deforestation, and environmental degradation has proved her right.)

In 1981, Brundtland was elected prime minister. Some questioned whether a woman could lead a nation of 4 million. She had no doubts: "Certainly we made political history," she recalled. "I would be the first woman prime minister, and the youngest. I honestly felt that I was as capable as any of the men with whom I had been working in national politics."[25] She went on to serve two terms in office.

When she was 59, Brundtland became director-general of WHO, where she took on tough issues like smoking (new employees could only be hired by WHO if they didn't smoke) and abortion, another sensitive topic from which she didn't flinch. She didn't have patience for people who wasted time, or for people she perceived as hypocrites. "Morality," she chided some UN delegates at a conference in Cairo in 1994, "becomes hypocrisy if it means mothers suffering or dying in connection with unwanted pregnancies and illegal abortions of unwanted children."[26]

I especially remember how Brundtland took on the threat of SARS. By mid-March 2003, WHO had received reports of 85 suspected cases, even as the Chinese government was working hard to stifle publicity about this disease, which had been smoldering in Guangdong Province for months. WHO experts were convinced that they were dealing with a new and dangerous virus. New cases were accelerating, especially among health workers.

Before long, WHO had gathered concrete evidence of an urgent global threat. Brundtland took command, issuing a rare WHO worldwide health alert. She also took the bold step of breaking protocol to make the announcement simultaneously to the media, rather than first to health authorities. She did this even though some countries, particularly China, bristled.

The severity of the outbreak led Brundtland to issue the most stringent emergency travel advisory in the 55-year history of WHO. The move incensed some. Infuriated by the inclusion of his city in its travel advisory, and fearing potential financial losses, Toronto's then-mayor Mel Lastman appeared on CNN and angrily demanded to know what this organization was. "Who is WHO?" he asked, earning his designation as a laughingstock.[27]

After months of secrecy and weeks of delay in allowing a WHO team into

Guangdong, China finally acceded to the WHO request to investigate what was happening. The findings were so disturbing and the discrepancies with China's public statements so troubling that Brundtland again broke protocol by publicly criticizing China's leadership. "Next time something strange and new comes anywhere in the world," she urged heads of state around the world, "let us come in as quickly as possible." Within days of Brundtland's public rebuke, newly installed Chinese premier Wen Jiabao met with party leaders to hear their views on the SARS issue. Two days later, he addressed a national meeting on preventing SARS. In a complete about-face, China quickly moved to full reporting, embraced external expert assistance, and mobilized a national effort to rapidly contain SARS. New cases dropped precipitously.[28]

Thanks to Brundtland's bold actions, SARS was quickly contained and, experts believe, eliminated forever—before it could inflict widespread casualties. By its end in July 2003, the mystery disease had infected 8,098 people in 29 countries, eventually causing 774 deaths and billions in losses to the global economy. But without Brundtland's rapid action, SARS would have spiraled out of control. This highly contagious, virulent virus might still be with us today. "Determination, even courage, is of the essence," Brundtland has said. "Great vision and speeches alone are not what really count the most. Vision without a plan, or a plan without action, is not much to admire."[29]

Defeating Ebola in Liberia

Liberia is among the world's poorest countries. In 2014, the country had only recently emerged from 13 years of civil war and was just beginning to recover. A decade and a half of unrest had left hospitals and clinics severely damaged or destroyed. Roads, transportation services, and telecommunications had cratered. When Ebola struck, the destruction made it difficult to get patients to treatment centers or samples to laboratories. And because illiteracy was high and trust was low, people listened more to their local healers than public-health officials.[30] A more formidable set of challenges would be hard to imagine.

In March 2014, healthcare workers with Médecins Sans Frontières (MSF), working directly on the ground in Guinea, reported what was found to be a new Ebola outbreak. They soon learned that cases were showing up more than 124 miles apart, across West African country borders. MSF sent out a press release warning about the cross-border transmission, followed by another one a month later.

Dr. Joanne Liu, the international president of MSF, told me that when Ebola exploded, the organization found itself completely overwhelmed: "We didn't have as many 'firemen' as we wanted." Local health workers and volunteers were not trained to deal with Ebola. "Nobody was prepared," Liu said.[31] By early August 2014, the situation was completely out of hand. Liu traveled to West Africa and met with the presidents of the three most affected countries, Liberia, Guinea, and Sierra Leone. Ellen Johnson Sirleaf, the president of Liberia, confessed to feeling utterly overwhelmed. The situation was so dire that Sirleaf asked Liu to delay building an Ebola center that would be handed over to the government, because so many Liberian health workers had died that the nation did not have a large enough workforce to operate the center. Liu promised the shaken Sirleaf that she would do everything in her power to bring the world's attention to the situation.

Despite early warnings from Liu, WHO was too slow to respond to the outbreak. "Nearly everyone involved in the outbreak response failed to see some fairly plain writing on the wall," a WHO internal document noted.[32] Because the public-health systems in West Africa were so fragile, WHO should have had a stronger regional presence there. Reporting was slow, and it took too long for Director-General Margaret Chan to get the message. In September 2014, Liu finally appeared before the UN Security Council, informing them that the epidemic threatened the security of the region. MSF was building "crematoria instead of hospitals," she said. In early September, she gave a no-holds-barred speech to the UN members in which she demanded that their nations deploy civilian and military assets to deal with the emergency. The UN had a "historic responsibility to act now," she insisted. "To put out this fire, we must run into the burning building."[33]

Thus galvanized, the U.S. and other countries finally responded with money, supplies, health workers, and even military troops to tackle the emergency, which finally began to abate in February 2015. Without Liu's dogged insistence, the Ebola epidemic might have spread much further and killed many more than 11,000 people. But the needless suffering and death, as well as the massive social disruption and collapse of even the most basic healthcare services, cruelly demonstrated what happens when governments are not prepared for a health crisis. It was also an important lesson for WHO, which admitted that it had failed to respond as early as necessary and pledged reforms. "We have learned lessons of humility," Chan said in a statement. "We have seen that old diseases in new contexts consistently spring new surprises."[34]

*   *   *

Ellen Johnson Sirleaf is nearly 80 years old now. A Harvard-educated public policy maven with a long, distinguished, albeit occasionally checkered, career in Liberia's government, she and her impoverished country have never been strangers to trouble. Following a military coup in 1980, Sirleaf was briefly imprisoned, and then she went into exile. She and her people lived through back-to-back civil wars in which hundreds of thousands were killed. She's made many "damned if she does, damned if she doesn't" calls, including mistakes like having once supported the brutal dictator Charles Taylor. Her good calls included guiding Liberia through the scourge of Ebola after an initial mistake. She went on to become Africa's first female head of state. In 2011, she won a Nobel Peace Prize for her contribution to women's rights.

Like all good leaders, Sirleaf learned from her mistakes. As Ebola gripped the Liberian capital of Monrovia, Sirleaf ordered a strict but poorly executed quarantine of a huge slum. When police in riot gear showed up, they blocked all exits from the area. The public reacted with anger, storming the barricades and throwing rocks. In response, soldiers shot at people with live ammunition, killing one teenager.[35] Six months later, Sirleaf acknowledged that in her fear, she had made a terrible error. "We didn't know what we were dealing with. [Ebola] was an unknown enemy," she said in an open and honest interview with the *New York Times* editorial board. "People attributed it to witchcraft. We did not know what to do. We were all frightened. I was personally frightened." The quarantine, she acknowledged, had "created more tension in the society."[36]

When leaders learn deeply from their mistakes, they can also turn things around fast. Sirleaf declared a national emergency and moved quickly to install a high-level pandemic-response commander to lead the fight against the disease in Liberia. Tolbert Nyenswah, a lawyer with a degree in public health from Johns Hopkins University, was exactly the right person to do it.

Nyenswah, a no-nonsense professional with a broad brow, is obsessed with making things happen. On a hot day in October 2016, I joined him as he conducted a meeting with 40 members, who came from government, from donor organizations, and from nongovernmental organizations. Over and over, he asked for deliverables, timeframes, and results.

In 2015, with the help of the CDC, WHO, and others, Nyenswah set up an "incident management system" designed to coordinate all the activities needed to defeat Ebola in Liberia. These activities included logistics and case management; worker training and support; contact tracing; finding, transporting, and isolating patients; safe burials; surveillance; laboratory testing; and communicating with and mobilizing the public on a national, regional, and local level.[37] Nyenswah ran the organization from the top down, military style, as was appropriate during the emergency. There was one command center and one commander. Meetings were short. Those running the various operations learned from what they saw and adjusted the battle plan as they went.

"The most important element to stop the spread of this disease is to stop the transmission at the community level," Nyenswah said in an interview at the height of the crisis. "This can be done through distributing hygiene kits to each household, providing health education in every community, and social mobilization throughout the entire country."[38] But the pivotal factor that made the difference between success and failure in Liberia may well have been Sirleaf's ear. Nyenswah reported directly to the president, who now clearly understood the urgency of the situation and empowered him to do whatever was necessary to coordinate the various response units and hold them accountable.[39]

Racing to the Fire

Let's say your kitchen stove has caught fire and you can't put it out. Now the flames are licking the walls and the ceiling. You call the fire department, but instead of sending a team to put out the blaze, the person who answers the phone either says, "Are you sure? Have you studied it enough?" or "Not our responsibility, try the police. Or City Hall." Alternatively, they might say, "Thanks for letting us know, but we're too occupied with the upcoming election to help you. Good luck."

Looking back on the history of epidemics over the ages, and especially over the last 100 years, it's screamingly obvious that every minute matters in responding to an outbreak. Dithering and denial on the part of those who should be protecting us kill people—sometimes in devastating numbers. If a new, deadly pandemic exploded today, would leaders continue to argue, deny, and defer while deaths mounted? Would they persist with their plodding, piecemeal approach? Or would they put the needs of humanity first and refuse to let anything get in their way?

Just as real firefighters understand that responding to an alarm within five minutes is crucial in preventing a house or even a neighborhood from being engulfed by flames, the most effective leaders understand that rapid response makes all the difference between life and death. D. A. Henderson, Peter Piot, Gro Brundtland, Ellen Johnson Sirleaf, Tolbert Nyenswah, Joanne Liu, and other visionary and courageous leaders led like the house was on fire. They put scientific evidence ahead of parochial and political interests. But beyond that, the common denominator they shared was courage. All of them stood up to the status quo, refused to take no for an answer, and put the health and well-being of the public above all else. If we are to end epidemics, we need such courageous and dogged leaders at all levels and in every sphere of society.

CHAPTER 7

RESILIENT SYSTEMS, GLOBAL SECURITY

Strong national public-health systems and robust international agencies can ensure health security for all.

We need resilient national public-health systems to prevent, detect, and respond to local outbreaks and avert global pandemics. National governments, the private sector, communities, and faith-based organizations have been enormously successful when they work in concert to fight disease. Even the poorest nations, such as Liberia and Ethiopia, prove that it's possible to do so. And on the global level, leaders of all stripes are coordinating in ways they never have before.

The stunning, ancient Buddhas of Bamiyan were one of the great mountainside sculptures. Standing nearly 115 feet high, they were carved from sandstone cliffs in the Bamiyan Valley of central Afghanistan in the sixth century, before Islam became established in the region. The two giant Buddhas were marvels of beauty and craftsmanship. In March 2001, in one outrageous act, Taliban militiamen blew them up.[1]

After coming to power in the 1990s, the Taliban also reduced public health to rubble. By September 1997, women were not allowed to work in Kabul's 22 hospitals. There were just 35 beds in the single facility where women were allowed. There was no electricity, water, or surgical equipment.[2] Nine out of ten women gave birth without any kind of medical assistance.

A decade ago, I met a gentle Afghani doctor who arrived in Bamiyan City just after the Taliban had been driven out by U.S. military forces in 2001. Dr. Ihsan Ullah Shahir found few health facilities and fewer workers. Many staff members had simply run away. During a visit to Bamiyan Province in April 2007, Dr. Shahir shared with me the experience of driving home one day from the wreckage of the Bamiyan hospital. He was totally overwhelmed. "I felt like everything was on my shoulders and couldn't bear it," he said as he started down the road to Kabul. "I was 100 percent convinced I would leave."

Shortly after this crisis of conscience, he attended a Management Sciences for Health (MSH) leadership-development program in Egypt, where he regained his courage.[3] He returned to Bamiyan, determined to restore health care in the district. He established a program to train 20 young women a year to be community midwives, enlisted scores of community health workers, and began putting health facilities back together. Over the next decade, with the support of other Afghans, USAID, and others in the international community, his country experienced dramatic improvements in services for millions of mothers and children, and remarkable reductions in maternal and child mortality.[4, 5, 6]

*   *   *

Since MSH was founded in 1971, we have worked shoulder to shoulder with local colleagues to strengthen national health systems in challenging places, from post-Taliban Afghanistan, to post-apartheid South Africa, to post-earthquake Haiti, to post-Ebola Liberia. I have been continually inspired by the resilience of those who have experienced misery and death firsthand and who remain in their countries to dedicate themselves to creating a better, healthier future for their nations and their children. Nomathemba Mazaleni, a South African nurse, fought against apartheid, then led MSH's USAID-supported program to reshape health care to serve all South Africans. Dr. Bernice Dahn, a Liberian physician, helped defeat Ebola and is now rebuilding her country's health system as minister of health. And Dr. Shahir is a walking, talking symbol of resilience, which he believes is all about facing challenges and solving problems. Facing and overcoming obstacles, he told me, "touches the heart; it brings people together."

Strong, resilient health systems are the second element in The Power of Seven. When you think about something that is resilient, you may conjure up a palm tree, whose rambling roots and wiry trunk enable it to bend in gale-force winds but not break. Psychologically speaking, resilience is the mental ability to recover, adapt, and triumph in the face of adversity, trauma, and tragedy. In the natural world, resilience means growing back better, like a forest recovering from a fire, its floor sprouting with new green shoots.

Likewise, a resilient national public-health system is like a mighty ship that can weather a terrible storm; it stays afloat amid battering waves and doesn't shatter apart. If a country has a solid public healthcare infrastructure to begin with and is well prepared for an emergency, then doctors and nurses can respond to a crisis with early detection and rapid response, even in remote communities. When an outbreak strikes, all kinds of well-prepared forces rush in to keep sickness and death to a minimum and ensure that the rest of the population receives standard medical care in the midst of the emergency. A truly resilient public-health system, experts say, delivers a "resilience dividend"—that is, both everyday benefits and positive health for everyone on an ongoing basis.[7]

National governments are responsible for protecting their citizens, but they can't succeed by fiat. International organizations like WHO, scientific organizations like the CDC, economic organizations like the World Bank, private-sector companies, faith-based organizations, and thousands of NGOs also help in a crisis and keep essential services operating. But most crucially, a health emergency is only overcome by committed local communities and health workers who are working with timely information and appropriate equipment and who are unequivocally supported in their tasks.

A resilient health system is one that "learns." If mistakes are made, leaders and medical professionals adapt quickly so that the country can return to normal as quickly as possible.[8] Organizational scholars note that a "learning organization" is one that encourages people to absorb lessons from mistakes and to take intelligent risks, to be open about what they are learning without fear of reprisal or being made wrong, and to constantly improve and innovate in a challenging environment.[9] When it comes to a fast-moving public-health crisis, a national government can't be too nimble when it comes to adapting because doing so is a matter of life and death. And when a crisis hits, having a national early detection–early response system in place makes all the difference, as the case of Nigeria that follows shows.

Integrating Resilient Health Systems and Health Security

Resilient national health systems based on universal health coverage are the foundation for national and global health security.

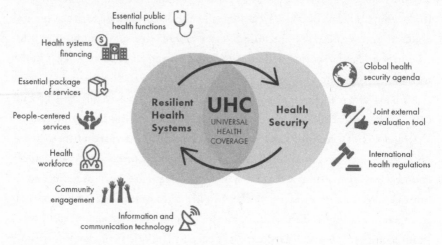

SOURCE: Adapted from Health security and health systems strengthening—an integrated approach. World Health Organization. 2017. http://www.who.int/ebola/health-systems-recovery/en/ (accessed 1 May 2017).

We can have the technology and knowledge available to heal the sick, but in the absence of strong health systems, we will continue to see AIDS and other epidemics cause needless illness, suffering, and death, as well as economic devastation. We can either enable people and countries to thrive or continue to lurch from one public-health crisis to another.[10]

Nigeria: When a Doctor, and a Government, Respond

In July 2014, Patrick Sawyer, a Liberian-American lawyer who had been exposed to Ebola in Liberia, traveled to Nigeria for an important regional conference and collapsed in the Lagos airport. At the time, doctors at all the government hospitals were on a labor strike. The only hospitals that remained open were private ones like that in which Dr. Ameyo Adadevoh worked. The doctor who first saw Sawyer initially diagnosed him with malaria; Sawyer claimed he'd had no contact with anyone suffering from Ebola. But after seeing him on her rounds the next day, Dr. Adadevoh suspected Ebola. After a test for Ebola came back positive, she knew exactly what to do: she created an isolation area in her hospital to continue Sawyer's treatment and to protect her staff.

Adadevoh's battle to protect herself and others from infection wasn't easy. The hospital wasn't equipped with the proper protective gear, correct protocols for Ebola treatment, or a real isolation unit. Adding to the challenge, the Liberian government officials were pressuring the Nigerian government, insisting that the doctor discharge Sawyer so that he could attend the conference. But Adadevoh held her ground and refused to let him go. Four days later, Sawyer died of Ebola. Ten days later the doctor herself became ill and was taken to a poorly equipped, makeshift isolation ward, where she too died.

Had Adadevoh not stood up to the government, Ebola might have gripped Nigeria because of the doctors' strike and the government's lack of preparedness. But thanks to her courageous actions, Ebola in Nigeria was limited to just 19 cases and seven deaths, including hers. Nigeria was declared Ebola-free in October 2014, even as the epidemic raged on in West Africa. That's an amazing feat in a country of more than 180 million people.

Prevention also involves locating everyone who has been exposed ("contact tracing"). As tragic as Dr. Adadevoh's death was, it became a catalyst for Nigeria to mobilize against Ebola. And the country did a marvelous job of contact tracing. Nigeria was fortunate, because in 2012, the Bill and Melinda Gates Foundation had built an emergency command center to detect polio cases. The disease surveillance system at the center was now deployed to look for new Ebola cases. Nigeria mobilized a rapid-response team of 100 Nigerian doctors trained in epidemiology.

After Ebola struck, the government moved 40 of the Nigerian doctors to a central hub that coordinated Nigeria's health ministry, WHO, UNICEF, the CDC, Médecins Sans Frontières, and the International Committee of the Red Cross. In what the WHO called "a piece of world-class epidemiological detective work," the government ended up tracking 100 percent of all potential Ebola contacts in Lagos, Nigeria's largest city, where Sawyer landed, and 98 percent of contacts in Port Harcourt, where his nurse visited family.[11] Nearly 1,800 health workers were rapidly trained and armed with protective gear. Safe wards were set up with enough beds and access to chlorinated water. In total, health workers made 18,500 face-to-face visits to check the temperatures of 900 possible contacts.

Nigeria wasn't perfect in its response to Ebola. It took too long for the government to act, and the doctors' strike slowed response too. Niniola Soleye, an employee of MSH and the niece of Dr. Adadevoh, wrote that her beloved aunt paid with her life because the Nigerian health system had been unprepared to deal with Ebola. "The system has since caught up, and Nigeria is today a model for other countries," Niniola wrote. "But the loss of such a gifted doctor and family anchor is incalculable." The story of her aunt was a vivid reminder to me that every death is personal, that we are all connected, and that there are terrible human consequences when health systems fail the people they are supposed to serve.[12]

As the story of Ebola in Nigeria demonstrated, finding and treating the sick before the outbreak has a chance to spread is crucial. But Nigeria wasn't the only country that prevented a local Ebola outbreak from becoming a national public-health emergency. In Senegal, "patient zero" was admitted to the hospital, having lied about his travel history. A week later, doctors found out that he had come from Guinea, and had him tested for Ebola. Senegalese officials closed the country's borders and tracked 67 people who had been in contact with the patient, all of whom underwent voluntary quarantine and twice-daily monitoring by Red Cross workers. None ended up contracting Ebola; even patient zero survived.[13]

These nations clearly showed that a good early detection–early response system—backed by enough trained health workers, equipment, facilities, and a public education campaign—can stop even the most infectious disease.

Ethiopia's Fight against AIDS: The Power of a Health Systems Vision

When local disease outbreak like Ebola in Nigeria or a global pandemic like the 1918 Spanish flu is not brought to a swift end, something far worse happens: it becomes embedded in human populations ("endemic" in epidemiological language), as happened with AIDS. Once a disease becomes endemic, it requires an even longer and vastly more costly response.

Before 2005, HIV/AIDS was a death sentence in the East African country of Ethiopia, the most populous landlocked country in the world. Those who worked in Ethiopia for MSH reported that hospitals overflowed with the dying. When someone died, the family would collect money for a funeral from friends and neighbors. In some communities, the collections—and the funerals—proceeded nonstop. "Roadside coffin sellers in Addis Ababa were plentiful," said Dr. Haile Wubneh, MSH's then–deputy director for the USAID-supported HIV/AIDS Treatment, Care, and Support project. "Saturdays would have been funeral day—sometimes one funeral after another."[14]

In 2004, Ethiopia had just started receiving U.S. funding to make testing, counseling, and ARVs widely available.[15] But it took a long time for the benefits to reach most people. By 2005, just 10 percent of people living with HIV in Ethiopia were on ARVs, which reduces the HIV viral load and likelihood of transmission.[16]

Initially, getting ARVs meant paying for one's own HIV medications at a cost of $289–$346 per month. This was later reduced to $28 per month.[17] But Ethiopians had, on average, only $42 in their pockets each month—hardly enough to cover the cost of drugs, let alone ancillary costs like transportation to clinics or laboratory fees.[18] Once at a treatment facility, people often encountered long lines and a fatigued, underpaid medical staff.[19] And in their communities, HIV-positive people faced stigma and ostracism. It was also tough for them to buy enough food, either because they were too ill to work or had no income because they were fired, or both.

It's hard to believe that today, Ethiopia has an enviably efficient and effective country-wide public-health system—one that not only turned a public-health emergency into a manageable chronic disease[20] but that provides a blueprint for an integrated national public healthcare system. What led to such a dramatic shift?

Ethiopia's Top-Down, Bottom-Up National Health Strategy

Samuel Tadesse was diagnosed with HIV in 2004. In search of a miracle, he traveled to Tsadkane Monastery, one of the largest holy water springs in Ethiopia. Samuel decided to join the growing group of people who lived at the well. He prayed, drank, and bathed in holy water and ate one serving of dried barleycorn flour each day. He waited for faith to displace despair, but day after day, year after year, more and more people found their final resting place in Samuel's arms. He came to believe that living at the well meant dying at the well. Sick as he himself was, he felt compelled to care for the sick and dying who visited, so he began working to raise money for food, blankets, and water.

A mere four years later, much had changed. A few miles away from the well, a new treatment center provided free testing for HIV, free counseling, and free ARV treatment. Alongside the treatment center, a bakery, restaurant, and a seed-oil extraction mill helped patients earn money, learn a trade, and eventually reenter their communities.[21]

Across the country, fundamental religious practices and ideologies were shifting. Leaders in the Ethiopian Orthodox Church were now stressing the importance of taking ARVs along with holy water. They preached the importance of referring people to a health facility for care and treatment, and how to prevent mother-to-child transmission of HIV.[22] HIV-positive mothers were giving birth to virus-free babies and, instead of dying, people were feeling better and living longer.

*   *   *

Fundamentally, Ethiopia's turnaround had to do with strong leadership. In each era of global health there has been an action-oriented pioneer and thought leader among the world's ministers of health—a person I have thought of as a de facto "dean." From the mid-1980s to the mid-1990s, that dean was Professor Olikoye Ransome-Kuti from Nigeria, who was a visible, vocal champion and driver for primary health care. From the mid-2000s to the mid-2010s, the dean was Dr. Tedros Adhanom Ghebreyesus of Ethiopia. Dr. Tedros, as he is called, used his authority, influence, and vision to radically improve health care in Ethiopia and to advocate among international policymakers and funders for strengthening health systems. In May 2017, Dr. Tedros's leadership and achievements received the ultimate recognition when he was elected director-general of the World Health Organization, succeeding Dr. Margaret Chan.

Dr. Tedros was appointed minister of health in 2005 by the newly elected prime minister of Ethiopia, Meles Zenawi. The prime minister's goal was to make Ethiopia a middle-income country by 2020.[23] He considered HIV a national emergency and a barrier to economic growth. For his part, Tedros deeply understood the crisis. He had been running the regional health bureau in Tigray, where there were often fewer than 200 hospital beds per 1 million people and one physician per 30,000 people. So in 2005, he launched a plan to improve access to care and provide free ARV treatment.[24, 25]

To combat HIV, Tedros's main strategy was to decentralize HIV care and treatment. Hospitals that provided ARV treatment were often difficult for most people to reach, so the government built a set of nearly 300 coordinated local healthcare centers. These centers integrated HIV treatment into services that medical staff were already providing, such as maternal, newborn, and family planning.[26] The centers became a one-stop shop for holistic, nondiscriminatory care for people living with HIV.[27] Tedros's plan was relatively well funded. In 2006, Ethiopia received nearly $2 billion in development, $84 million of which was from the U.S. President's Emergency Plan for AIDS Relief (PEPFAR).[28, 29] It was also well supported by internationally known funders like the Clinton Foundation.

Key to the success of Tedros's integrated public-health strategy was deep penetration into local communities. The government trained and deployed new types of health workers to community and regional positions. This ensured quality of services and coordination of care. For example, HIV case managers who were themselves HIV positive worked closely with patients, helping them stick to their ARV regimens and providing support and advice. If someone stopped treatment, case managers traced patients through community-based health-extension workers and community mobilizers. Data clerks shared information about missed appointments with case managers and monitored patient outcomes and emerging needs. Healthcare providers could tap patient data to make evidence-based decisions about patient care. And health center "mentors" conducted on-site visits to local health centers to ensure that providers were complying with national standards.

Fighting AIDS on the Local Level

Ethiopia's outreach effort particularly targeted women who could pass the HIV virus on to their babies.[30] One community support service that started in 2005 is the Mother Support Groups (MSG), committed to helping mothers give birth to HIV-free babies.[31, 32] The groups are run by "Mother Mentors" who are themselves HIV positive and who advise women about their options and help them stick to their regimens. The Mother Mentors also work with husbands and fathers to teach them how to keep their babies safe from HIV.[33]

One of the mothers who attended an MSG was Mearg, an HIV-infected mother who lived with an unemployed husband, a ten-month-old son, and an eight-year-old HIV-positive daughter. She was desperate to generate income, so the Mother Mentors worked with Mearg to establish a small sheep and backyard vegetable farming business. After Mearg earned enough income to support herself and her children, she disclosed her HIV-positive status to her community.

From that point forward, she was considered a role model for other HIV-positive mothers, and Mearg paid it forward. She encouraged others to get HIV testing and coordinated community-wide efforts to support orphans who were abandoned because they were HIV positive.[34]

While HIV is still a priority issue for Ethiopia's ministry of health, it's not the national emergency it once was. PEPFAR funds have shifted directly to the government and to institutions responsible for clinic-based services. Ethiopia's government has also invested heavily in "train the trainer" and mentorship programs. For example, a clinical mentorship program trains current ARV providers to become clinical mentors for their peers, who in turn provide training to their colleagues on integrating HIV treatment into services like antenatal care and tuberculosis.

Today, the public-health situation in Ethiopia is improved practically beyond recognition. It now has a top-to-bottom public-health system that should be the envy of the rest of the world. In this system, everyone from the top of the government to the poorest person gets access to health care through a thorough, aggressive system that includes not just hospitals and health clinics but community workers and volunteers who are in charge of looking out for others. Ethiopia's current public-health system integrates AIDS care with overall public health. It makes disease prevention and treatment the cornerstone of its system. And it has built a solid supply chain to support that system. It's the very definition of what an integrated and resilient public healthcare system should look like.

When the Private Sector Steps Up

Stopping epidemics is not just a government responsibility, as is the common assumption. It also requires a big lift from the private sector, where multinational corporations play a crucial role in protecting communities.

Tire manufacturer Firestone, for example, managed to stop Ebola in its tracks when the virus threatened some 80,000 people in the Liberian town of Harbel, where Firestone operates a gigantic rubber plantation. After an employee's wife showed up with the disease in the early, springtime phase of the epidemic, she was cared for in isolation in the company's treatment center. Nobody knew anything about Ebola, but the medical staff at Firestone's facility learned fast and improvised—discovering, for example, that the hazmat suits designed to clear up chemical spills served perfectly well to protect themselves.

When a more virulent wave of the disease showed up in late summer, Firestone went into full emergency mode, enforcing a strict "no visitors" policy, monitoring those who came and went, converting their trucks into ambulances, and giving its time, money, resources, and resolve to the crisis. It built a health annex and quarantine centers, and sent teachers (whose schools had been shut down) door-to-door to teach children. None of Firestone's roughly 8,500 employees and 71,500 family members got sick.[35, 36]

*   *   *

As Ebola threatened the Liberian operations of the mining company Acelor-Mittal, Dr. Alan Knight, the general manager for corporate social responsibility, realized that protecting the firm's employees in Liberia wasn't enough. "We had done as much as we could do to protect ourselves, but I realized that the risk management stance we had taken was very self-serving," he says. "And we hadn't spoken to other companies facing the same challenges as we were. So we invited people who had offices in London to see what we could learn from each other."[37]

Knight reached out to other companies to found the Ebola Private Sector Mobilisation Group (EPSMG), 11 companies that had banded together to share information and best practices, such as how to set up screening mechanisms. The network—which Knight describes as a "hub" rather than a formal organization—provided millions of dollars' worth of products, labor, and logistics support. At its peak more than 100 companies, nearly 70 public bodies and NGOs, and 600 individuals collaborated through the group.

Early on, the group sent a letter to WHO director-general Margaret Chan to demand action. It was unprecedented for a private-sector group to do such a thing, and she took it seriously. On a conference call with the group, she begged the companies to keep their businesses going and to do what they could to teach not only employees but also local citizens how to avoid catching the disease. "We understood that if every employer in West Africa did this for neighbors and family and kids, it would be a big intervention," Knight recalled. "So we all agreed to do it."

When Knight was invited to a special meeting on Ebola at the UN, he made it clear that the private sector could do more than just donor dollars. In-kind donations were crucially important. "Business can offer a lot more than whopping big checks. We can offer the key to the bulldozer, invitations to eat in the canteen, and so on. We need the world to stop treating us as donors and more as operational partners." For its part, Knight says, the private sector must understand the power of its role to help communities. "Companies can have a lifelong conversation with people," he says. "In your role as an employer of citizens, you have the ability to talk about intimate things like protecting against HIV and caring for the dead."

How Faith-Based Health Services Help

Caring for the sick is a central tenet of the great world religions. In fulfilling their promise to serve the most vulnerable, religious people are the first in line to help when there is little other aid or protection for people. It's difficult, often dangerous work. In Liberia, life for workers in the faith community has been hazardous for generations. During Liberia's civil wars, millions of people were displaced, and the healthcare infrastructure was destroyed. Approximately 250,000 people were killed during the fighting. The Catholic Church provided food, shelter, and hope to people who had lost everything.

Sister Barbara Brilliant is a radiant, take-charge American nun in her sixties who has worked in Liberia for 40 years. She, too, is another walking, talking symbol of resilience. In addition to building a nursing school in Liberia, she has protected the most vulnerable people through brutal dictatorships, civil wars, and most recently the devastation of Ebola in her beloved adoptive country. Through all these years, Sister Barbara has held to her deep faith.[38]

During the peak of the Ebola crisis, Catholic hospitals served on the front lines. The minute Ebola showed up on the news, Sister Barbara got hold of 36,000 gallons of bleach and as many sets of protective gear as she could possibly find—including raincoats—and got everyone in Monrovia's Catholic hospitals and clinics trained in the facts about Ebola. The church's biggest hospital shut down after several of their top doctors and administrators succumbed to the virus. Even in the worst days of the outbreak, the committed staff managed to keep 15 of its 18 hospitals and clinics open. The church worked to train community volunteers to educate people to protect themselves from the virus. They distributed buckets of diluted chlorine for hand-washing outside buildings. They helped set up Ebola-specific treatment centers. They taught people to bow to greet each other from a distance instead of embracing or shaking hands.[39]

For her, the biggest battle was the one against fear. "During the war," Sister Barbara has written, "you could at least hear the bullets." But Ebola was a silent killer that could strike anyone, anytime. The level of fear she experienced from her staff was unlike any she had ever seen. She kept reminding them that they had gone through 13 years of civil war. They ran, they suffered, they hid, they saw people die. Why worry about a little Ebola virus? By arming her frightened staff with the facts and instituting a strict "no touch" policy, they were able to stay alive. Even the sisters did not touch each other for a year. Not even the kiss of peace.

WHO and the World

In the end, West Africa and the world beat back Ebola through the efforts of people like President Sirleaf, Dr. Joanne Liu, Dr. Adadevoh, Alan Knight, and Sister Barbara. And, as horrific as the outbreak was, it proved to be a stunning call to action for WHO and the world.

In the prologue to this book, I described my sense of shock and horror at the gravity of the West African Ebola outbreak. I kept asking: Why? Why didn't we know the Ebola virus was already in West Africa and that it could cause a massive problem? Why did it take months to confirm that the Ebola virus was the cause of the outbreak? Why did leaders fail to act on increasingly alarming warnings coming from Africa? Why was there no coordinated three-country action plan? Why did the affected countries make the same panic-generating communications mistakes that had occurred during the AIDS epidemic 30 years earlier? And why, after 22 outbreaks had occurred over 40 years, was there still no Ebola vaccine?

The simple and inexcusable truth was this: nobody was in charge. The fight against Ebola was like fighting a war without a general or a strategy. The metaphorical infantry, artillery, air force, and navy were all under separate commands. The UN was responsible for information sharing and health diplomacy. The WHO issued a global alert, provided technical advice, and supported medical aid in the affected countries. The World Bank provided funding. Médecins Sans Frontières fought on the front lines of treatment. The CDC also offered expertise. But no single individual or organization had either anticipated such an epidemic or taken charge of organizing a collective response.

Maddeningly, the Ebola epidemic was hardly the first time a virus accelerated out of control because there was no unified global leadership. Protecting a community—or even a nation—is a piece of cake compared to getting the entire world to fight epidemics on a coordinated level. When countries have weak health systems, epidemics are much more likely. What would it take to build a coordinated international response that provides the people, medicines, vaccines, supplies, and funding that countries need to succeed against an overwhelming epidemic?

Since its creation in 1948, the Geneva-based World Health Organization has been the United Nations body responsible for protecting international public health. WHO's rules are called the International Health Regulations (IHRs). With 194 member countries, WHO is the only body with the mandate to establish international requirements for preventing, reporting, and controlling epidemics through the IHRs.

These rules have the force of international law to prevent the spread of disease across international boundaries, while avoiding "unnecessary interference with international trade and traffic." The current regulations empower WHO to declare a global health emergency (or a "public health emergency of international concern"), as it did in the case of the pandemic influenza in 2009, the polio outbreak in 2014, and the Ebola pandemic in West Africa that same year.

The IHRs were first published in 1951. In 1995, after outbreaks of cholera in Peru, plague in India, and Ebola in Africa, the World Health Assembly resolved to revise and strengthen the IHRs. It took the 2003 SARS outbreak to force action on this commitment, so the current IHRs were not approved until 2005. The IHRs looked great on their 90 pages of paper, but they had no enforcement teeth and failed to get adequate support from national leaders. As a result, when Ebola struck in 2014, only one in three countries worldwide—and not a single country in Africa—had fully implemented the IHRs. Gallingly, in the two decades since the world's health leaders identified the need for strong IHRs, the world remained vulnerable to catastrophic epidemics.

Even before Ebola hit the headlines, however, the U.S. CDC, State Department, and others in the U.S. government were strategizing about how to accelerate implementation of the IHRs. They recruited Bonnie Jenkins for the task. With a modest yet determined style that makes her a natural coalition builder, Jenkins was the first African American woman specialist in biosecurity for the U.S. government. Described by her law school roommate as "intellectually, emotionally, and physically fearless," Jenkins brought together WHO, the World Organization of Animal Health, and the Food and Agriculture Organization to ensure that all the pieces of the puzzle—from discovery of disease in animals and transmission to humans to public health—came together to create a new, broadly applicable set of guidelines.[40]

With leadership (and a tight deadline) from the Obama White House, Jenkins and her colleagues worked feverishly to launch the new Global Health Security Agenda (GHSA) in February 2014. The GHSA is a multisector, multi-partner approach to "build countries' capacity to help create a world safe and secure from infectious-disease threats and elevate global health security as a national and global priority."[41] The core of the GHSA is a set of 11 action areas based on the IHRs that aim to strengthen nations' abilities to prevent, detect, and respond to infectious-disease threats. By early 2017, 70 countries had signed on to it.

Jenkins takes pride in having the lead in engaging nongovernmental stakeholders as well. The GHSA Consortium consists of more than 100 universities, foundations, and research labs; the GHSA Private Sector Roundtable consists of more than a dozen multilateral and national companies; and the GHSA Next Generation Network features rising young professionals in health security.

This global health security push includes a process for individual countries to sign on to a national action plan for health security (GHSA Roadmap), with a national scorecard to publicly report progress. As of early 2017, 93 countries had embarked on the process across key performance areas within prevention, detection, and response.[42] In championing the success of the first two years of the GHSA, former CDC director Dr. Tom Frieden noted that "[i]n Cameroon . . . an outbreak of avian influenza was rapidly recognized and stopped, with the emergency team in place within 48 hours, compared with a response to past emergencies that took 8 weeks or more to organize. In Uganda, outbreaks of cholera, meningitis, and yellow fever have been rapidly identified and stopped. And in Tanzania, GHSA enabled a more rapid and more effective response to cholera."[43]

In three short years, from 2014 to 2017, the GHSA catalyzed a level of national and international action toward health security and IHR implementation far beyond what had been achieved in the preceding two decades.[44] And this has been achieved with a remarkable degree of shared commitment, participation, transparency, and level of rigor. Much of the success is due to

Three Lines of Defense Against Epidemics

Active prevention, early detection, and rapid response are the three lines of defense to keep local outbreaks from becoming devastating epidemics or global pandemics.

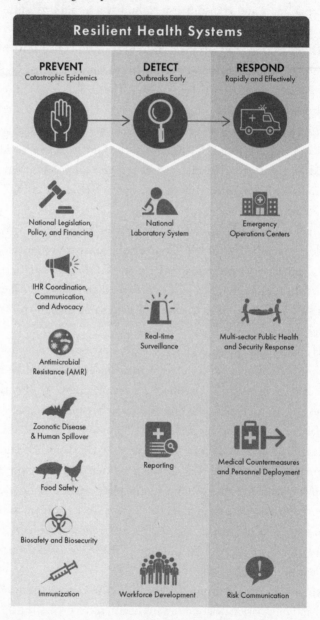

Resilient Health Systems

PREVENT
Catastrophic Epidemics

DETECT
Outbreaks Early

RESPOND
Rapidly and Effectively

National Legislation, Policy, and Financing

National Laboratory System

Emergency Operations Centers

IHR Coordination, Communication, and Advocacy

Real-time Surveillance

Multi-sector Public Health and Security Response

Antimicrobial Resistance (AMR)

Zoonotic Disease & Human Spillover

Reporting

Medical Countermeasures and Personnel Deployment

Food Safety

Biosafety and Biosecurity

Immunization

Workforce Development

Risk Communication

SOURCE: Adapted from International Health Regulations. World Health Organization. 2005. www.who.int (accessed 7 July 2017); Joint External Evaluation Tool: International Health Regulations. World Health Organization. 2016. www.who.int (accessed 7 July 2017); Action Packages. Global Health Security Agenda. 2017. www.ghsagenda.org (accessed 7 July 2017).

the spirit of collaboration and shared purpose exemplified by Bonnie Jenkins and countless other dedicated colleagues like her who are committed to a safer world.

Monitoring National and Local Readiness in the U.S.

As a champion for the International Health Regulations and global health security, the U.S. was one of the first countries to use the 2016 WHO Joint External Evaluation tool to assess its own capacity to prevent, detect, and rapidly respond to public-health threats. It scored well on nearly all 48 indicators, as might be expected from its resources and internationally recognized expertise. Even so, areas for improvement were identified, including laboratory services, senior-level expertise in some core capacities, and coordination in public-health systems decentralized to the state and local levels.[45]

In 2013, the U.S. had also established the National Health Security Index, which provides a model for local public-health performance monitoring. Despite recent improvements, 20 U.S. states in the south and mountain west continue to fall behind, including those most at risk for mosquito-borne illnesses like Zika. The 2016 index demonstrated that even in one of the world's richest countries, there are large, persistent inequities among states that must be addressed to ensure that all are protected from infectious-disease outbreaks and other health threats.[46]

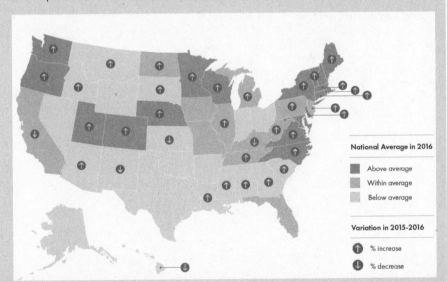

Adapted from National Health Security Preparedness Index: Summary of Key Findings. National Health Security Preparedness Index. 2017. http://nhspi.org/wp-content/uploads/2017/04/2017-NHSPI-Key -Findings.pdf (accessed 19 April 2017).

Strengthening Health Systems Around the World

If there is one overarching lesson to be learned from the struggle against epidemics, it's that health systems, particularly in poorer countries, must be made much more resilient. This means that healthcare workers, institutions, and the general public have to be as prepared as possible for a public-health emergency. None of this is easy, because it first requires being aware of a potential threat in the first place and targeting resources to it, which demands strong surveillance. It also requires having a solid, well-supplied, accessible, and affordable primary-care foundation, so that people don't have to travel for days or wait for weeks to see a doctor. And because leaders and professionals at different levels often have conflicting or overlapping goals, local, national, and international organizations need to know who is doing what, where. It's also crucial to have a strong, well-trained, and committed healthcare workforce and a public that is well informed and responsive. Finally, we need to be financially fair: some kind of universal healthcare coverage would prevent people from going into medical debt and encourage them to seek regular care.

Fortunately, thanks to the efforts of so many at the local, national, and international levels, there is much to hope for. We just need to do a better job, faster, before the next pandemic strikes.

CHAPTER 8

ACTIVE PREVENTION, CONSTANT READINESS

Vaccines, mosquito control, and other preventive measures will stop killer diseases before they spread. Constant readiness to respond will save lives.

Prevention remains our most valuable strategy to save lives and livelihoods in the face of epidemic threats. Top-priority actions include promoting personal hygiene, controlling transmission of mosquito-borne diseases, attacking the sources of new and reemerging diseases from the bush and barn, and ensuring that needed vaccines are developed, affordable, available where and when they are needed, and accepted by everyone. Disruption of health and other essential services can pose a greater threat to human life and well-being than an epidemic or pandemic itself. Most health systems and many businesses worldwide are not prepared. They can be and they should be.

In the mid-nineteenth century, when microbes were yet to be discovered and the germ theory of disease was decades away, a physician named Ignaz Semmelweis worked in Vienna's General Hospital. The hospital had two maternity clinics; one was attended by medical students who moved straight from autopsy rooms to the delivery suite. In that clinic, 10 percent of the women died of postpartum fever. The second clinic, attended by midwives, had a maternal mortality of only 2 percent. Semmelweis was puzzled by this, but he got a clue when a colleague, Jakob Kolletschka, was accidentally cut by a student's scalpel while performing an autopsy; he subsequently got sick and died. Kolletschka's own autopsy showed a pathological condition similar to that of women who died from puerperal (childbirth) fever. Semmelweis was unawave of microbial pathogens, but he concluded that some "unknown cadaverous material" caused the fever, so he instituted a policy of washing hands with chlorinated lime for those leaving the autopsy room. The rate of maternal mortality dropped tenfold.[1] As scientific knowledge has progressed, we've learned that the simple practice of hand-washing is one of the most important elements of infection control.

Since Semmelweis's discovery, time has tested and proven three lines of defense in stopping local disease outbreaks: prevention, early detection, and rapid response. Prevention through self-protection is our most lifesaving, cost-effective course of action, but crucial gaps remain, especially in the areas of mosquito control and vaccination. Early detection of pandemic threats and disease outbreaks is vital to our ability to mount threat-specific defenses. Yet, too often, we're surprised when we shouldn't be. Our early warning systems are not good enough and we are still too slow in detecting and reporting local outbreaks. And finally, stopping the spread of disease once it strikes requires rapid action on the part of citizens, public-health leaders, and governments alike. We need early detection and early, well-coordinated response from the powers that be, and on several levels.

For generations since Semmelweis's discovery, public-health experts have known how to prevent human infection, and most of what they have discovered comes down to you and me as individuals. We first must be self-protectors. If we're lucky enough to live in a country where we learn from childhood about the importance of washing our hands after using the toilet or before eating a meal, we also know about taking other preventive measures to protect both ourselves and others. We cover our mouths when we cough or sneeze. (If we're really informed, we cough into our sleeves rather than onto our hands, which can spread germs to anything we touch.) If we're sick, we stay home, monitor our temperature, drink fluids, and rest. If there is an outbreak of flu or measles where we go to school or work, we try not to go there until the threat subsides. We get ourselves and our children immunized.

But to stop an epidemic in its tracks, we need to do much more. This is why active prevention and constant readiness are the third elements in The Power of Seven. We need to thump incessantly on the doors, ceilings, walls, and floors of public and private leaders to make sure that other protective measures such as vaccines are in place; that those in charge of detecting disease early have all the support they could possibly need; and that local, regional, and national leaders have emergency public-health programs ready for the onslaught.

Preventing Disease from Mosquitoes

Mosquitoes are the most dangerous creatures on earth for humans. Each year their tiny bites infect more than 700 million people worldwide and kill more than a million, half of whom are children in Africa. These flying syringes are capable of transporting and injecting into our bloodstreams more than a dozen different killer diseases. And they have proven extremely challenging to control.

There are three main groups of dangerous mosquitoes, each of which includes many species. *Anopheles* mosquitoes are responsible for malaria—one of the top killers of all time. *Aedes* are the ones that spread the Zika, dengue, yellow fever, and chikungunya viruses. Mosquitoes from the *Culex* genus, which are found worldwide except in the extreme north, carry West Nile fever, Japanese encephalitis, several other encephalitis viruses, and filariasis.

Most *Anopheles* like to feed on humans at night during our sleep, though some species prefer their blood meals at dusk or dawn. *Aedes* are urban creatures that are daytime biters (most active two hours after sunrise and several hours before sunset), thrive in populated areas, prefer human blood, and will bite several people in a short time. An *Aedes* mosquito can be trickier to control than an *Anopheles* mosquito; it feasts on a variety of nonhumans, as well as people, and eats more often than other mosquitoes do. Thanks to global warming and deforestation, this creature is now burgeoning on all continents, including Europe and at least 30 U.S. states. As a result, more than 3 billion people are at risk for *Aedes*-borne infections like Zika. As of early 2017, 85 countries from every continent except Antarctica had reported recent cases of Zika, with person-to-person sexual transmission occurring in more than a dozen countries.[2] Millions of men and women and their families are at risk of becoming infected. And vacationers and conference attendees from Miami to North Borneo are advised not to have unprotected sex for at least two weeks after returning home.

Another devastating *Aedes*-borne virus is yellow fever. International travelers carried the virus into Asia from Africa in 2016, putting nearly 2 billion unvaccinated people at risk. While most yellow fever infections are mild, the virus can be fatal: About 15 percent of victims develop a severe form of the virus that leads to liver damage (the name "yellow fever" comes from jaundice). Of those who contract the severe form of the illness, 20 to 50 percent die. Yet another *Aedes*-borne virus, dengue, has seen a 30-fold increase over the last four decades, up to the current level of 400 million annual infections. Up to a quarter of those who get infected develop agonizing dengue hemorrhagic fever.[3]

*   *   *

Preventing mosquito-borne disease requires massive efforts on the part of individuals, communities, and governments. The good news is that concerted campaigns pay off enormously. For example, in a pioneering, eco-friendly study called the *Camino Verde* (Green Way), 150 communities (85,000 residents in nearly 20,000 households) in Nicaragua and Mexico joined together to assess the impact of chemical-free mosquito control. In one experiment, half the communities (the experimental groups) took steps to clean interior walls of buildings, cover breeding sites, hold awareness events like puppet shows and basketball tournaments, clean up vacant lots, and add mosquito-eating fish to water-storage containers. Because of these efforts, the mosquito population was reduced, and dengue infections in children dropped by an average of 30 percent.[4]

The battle against malaria by the Sri Lankan government is especially worth mentioning. The island country suffered a million cases of *Anopheles*-borne malaria per year through the 1940s. After officials began using DDT to kill the bugs, the number of malaria cases dropped to 17 by 1963—a success story by any measure, but unfortunately short-lived, as the bugs developed resistance to DDT.[5]

Following a decades-long civil war, the government (except rebel-held areas in Sri Lanka's northeast corner) ran out of money and was forced to rely on help from outside donors to renew the attack on mosquitoes. Thanks to those donations, the government in the year 2000 began deploying a combined strategy consisting of indoor spraying, bed nets, rapid diagnostic kits, screening citizens' blood, and a national electronic reporting system. The government also set up mobile clinics near mines and logging camps. In 2016, WHO declared the country of 20 million free of malaria.[6] That was an amazing feat.

What Sri Lanka proved possible in Southeast Asia had a precedent in

North America. In less than four years (July 1947 through the end of 1951), a cooperative undertaking by state and local health agencies in 13 southeastern states and the U.S. Public Health Service eliminated malaria by spraying insecticides on the interior surfaces or entire premises of more than 4.6 million rural homes, as well as draining standing water and removing mosquito breeding sites.[7] Unfortunately, access to global travel has compromised that achievement. Today, 1,500 to 2,000 cases of malaria still occur in the U.S., nearly all among recent travelers from other countries. Occasional local outbreaks where malaria-transmitting mosquitoes are still present remind us that malaria could return in the U.S.[8]

The global fight against malaria reached a tipping point in 1998 when the newly elected WHO director-general, Dr. Gro Brundtland, along with leaders from UNICEF, United Nations Development Programme, and the World Bank, launched the Roll Back Malaria Partnership. The partnership galvanized a global campaign that mobilized scores of public and private organizations in more than 30 countries. This has led to a 60 percent reduction in worldwide malaria deaths since 2000, thanks to a combination of insecticide-treated bed nets, antimalarial drugs, and environmental measures.[9, 10]

Building on this stunning progress, Bill Gates and Ray Chambers (a wealthy fellow businessman and UN special envoy) announced the creation of the End Malaria Council at the 2017 World Economic Forum in Davos, Switzerland. By mobilizing influential public- and private-sector leaders, Gates and Chambers hope to eliminate malaria across the globe by 2030.[11] In speaking of this effort, former Tanzanian president Jakaya Kikwete—who lost a brother to malaria in childhood—observed that "ending malaria was once an impossible dream. It is now within our reach. It will take strong leadership and serious financial commitments, but I believe we can make history and end this brutal disease once and for all."[12]

While substantial progress has been made against diseases borne by *Anopheles*, preventing disease from the *Aedes* mosquito is proving more challenging. Since the 1950s, various combinations of DDT applications, indoor residual spraying, and intensive efforts to control breeding sites have achieved dramatic reductions in *Aedes* mosquitoes in Latin America, Cuba, and Singapore. However, when officials relaxed those control efforts, the mosquitoes sprang back.[13] As I will describe in chapter 10, bringing *Aedes*-borne disease under control and preventing another unexpected and devastating surprise like Zika will require a major innovative breakthrough.

Preventing Diseases from Jungle and Farm

Mosquitoes bite us, but we humans bite other creatures. As I've shown in chapters 2 and 3, the human desire to eat wild or domestic animals also exposes us to all kinds of pathogens. When people live in squalor, disease spreads. So, what can we do to reduce the chance that a pathogen from a jungle or domestic animal brings a new epidemic into the world?[14] The answer is to make it harder for diseases to jump from animals to humans.

One way is to support initiatives that limit people's dependency on bushmeat in places where survival depends on it. One such effort, in Kenya, aims to offer rural residents an alternative to hunting bushmeat by providing a source of income. In this example, an 80,000-acre cattle range located between Kenya's largest national parks was failing. An organization called Wildlife Works developed a new use for the range. In exchange for removing squatters and snares from the land, the group was given permission to build an "EcoFactory" where workers now produce designer T-shirts to be sold in the U.S. and Europe. Today, sales of the T-shirts finance development projects and support 56 full-time jobs. Those 56 workers are no longer hunting bushmeat, and therefore they, their families, and their villages are safer.[15]

"Protein projects," another alternative to bushmeat, introduce other clean sources of nutrition. The Heifer Project, for example, provides rural families in developing nations with meat animals such as rabbits, chickens, cane rats, and snails, and products such as milk, cheese, and eggs. After the older animals mate, their babies are passed on to other families, thus spreading the community wealth. The Heifer Project also helps form farm cooperatives to supply volume orders for restaurants and offers training in animal husbandry, meal preparation, and marketing.[16]

We can also support programs that stop industrialization and deforestation in jungle areas.[17] Some countries are establishing protected areas, and some companies have agreed to moratoriums on buying soy or beef raised on deforested land. A UN program called REDD+ (the United Nations Collaborative Programme on Reducing Emissions from Deforestation and Forest Degradation in Developing Countries) offers financial incentives to developing countries for reducing deforestation. Today, 80 percent of original Amazonian forest is still standing because people haven't cut it down yet—in part thanks to forest protections, moratoriums, and the REDD+ program.[18]

In developed nations we can also work for change among industries involved in resource extraction, livestock production, and trade. A focus on livestock alone would help mightily. Reducing the risk posed by farm animals requires us all, as individuals, to fight factory farming on a variety of levels. Beginning with our personal food choices, we can vote with our mouths: If we choose to eat meat or dairy products, we can eat them less often, and buy our food from places that don't rely on factory farm sources (goodbye, McDonald's and Burger King). If we live in agricultural areas, we can organize our communities and vote for candidates who oppose factory farming. If a factory farm wants to settle in your area, you can work to prevent the company from getting or extending permits. You can also take to social media and write to newspapers and magazines to decry factory farms.

Vaccines: Our Most Powerful Protection

Just after Thanksgiving 2005, a healthy 17-year-old boy from Sheboygan County, Wisconsin, was helping his brother-in-law butcher pigs at a local slaughterhouse. Three days later he came down with the flu. He fully recovered, but lab tests showed he carried an unusual H1N1 influenza virus— a mosaic of genes from wild birds, humans, and pigs.

Four years later, in early 2009, a closely related H1N1 virus caused an influenza outbreak in La Gloria, Mexico, east of Mexico City, just down the road from a factory farm that raised a million pigs in 2008. We can only guess at the pathway that connected the Wisconsin and La Gloria H1N1 flu virus. New cases of H1N1 quickly showed up in Mexico City and almost simultaneously in southern California. Within weeks, WHO had received confirmed reports of H1N1 in Europe, the Middle East, and the Western Pacific. The new virus sprinted across the globe and within a month reached 46 countries.[19]

The virus was a different strain of the same H1N1 that caused the 1918 global influenza pandemic, and influenza experts feared the worst. On April 25, 2009, following a meeting of the WHO Emergency Committee, WHO director-general Margaret Chan declared the outbreak an international public-health emergency and advised countries to be on the lookout for unusual outbreaks of influenza-like illness and severe pneumonia.[20]

The good news was this: within a month of declaring the emergency, scientists working with WHO had identified the virus. Samples were immediately sent to prospective manufacturers, and a massive vaccine-production effort began. (Vaccines had been developed for H5N1 influenza, but none had been developed for this particular strain of H1N1.) In short order, 11 vaccines were prequalified for use. Ultimately, WHO deployed 200 million doses of vaccine to 77 countries around the world. Roughly 36 percent of the people in those countries were vaccinated.[21] Researchers estimated that the vaccine prevented as many as 1.5 million cases, 10,000 hospitalizations, and 500 deaths in the U.S alone.[22, 23]

*   *   *

Despite the success of WHO's initiative, H1N1 still had serious effects worldwide. In many ways, the H1N1 pandemic was a dress rehearsal for a pandemic of influenza of the magnitude predicted by Bill Gates and infectious-disease experts such as Michael Osterholm. By the time the H1N1 pandemic ended in 2010, as many as 200 million people had been infected, and an estimated 575,400 people may have perished worldwide. The pattern of illness was disturbingly like the 1918 epidemic. Mortality was highest among pregnant women, children, and young adults.[24] Of those who died, 80 percent were under 65 years of age.[25] By comparison, the regular flu season is most lethal to the elderly, who account for 90 percent of the deaths every year.[26]

As a doctor, I know that nothing can protect people against illness as effectively as a vaccine. It is the single most cost-effective public-health tool we have. Without vaccines, smallpox would still be killing people, and polio would be crippling millions. Before the introduction of routine childhood immunizations in the 1950s, epidemics of measles, pertussis (whooping cough), diphtheria, rubella, polio, and other infectious diseases killed, disabled, or produced birth defects in millions of children and adults. Since the 1960s, these immunizations have saved an estimated 2.6 million lives a year and have doubled the average life expectancy for millions more in the twenty-first century. Vaccines also save lives when used selectively in high-risk areas, during local outbreaks, and in specific situations (such as an outbreak of rabies).

When it comes to preventing epidemics, there are five critical questions: (1) Do we have a proven vaccine? (2) Can we produce the needed vaccine quantities quickly enough? (3) Can a country obtain enough vaccine through purchases or donations? (4) Do countries have the capacity to distribute and administer the vaccine? (5) Will people accept the vaccine?

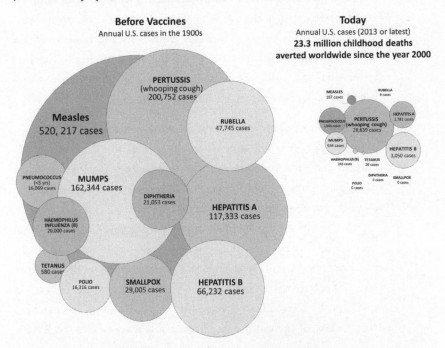

Vaccines Work

(Size of bubble proportional to number of cases)

Before Vaccines
Annual U.S. cases in the 1900s

Today
Annual U.S. cases (2013 or latest)
**23.3 million childhood deaths
averted worldwide since the year 2000**

PERTUSSIS
(whooping cough)
200,752 cases

Measles
520, 217 cases

RUBELLA
47,745 cases

PNEUMOCOCCUS
(<5 yrs)
16,069 cases

MUMPS
162,344 cases

DIPHTHERIA
21,053 cases

HAEMOPHILUS
INFLUENZA (B)
20,000 cases

HEPATITIS A
117,333 cases

TETANUS
580 cases

POLIO
16,316 cases

SMALLPOX
29,005 cases

HEPATITIS B
66,232 cases

MEASLES
187 cases

RUBELLA
9 cases

PNEUMOCOCCUS
1,900 cases

PERTUSSIS
(whooping cough)
28,639 cases

HEPATITIS A
1,781 cases

MUMPS
534 cases

HEPATITIS B
3,050 cases

HAEMOPHILUS (B)
243 cases

TETANUS
26 cases

DIPHTHERIA
0 cases

SMALLPOX
0 cases

POLIO
0 cases

SOURCE: Adapted from BlueLIFE. Virus protection. BlueLIFE. 2014. http://lapdbluelife.com/virus
-protection/ (accessed 14 April 2017). (map) Hyman M, Nurses C, Smith M et al. 13 vaccines that save lives
around the world (infographic). Health Essentials from Cleveland Clinic. 2014. https://health.clevelandclinic
.org/2014/01/vaccines-that-save-lives-around-the-world-infographic/ (accessed 14 April 2017). (table) Data
from: Centers for Disease Control and Prevention. Parents' Guide to Childhood Immunizations. Centers
for Disease Control and Prevention. 2011. http://www.cdc.gov/vaccines/pubs/parents-guide/default.htm
(accessed 15 August 2011). Centers for Disease Control. Impact of vaccines in the 20th & 21st centuries.
Centers for Disease Control and Prevention. 2011. www.cdc.gov/vaccines/pubs/pinkbook/downloads
/appendices/G/impact-of-vaccines.pdf (accessed 15 August 2011).

I attempt to answer each of these five questions here.

1. *Do we have proven vaccines for every major epidemic threat?*

   Not yet, and for a few pathogens, perhaps we never will. On the positive side, in addition to the vaccines commonly used for childhood
   illnesses, there are more than two dozen infectious diseases for which
   vaccines are available, including seasonal influenza, pneumococcal
   pneumonia, yellow fever, hepatitis A and B, Japanese encephalitis, anthrax, and rabies.[27] Maddeningly, some major gaps remain. The biology of viruses, including HIV (the virus that causes AIDS), dengue
   fever, and malaria, has bedeviled vaccine developers for decades, so no

proven vaccine yet exists for these diseases. An effective vaccine for several common strains of Ebola became available in 2016, unfortunately too late to help the millions of sufferers and survivors in West Africa. As of this writing, vaccines are not yet available for Zika, MERS, and several other viruses of pandemic potential. (Vaccines for seasonal and pandemic influenza, a challenge of its own, is something I'll discuss in chapter 10, on innovation.)

2. *If an epidemic strikes, can we produce enough vaccine quickly?*
The short answer is no, because vaccine-production methods are antiquated and vaccine-production surge capacity is inadequate. Most vaccines are grown in chicken eggs, a process that takes months and requires specialized production facilities.

One of the core principles in combating epidemics, as I note throughout this book, is that time matters a lot. In many respects, the development and large-scale production of the H1N1 vaccine were unprecedented. Had the H1N1 vaccine already existed in April 2009, thousands of lives could have been saved. Researchers estimate that if the vaccine had been available even two weeks earlier, it would have reduced deaths by 25 percent. Two months earlier than that and deaths would have been reduced by more than half.[28]

As of 2015, the production capacity of pandemic influenza vaccine is 6.4 billion doses. This represents enough vaccine to immunize just over 3 billion people with two doses, or 43 percent of people around the world. If we get lucky, and one dose of the vaccine offers sufficient protection as it did in the 2009 H1N1 pandemic, then we could cover 86 percent of the current population.[29] Practically speaking, that's the best we're going to be able to do.

International agencies like WHO; Gavi, the Vaccine Alliance; and the World Bank, as well as national governments and pharmaceutical companies, should do much more to ramp up rapid production and supply chain capacity in the event of an emergency. Today, in the absence of a universal flu vaccine, it might take a year to get another vaccine up and running and distributed—and in the interim, millions could die.

3. *Can countries obtain enough vaccine through purchases or donations?*
    Too many vaccines aren't affordable. In 2015, MSF accused Glaxo-
    SmithKline and Pfizer of overcharging nonprofits for new vaccines
    that protect against pneumonia-causing bacteria. "The price to fully
    vaccinate a child is 68 times more expensive than it was just over a
    decade ago, mainly because a handful of big pharmaceutical compa-
    nies are overcharging donors and developing countries for vaccines
    that already earn them billions of dollars in wealthy countries," Ro-
    hit Malpani of MSF's Access Campaign told NBC News.[30]

    The problem is that pharmaceutical company shareholders are
    demanding, and market forces too often get in the way of public
    health. Drug companies have little incentive to develop new vaccines
    that offer protection over several years, because such vaccines can be
    even costlier and yield comparatively few returns (since people need
    the vaccine less frequently).[31] Pharmaceutical companies also like to
    exploit their monopolies, hence the high prices.

    To deal with the rising prices in the U.S., the *New York Times* re-
    ported, "Some doctors, who say they lose money on every vaccination,
    reserve their shots for longstanding patients." The *Times* took note of a
    survey of family-practice doctors, who "along with pediatricians are
    among the lowest-earning physicians, found that about one-third were
    considering giving up immunizations because of the expense." Another
    40 percent "do not offer at least some required childhood immuniza-
    tions."[32] That this is the case in the world's richest country is shocking.
    Refusing to inoculate people because of cost is, in my view, immoral.
    Fortunately, the U.S. government currently buys half of all vaccines for
    children and does so at deeply discounted prices.[33] It also provides in-
    formation on finding affordable vaccines.[34]

    To counteract the problem of vaccine access in developing
    countries, public/private partnerships like Gavi do everything they
    can to work with manufacturers to bring affordable vaccines to the
    poor. Another group, the Developing Countries Vaccine Manufac-
    turers Network (www.dcvmn.org), brings 40 different high-quality
    vaccines at affordable prices to the developing world. One such vaccine
    protects children against five diseases: diphtheria, tetanus, pertussis,
    hepatitis B, and Haemophilus influenza type b. Such combination

vaccines offer many benefits: they reduce the number of injections, vials, and visits while lowering costs at the same time.[35]

4. *Do countries have the capacity to distribute and administer the vaccine?*

Even if we had an effective vaccine against viruses like H5N1, we still couldn't ensure that enough people would receive it in time. Vaccination programs in developing countries are plagued by lack of cold storage for serum, by poor transportation, and by lack of reliable data-tracking systems.[36, 37, 38] That said, there are a few emerging bright spots. The University of Rwanda, for example, started Africa's first training on health supply chain management in 2015.[39] Students are paired with mentors from United Parcel Service, which teaches them to manage data and logistics and impart problem-solving and team-building skills. Similar programs are taking place across both Africa and Asia; a program in Benin expects to graduate 100 specialists by 2020.

5. *Will people accept the vaccine?*

Not everyone welcomes potentially lifesaving medicines. In fact, as you will read in the next chapter, vaccine rejection is surging in some countries and among some populations. In the event of a major epidemic, those who reject vaccines could be looking at a death sentence.

Early Detection Saves Lives

"It's tough to make predictions," the baseball-playing philosopher Yogi Berra once quipped, "especially about the future."[40]

Au contraire. Steve Kunitz, the professor who taught me about the ways domestic dogs could forecast plague among prairie dogs in Arizona, revealed to me the possibility of predicting disease by carefully following clues. I'm happy to report that disease prediction has advanced light-years since I sat in his class back in the 1970s. Instead of waiting around for disease to strike and responding to an epidemic after the fact, innovative scientists are rooting out viruses at their animal sources.

The Epidemic Intelligence Service (EIS) is a two-year service and training program of the Centers for Disease Control and Prevention.[41] EIS was founded in 1951, during the height of the Cold War, when the fear of biological warfare was first raging. "EIS is indeed the most important (and effective) U.S. government agency of which you have never heard," notes Mark Pendergrast, a freelance journalist and author of the 2010 book *Inside the Outbreaks: The Elite Medical Detectives of the Epidemic Intelligence Service.*[42]

Pendergrast's book documents how, behind the scenes and headlines, the EIS, mostly composed of young people, investigated many famous epidemics. "EIS officers pioneered the identification and control of hospital infections, learned that people could contract rabies from bats without being bitten, and helped to eradicate smallpox." He told an interviewer, "Do you want me to go on? I haven't mentioned solving listeriosis, identifying AIDS, finding Cryptosporidium in drinking water, battling rotavirus, multiple-drug-resistant tuberculosis, botulism, yellow fever, parasites, pesticides . . ."

The CDC still operates the EIS, though Pendergrast says it is perpetually underfunded. The good news is that it's been copied by similar programs around the world. Says Pendergrast, "EIS alumni have helped to start all of them."

Unfortunately, not all countries have yet developed outbreak detection systems as vigilant as EIS. The 1994 pneumonic plague outbreak in India was a spectacular disaster for that country's government. Reporters from the BBC were stationed there, unfurling the crisis for the horrified world even before the government had announced it, perhaps even before health officials in New Delhi knew what had happened. The government hesitated while WHO responded with a pathetic flurry of press releases. WHO's antiquated information system was built on a platform of phones and fax machines, and the organization could not answer questions from reporters and governments anywhere near quickly enough.

As is so often the case, crisis often leads to solutions. The Indian plague outbreak ultimately inspired researchers to develop new ways to discover and report disease before chaos erupts. Immediately after the disaster, technology began filling the information gap, beginning with ProMED, an internet-based outbreak reporting system. Using ProMED, health professionals could share information about emerging infectious-disease events via a moderated email list.[43]

*   *   *

As an epidemiologist who fought smallpox alongside D. A. Henderson and who has worked hard to eradicate polio, Dr. Larry Brilliant knows a thing or two about stopping epidemics. He's also a "brilliant" character with an eclectic biography. Once, he was cast as a doctor in a film about the hippies who followed the Grateful Dead. He has also run high-tech firms in Silicon Valley. Alongside Stewart Brand, he founded the Well, a Facebook precursor for the early "wired" population. His Seva Foundation has prevented millions of people in developing countries from going blind.

Brilliant received the $1 million TED Prize in 2006.[44] The prize goes to a leader with a big dream, and he wanted to use it to help stop epidemics. For Brilliant, the internet is a potential savior. Working with Google, he and his colleagues developed a system called Innovative Support to Emergencies, Diseases and Disasters (InSTEDD for short), which aims to improve early detection, preparedness, and response capabilities for global health threats and humanitarian crises. InSTEDD looks out for disease outbreaks via "web crawlers," software programs that search the internet for references to illness.

Brilliant also puts great faith in a system called the Global Public Health Intelligence Network, or GPHIN. GPHIN is a multilingual, early warning web crawler developed in Canada that continuously monitors global media and online sources to identify disease outbreaks, searching constantly for words or combinations of words using a complex algorithm. GPHIN has been amazingly successful. It can find 40 percent of the outbreaks WHO subsequently investigates and verifies each year, alerting authorities long before calls up the chains of command ever could.[45]

Here's how GPHIN helped stop the 2003 SARS epidemic. The WHO Emerging Infectious Disease unit was headed by Dr. David Heymann, a veteran of smallpox eradication and early Ebola outbreaks, and a good friend and colleague during our time together at WHO. At that time WHO rules forbade the use of information from any source other than its 192 member governments. But David knew that official sources could not always be trusted when it came to early detection and rapid response to outbreaks. He also knew that more than 60 percent of early outbreak reports came from the press, the internet, and other informal sources. So David looked for a reliable source of early epidemic intelligence. He found that in GPHIN, whose early alert of an unusual outbreak in China prompted the WHO epidemic investigation that led to Gro Brundtland's March 2003 international travel alert. Shortly after the alert, David assembled a virtual team of top-notch research institutions in

11 countries to identify the new virus, develop diagnostic tests, and define the public-health response—long before Chinese officials admitted to the disease's existence. As a result of the early action catalyzed by GPHIN, SARS was rapidly contained and has not been seen since.[46]

Since its inception, GPHIN has grown both more multilingual and more robust. It solves a plethora of problems in disease reporting. Because it doesn't rely on human connections for reporting, it's transparent, objective, and trustworthy. It also allows users to see details about what is occurring where on the international, national, regional, and local levels. With GPHIN, "[a]ll of a sudden, we had a very powerful system that brought in much more information from more countries," David said. "And we were able to go to countries confidentially and validate what was going on, and, if they needed help, we provided help. And we provided help by bringing together many different institutions from around the world that started to work with us."[47]

As promising as these technologies are, they aren't perfect in reporting disease early on because many people don't go to a healthcare provider when they feel sick. So, what could happen if people took into their own hands the responsibility for reporting disease, using their computers and cell phones?

An approach called "participatory epidemiology" brings the reporting system right to the people who are feeling sick. With participatory technology, people can report their symptoms directly to the system. Citizens and health officials can see disease clusters in real time and find out about participation in vaccine programs.[48] Flu Near You, a website in the U.S., has been tracking self-reported trends in the presence of flu-like systems from thousands of users (40,000 of them actively respond to weekly email updates).[49] Participants receive weekly email messages asking whether they have had a flu shot and whether they have experienced any flu symptoms. On the system, a variety of colored dots show where flu might be spreading (blue means no reported symptoms, orange represents some symptoms, and red indicates likely flu in the area).[50]

Elsewhere, in Thailand, a program called DoctorMe allows people to diagnose possible health conditions through a simple application on their smartphone; the data is then sent anonymously to Google, which analyzes the symptoms and location of the users.[51] DoctorMe found the first case of MERS, and it's considered one of the world's best detection systems.

Participatory Surveillance for Early Detection

Participation of citizens, communities, frontline health workers, and others in direct reporting of suspected outbreaks would save lives and livelihoods through earlier detection and earlier response.

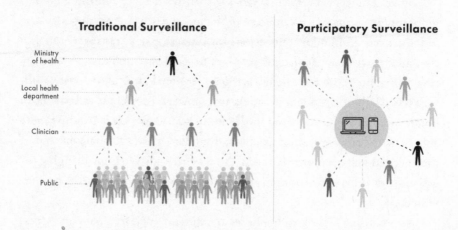

SOURCE: Wójcik O, Brownstein J, Chunara R, Johansson M. Public health for the people: Participatory infectious disease surveillance in the digital age. *Emerging Themes in Epidemiology* 2014; 11: 7. http://www.ete-online.com/content/11/1/7EMERGING THEMES.

Rapid Response: Stopping the Spread

Anyone who's caught a cold from a child knows that school environments are perfect incubators for the flu. And anyone who has dragged him- or herself to work while sick as a dog would probably prefer to stay home in bed, but too many workers don't have sick leave and feel they have to go to work anyway.[52] Just imagine if one of these children or workers came to school or work sick with something like H5N1.

If people won't stay home of their own accord during a deadly epidemic, they may be forced to do so by public-health officials. Since an effective flu vaccine can't be produced until four to six months after a virus spreads, what epidemiologists call "social distancing" is probably the most effective method of preventing transmission. Social distancing is the practice of closing schools or public areas like shopping malls during an epidemic for as long as necessary. Businesses would have to tell sick employees to work from home, or set up flexible shift plans.[53]

Social distancing is never popular, but it works. In 2012, scientists at McMaster University in Ontario, Canada, found compelling evidence that closing schools is an effective way to control flu epidemics. They found that school closure reduced flu transmission among school-age children by more than 50 percent (seasonal changes in weather also had a significant effect).[54]

In severe conditions, the more draconian strategy of quarantine may also be necessary. From the time of the Black Death to the first pandemics of the twenty-first century, public-health officials have resorted to quarantine to reduce contact between the sick and the healthy. During the fourteenth-century plague in Europe, city-states installed armed guards at entry points.[55] Once, while enjoying an evening meal with a resident of Bellagio in the Lake Como area of Italy, I learned how separating the sick from the well prevented disease from spreading during those deadly years. Residents in my companion's town, located on a peninsula separated by forest and water on three sides, discovered an interesting way to keep residents healthy. People living on the mainland wanted bread that Bellagio produced, so the people in the isolated town would leave the bread on a boulder just offshore in the lake. In exchange, people from the mainland left coins in a sanitizing jar of vinegar. No one in Bellagio got the plague.

More recently, public-health authorities quarantined more than 100 people with tuberculosis in New York City between 1993 and 1995 to ensure they were taking their medicine and following other protocols. To prevent the spread of SARS, Canada quarantined about 30,000 people in their Toronto homes. While some experts debate whether such an extreme measure was actually effective at limiting the spread of the disease,[56] the CDC reported that, during SARS, "the use of quarantine, border controls, contact tracing, and surveillance proved effective in containing the global threat in just over three months."[57]

As a strategy, quarantine is always a last resort. As the CDC notes, quarantine raises all kinds of political, ethical, and socioeconomic issues and requires a careful balance between public interest and individual rights.[58] It only works well if accompanied by regular, transparent, and comprehensive communications that balance the benefits of quarantine against the risks, and by carefully guarding the needs and rights of those held in isolation.

Protecting Routine Health Care

"War is unhealthy for children and other living things." I remember those words from a 1960s-era poster that protested the Vietnam War. It's true in more ways than one. In the Revolutionary War, 17,000 soldiers died from disease, more than twice the number who died from battle wounds. During a war, soldiers and civilians have historically been just as—or more—likely to die from disease as to die from battle. In the American Civil War, two-thirds of the 620,000 soldiers who died succumbed not to battle wounds but to diseases like dysentery and typhoid.[59] In World War I, American soldiers exposed to smallpox in Spain brought it back home.

Like a war, a major epidemic can shred routine health care because all the fire hoses are trained on it—leaving children without immunizations, women without maternal care, and those who suffer from chronic diseases like diabetes without access to lifesaving drugs. During the Ebola epidemic, fear among staff and patients closed many health facilities for weeks. Deaths of healthcare workers compounded the problem. With many facilities closed and fewer doctors and nurses available, women were giving birth in the streets without help.[60] And people also died of entirely preventable ills like diabetes and septic wounds.[61]

The first step in protecting routine health services is to rapidly and correctly identify the specific cause of the outbreak, so that healthcare workers can establish proper control measures and isolate suspected cases. Hospitals that set up Ebola treatment units in buildings separate from other inpatient and outpatient centers were better able to keep routine services intact. Periodic disaster preparedness exercises also help health staff to plan ahead and maintain high-priority services like labor and delivery and emergency care.[62]

Controlling International Travel

When Dr. Brundtland issued the WHO emergency travel advisory for China, Hong Kong, and Canada to stop the spread of SARS, she acted on her own judgment and authority. At that time, there were no established procedures for WHO to declare a health emergency. As a result of Canada's vigorous protest at not being consulted, WHO coined the term Public Health Emergency of International Concern (PHEIC) in 2005, when the International Health Regulations (IHRs) were revised. A PHEIC is "an extraordinary event which is determined to constitute a public health risk to other States through the international spread of disease and to potentially require a coordinated international response."[63]

WHO declares a PHEIC when a serious public-health incident requires immediate international action. In such an event, IHRs require UN member states to prevent and reduce the spread of disease.[64] The IHRs were specifically designed to protect public health while avoiding overly restrictive measures by governments and businesses that could disrupt economies, undermine emergency response efforts, and actually worsen the impact of an epidemic. A PHEIC allows WHO to coordinate response efforts and make decisions to contain and control an outbreak. WHO can also support research and development and speed the progress of diagnostic tests and vaccines. If deemed necessary to contain an outbreak, WHO can also impose travel bans to and from certain countries and can even mobilize NATO military personnel.[65]

Following the PHEIC for SARS, WHO declared PHEICs in 2009 for the influenza pandemic; in 2014, when polio was making a comeback; for Ebola in August 2014; and for Zika in 2016. In the case of Zika, Dr. Brundtland's successor, Dr. Margaret Chan, convened by teleconference 18 experts in epidemic disease.[66] First, they examined the relationship between Zika infection during pregnancy and microcephaly. (While not yet scientifically proven, a causal link was strongly suspected at the time.) The committee looked at a variety of factors, including the geographic spread of the mosquito that delivers the virus; the lack of a vaccine and fast, reliable diagnostic tests; and the fact that people in newly affected countries like Brazil had no immunity to Zika. Given all these factors, Chan accepted the advice of the committee and formally declared a PHEIC in February 2016.[67]

For Ebola, WHO recommended strict screening at airports, seaports, and land crossings for people coming from West African countries with active transmission of Ebola. But WHO did not recommend barring incoming travelers from these countries altogether, provided they had passed the exit screening.[68] (As it turned out, this recommendation was neither completely effective nor universally implemented.)

What more can WHO do to protect us? Given the increased risks, I would strongly urge more rigorous assessment screening measures for current and potential risks. In the meantime, if you are traveling internationally, the best advice is to consult the CDC and the European Centre for Disease Control and Prevention.[69]

Catastrophic Pandemics Are Not Inevitable

The epidemiologist Michael Osterholm asks this simple, smart question: "Just imagine if we had had three years' notice that Hurricane Katrina would happen on the day it did. What would have been done in that three-year period from the time they were notified to the day it happened?"[70]

Major epidemics, like big hurricanes, can be overwhelming, but today they are more or less predictable. To stave off disaster, we must devote ample resources toward active prevention, early warning systems, and rapid response. We need to make sure that basic preventive measures are in place. We must support vaccine research and development. We have to ensure that the disease detectives like Nathan Wolfe, Larry Brilliant, and the experts at CDC[71] get all the support they need so that they can help us. We can urge leaders at the governmental level, as well as those at our hospitals and clinics, to practice emergency readiness so that they can keep routine services going when the big one comes.

What can you and I do in the meantime? Public health starts with you and me. We can be vigilant, prepared, and quick to respond, which means taking individual responsibility for things within our power like washing our hands, covering our coughs, getting immunized, and so on. If we are to survive, we need to protect ourselves and support public-health epidemiologists and clinicians with everything we have for active prevention, early detection, and rapid response.

CHAPTER 9

FATAL FICTIONS, TIMELY TRUTHS

Trustworthy communications, close listening,
and local engagement are the best weapons
for fighting disease and quelling rumors, blame,
distrust, and panic.

When we communicate in ways that reflect people's needs, concerns, and voices in a trustworthy way, they respond to constructive guidance and help to limit the spread of disease. Consistent, fact-based information across all forms of media, including traditional media, social media, and entertainment channels, encourages community discussion and behavior change. But counteracting panic and resistance can't just be a top-down, government-issued effort, because trust in government is eroding everywhere. Rather, trust evolves from community leaders and public-health officials working in concert.

In September 2014, a team of eight health workers and journalists disappeared shortly after arriving in the southern Guinean village of Wome, not far from the place where the Ebola outbreak first erupted eight months earlier.[1] They had come to teach Wome's villagers how to protect themselves against Ebola. But instead of welcoming their helpers, the villagers attacked them with stones, clubs, and machetes, believing the workers to be spreaders of the disease. The attackers then slit the visitors' throats and dumped the bodies in the village cistern, where they were discovered three days later.[2]

The attack was not unique. In the space of a year, Red Cross teams in Guinea were attacked roughly ten times a month.[3]

History is rife with examples of groups that have fought back violently against public-health authorities. In 1894, people in a poor south-side community in Milwaukee, Wisconsin, attacked police and ambulances during a city-wide smallpox outbreak.[4] Mobs wielded household items from baseball bats to potato mashers, anything that would serve as a weapon. People tossed pots of scalding water on the horses pulling the ambulances. Rioting went on for a month. Citizens were so fearful of health authorities that they hid the sick, which naturally increased the rates of infection within households.

Well over a century later, a similar mentality reared its head during the Ebola epidemic.

*   *   *

In the face of an epidemic, terror, blame, rumors and conspiracy theories, distrust of authorities, and panic can take hold simultaneously. This is why establishing and maintaining trust through honest, clear communication is paramount. History continues to show us that health communication lies at the heart of epidemic control, yet staffing for such communication is usually tacked onto health budgets as an afterthought, at woefully inadequate levels.[5]

Trustworthy public-health communications are an essential part of The Power of Seven because public trust is a crucial element in preventing and in containing an epidemic.[6] Trust is built on both the good intent and the credibility of the person conveying information, as well as on the confidence in that person's ability to deliver results.[7] Trust can prevent horrific acts of public outrage, chaos, and violence. Trust enables people to accept the reality of an invisible and mysterious attacker, and to change deeply established behaviors.

The Psychology of Fear and Distrust

Why would people at risk of a deadly disease turn on those who come to help? As behavioral economists have demonstrated, we humans aren't as logical and rational as we like to think we are.[8] In fact, our brains haven't evolved much since the Stone Age.[9] Like other animals, we feel before we think. When faced with risk—whether the risk is real or not—we feel endangered.

We simply cannot think straight when we're fearful. We overreact. The Stone Age part of our brains, the amygdala, initiates a fear response and overrides the more rational frontal cortex; fear trumps intellect. And whether the goal is to sell guns or beauty products, experts in marketing and media understand that, because it kidnaps our brains so effectively—fear sells.[10, 11] Some in the news media may deliberately fuel fear because it increases readership, viewers, and advertisers. *Politico* reporter Tara Haelle wrote, "No media outlet—this one included—has managed to restrain itself in reporting the facts [about Ebola] without trumping up the overall story of the virulent disease."[12] As more and more media outlets break new stories around the clock and experiment with riveting news angles, the cumulative effect makes people feel afraid even in the absence of personal risk.

During the Ebola epidemic, author and journalist Maryn McKenna called this common phenomenon "Ebolanoia"[13] and tracked public response to it in the U.S. The stories McKenna followed were not pretty. Individuals and businesses wrongly identified in news stories as having been exposed to Ebola suffered from stigmatizing overreactions. False rumors caused a small, long-standing, family-owned bridal shop in Ohio to close. Rumors forced healthy school personnel and students in North Carolina and Texas who had visited West Africa to stay out of school, even though they were thousands of miles from the nearest Ebola outbreak. Misinformation fomented harassment of African-born students as well as other acts of fear and discrimination.[14, 15, 16]

Where fear reigns, trust in "authority" devolves. During an outbreak, in the absence of facts from highly trusted sources, people fill in the blanks with stories to make sense of what is happening. Those stories can often spread far faster than the disease itself. In Guinea, rumors spread that Ebola was mere propaganda to raise more money for the government. Red Cross workers supposedly spread disease and plotted to steal body parts from the dead to sell.[17] Stories like these went unchallenged.

In his book *An Epidemic of Rumors*, Jon D. Lee details the common characteristics of rumors that attend epidemics.[18] One of the most common responses is a belief that an untrustworthy government has concocted the outbreak in an effort to grab power.[19]

Such a response is hardly surprising when authorities ignore and abuse people's civil rights, as they often do. Poor citizens who resisted health authorities in the nineteenth-century smallpox outbreak in Milwaukee had every reason to distrust them. Health officials believed a myth that the homes of the well-off were large enough for household members to keep a safe distance from a sickbed. They tried to forcibly haul away people in poor immigrant communities to a quarantine facility but allowed the wealthy to remain at home, even though smallpox was class-blind and killed rich and poor alike.[20] The poor wanted to tend to their sick at home, just as the wealthy did. When people in the community defended their turf, they did not see themselves as a savage mob—they believed they were protecting their families from outrageous violations of their civil rights. They thought they might never see their loved ones again if the sick were taken away. It didn't help when the health commissioner said, "I am here to enforce the laws, and I shall enforce them if I have to break heads," or that the police drew their guns on the protestors.[21] Stigmatizing the community members as superspreaders of disease only created more suffering. (In the end, 1,000 Milwaukeeans were infected and more than 200 died.[22])

Unfortunately, we're living in a time when distrust in government and institutions around the world is at an all-time high.[23] When authorities are untrustworthy or suspect, public fear increases.[24] David Ropeik, a former TV journalist who has written about the psychology of fear, observes that trust, or the lack of it, is pivotal. Most people have a set of basic questions for which they want clear and truthful answers. "When an outbreak starts and people feel freshly threatened, they are more likely to put trust in their public officials, but once rumors take hold and the public starts asking questions, trust can erode quickly," he says.[25] Those who already mistrust the government or public institutions raise fear by instilling doubt. Whom do we trust more, our neighbors or "them" (WHO, government, Big Pharma, and so on)? What are "they" selling? And how much of what "they" are selling has to do with the actual risk? When we revert to our Stone Age brains, it's everyone for him- or herself.

The Leadership-During-Crisis Tightrope

Given the level of fear during an epidemic and the need for public trust, even the most honest and well-intentioned government officials have a tightrope to walk. On one hand, they need to keep the public calm; on the other, they must also give the public a factual and realistic understanding of the risks. Leaders of major institutions and private-sector companies must also be prepared for crisis communication. When officials underreact to threats, they lose enormous trust and incite anger, as we saw with the story of SARS in chapter 6. As Ropeik explains, "The instinct is to calm people down and play down the scariness, but if you over-reassure and things get worse, trust goes down the toilet."

Here is the tightrope: "People want the truth, even if it is worrisome," Baruch Fischhoff, an expert in pandemic risk communication at Carnegie Mellon University, noted in testimony before the U.S. Congress. "They want to know what they are up against, in order to have the best chance of figuring out what to do. As a result, candor is critical in risk communications."[26]

In 1997, Dr. Barbara Reynolds was the CDC's first communications professional to travel outside the U.S. to respond to a health emergency. The occasion was the Hong Kong bird flu outbreak. She saw that health officials had no footing in crisis communication, and she has since devoted her career to preparing leaders to be better spokespeople during a serious outbreak.[27] She has been unstoppable in her mission. Dr. Reynolds's communication expertise has been used in the planning and response to pandemic influenza, vaccine safety, emerging disease outbreaks, and bioterrorism.[28]

"Being afraid the public will panic is never a reason not to communicate. Not knowing is scarier than knowing," says Reynolds, which is why it's important to get ahead of the story before people's uninformed fears take over.[29]

Reynolds teaches the following principles, published in the 58-page downloadable guide *Crisis, Emergency and Risk Communication*, to public officials to help people through a crisis[30]:

+ *Be first.* If the information is yours to provide by organizational authority, do so as soon as possible. If you can't provide the information, then explain how you are working to get it.

+ *Be right.* Give facts in increments. Tell people what you know when you know it, tell them what you don't know, and tell them you will share relevant information as it becomes available.

+ *Be credible.* Tell the truth. Do not withhold information to avoid embarrassment or the possible "panic" that seldom happens. Uncertainty is worse than not knowing. Remember, rumors are more damaging than hard truths.

✦   *Express empathy.* Acknowledge in words what people are feeling—
   it builds trust.

✦   *Promote action.* Give people things to do. It calms anxiety and helps
   restore order.

✦   *Show respect.* Treat people the way you want to be treated, even if
   you must communicate hard decisions.

Reynolds believes most people can cope with almost anything as long as
they feel that the powers in charge are leveling with them in clear, plain, jargon-
free language. Citizens can handle fearful uncertainty if they feel respected, if
they are given choices of productive things they can do, if they are being kept
informed of an emerging situation, and if they are told what officials are doing
to find answers and keep them safe.

Being right is not always as straightforward as it seems, especially with an
entirely new disease. In the early years of the U.S. epidemic, for example, AIDS
became known as the "4H disease" because of its association with heroin
users, homosexuals, hemophiliacs, and Haitians. In New York City, Haitians
faced horrible discrimination. Only after good epidemiology showed that being Haitian was not itself a risk factor for AIDS did things get better for that
population.[31]

It is possible to walk the tightrope by advising the public of appropriate
cautionary action. In August 1999, New York City hospitals began seeing
deaths from a mosquito-borne disease initially diagnosed as St. Louis encephalitis. Some officials wanted to wait for more data before making the information public, while others argued that during a long, warm holiday weekend
people would need to protect themselves against mosquito bites. The diagnosis turned out to be wrong (the disease was West Nile fever), but warning the
public turned out to be the right decision.[32]

Walk in Their Shoes

The tragedy of the killings of Red Cross workers in Guinea underscored locals' long-standing distrust of outsiders. The "outsiders" in this case, health officials and medical personnel working hastily to stop the epidemic, assumed

villagers would perceive them as trustworthy and comply with official advice.[33] Instead, the officials' ignorance of the villagers' beliefs, needs, and fears worsened the situation. Like too many white colonists and missionaries before them, the Red Cross workers had an agenda that went counter to the culture. The Red Cross officials knew the science: corpses of Ebola victims are extremely infectious. Touching them would quickly spread the disease, a message they came to warn about. But the outsiders didn't understand that for Guineans, bathing a corpse is a sacred act that ensures the dead will leave this world in peace.

The Red Cross had come armed with medical knowledge and frightening hazmat suits, but they lacked the cultural knowledge that could have saved their own lives, not to mention the lives of so many others. Had they walked "a mile in the villagers' shoes," as the saying goes, the outcome might have been very different.

If we put ourselves in the villagers' place, we can understand. Many of the dead were small children; what mother could hold herself back from cradling and preparing her child for the next world? The white strangers in masks and plastic defied the beliefs that held their lives together from birth to death, and ignored the most basic impulses of the human heart.

When outsiders begin by understanding and honoring the native culture, they can find sensitive approaches that honor a culture's traditions while enabling changes that ensure safety. For example, in June 2014, a pregnant Guinean woman died, her corpse teeming with Ebola virus. Villagers refused to allow a group of responders in hazmat suits to bury the woman, insisting that her fetus be removed first. Otherwise, they argued, her soul would wander for eternity and never reach the village of the dead. But the people in the hazmat suits insisted that the woman's blood was too infected to allow cutting into the body.

"For the population of Forest Guinea, resistance [to the authorities] became a way to reclaim their very essence, to assert their cultural identity and to defend their beliefs," wrote Julienne Anoko, a Cameroonian anthropologist with WHO.[34] Anoko understood the villagers' customs and grievances. She searched for a way to make reparations to the spirits. She found an old man who knew how to perform a reparation ritual and instructed the villagers to gather a goat, twelve yards of white tissue, salt, oil, and rice. The burial ceremony began at sunset with the distribution of smooth kola nuts, symbols of respect. On the other side of the village (but culturally, a world away), the burial workers in their sweltering plastic suits hygienically laid the pregnant woman to rest.

Anoko's work demonstrates the importance of listening to the fears of people who feel threatened. Fundamental to effective communication is listening to your audience.[35] Even if the patient's fears are illogical, those concerns need to be acknowledged and addressed for everyone's safety. Once public-health workers listened to the concerns underlying the villagers' fears, they were able to find a solution that met their needs as well as the need for safe disposal of Ebola-ridden bodies.

"Instead of asking for more beds," MSF's Claudia Evers, the Ebola emergency coordinator in Guinea noted, "we should have asked for more sensitization activities."[36] If public-health officials want to be heard, they need to understand the context in which a disease is circulating before behaving in the same old "move-over, we're here to fix the problem" ways.

Messengers, Messages, and Local Hands on Deck: Lessons from Sierra Leone

The Ebola outbreak reinforced the basic epidemic communication principle that top-down, government-issued disease prevention too readily glances off its target audience. Messages delivered from on high didn't engender the community's trust in this case; people overwhelmingly refused to adopt sound, official health advice. The good news is this: when government works *together* with local efforts, everything changes.[37]

An example comes from Sierra Leone, one of the poorest places in the world.[38] The country suffered more than 14,000 Ebola cases—more than any other affected nation.[39] "Ebola . . . attacked us with a ferocity that stunned the world,"[40] said President Ernest Bai Koroma. The country's first Ebola case was reported in May 2014. Over the next several months, the disease spread throughout the country. Every week the number of new cases rose, despite early public-health efforts.

Finally, in October, in a brilliant move to achieve zero new Ebola cases while treating the sick, President Koroma established the National Ebola Response Centre (NERC) as the command and operations hub for the battle against Ebola. NERC officials created core teams, called "pillars," at the national and district level. These teams were responsible for social mobilization, surveillance, case management, burials, logistics, psychosocial support, child protection, and food security.[41]

One of the people deeply involved in NERC's social mobilization effort was Mohammad B. Jalloh, a public-health leader who had spent 37 years working with both the Sierra Leone government and UNICEF. Under his watch, national immunization coverage in Sierra Leone skyrocketed from 6 percent in 1986 to 80 percent in 1990, and he guided similar campaigns in 30 countries.[42] A passionate, animated social scientist, Jalloh has led Focus 1000, his own local public-health nonprofit, from a modest office near the ministry of health in the capital Freetown since 2012.

When the Ebola crisis hit, Focus 1000 helped lead a social mobilization group called the Social Mobilization Action Consortium (SMAC) to engage Sierra Leoneans from every corner of the country in ending the crisis.[43] At first, people flatly denied the reality of the frightening new disease. When a local driver chauffeured a viral emergency specialist through Freetown, the driver insisted, "There is no such thing as Ebola,"[44] even as people throughout his country clearly were in its throes. Barely a month after Sierra Leone's first Ebola case, Focus 1000 conducted the first of four community surveys to understand the prevalence of denial and to assess changes in knowledge, beliefs, and practices. To gather the data, Jalloh put coordinators on bicycles and sent them to meet with households, village chiefs, and religious leaders to understand why people were continuing to engage in risky behaviors like hand-washing corpses and hiding the sick.[45]

Jalloh did his work quickly, and Focus 1000's efficiency paid off with both rapid data collection and real-time learning. The information enabled SMAC to continuously create, test, and revise messages that resonated with local communities. The aim was to correct misinformation and to provide comprehensive knowledge. They learned that some messages—such as "Ebola is real"—were finally penetrating deeply. People wanted to know how to protect themselves. So SMAC tested and then disseminated culturally sensitive messages about hand-washing, safe burials, and the importance of avoiding physical contact with others. One of the most dangerous misconceptions workers found was that people believed that if you got Ebola, you would surely die—after all, there was no vaccine to prevent Ebola and no medicine to cure it. (In fact, people had a 50 percent chance of survival with basic supportive care.) So why go to Ebola treatment units? Most people didn't realize at first that lives could be saved with oral or intravenous hydration and by treating complications.

Another dangerous misconception was that washing yourself with saltwater after midnight would protect you from getting Ebola.

Jalloh knew that success depended not only on sending the right messages but also on having the right messengers to spread them. He knew that by delivering SMAC's lifesaving information, trusted local leaders could play a critical role in breaking through myths and denial about Ebola. The agency focused its initial efforts on enlisting religious leaders to help people reconcile their spiritual beliefs with the need to practice disease prevention.

To do this, Focus 1000 talked with the religious leaders—the imams, pastors, and traditional healers—about ways to stop Ebola. These conversations won the religious leaders' trust. In turn, they scoured their holy texts for references that would validate the official health measures.[46] The messages became contextualized with relevant biblical scriptures and Quranic dictates that permitted widespread Ebola prevention. In the northern town of Magburaka, one villager told Jalloh, "I heard all these things on the radio. But I didn't believe until Abu Bakarr Conteh [a powerful local sheik] said them." The religious leaders delivered the messages of Ebola prevention via sermons, in village settings, mosques, and churches.

Having brought religious leaders on board, Focus 1000 then turned to mobilizing the 4,000-strong Sierra Leone Association of Market Women. Market women are powerful forces at the center of everyday life and commerce in the country's towns and villages. People go to market as much to congregate as to buy. "If there is any place for touching, it's the market," Jalloh told me. Each market has a "mammy queen," a widely respected leader. Empowered with messages road-tested by Focus 1000 and echoed by the religious leaders, the mammy queens banded together to teach their customers—and through them the entire community—how to stop Ebola. The mammy queens demanded that no one touch during market days; during the peak of the crisis, they suspended markets entirely.

Finally, Jalloh engaged the roughly 40,000 traditional healers throughout the Sierra Leone Indigenous Traditional Healers Union, whom the government had initially excluded from the Ebola response. It took three months, but once convinced, the group undertook its own national campaign called "Bush to Bush" to ensure that traditional healers in Ebola hotspots would refer the sick to treatment units and halt unsafe secret burials.[47]

*   *   *

Jalloh and his colleagues followed what proved to be a highly successful four-part strategy: (1) ensure that social mobilization and crisis communications are part of a unified emergency response that stretches from villages to the president; (2) base messages not only on the most current public-health science but also on an understanding of local beliefs, customs, and traditional responses to illness; (3) listen to community responses and adapt them as the epidemic evolves; (4) and, most critically, ensure that everyone is getting the same information by engaging all stakeholders as messengers, from the president to national and local health officials, to local sheiks and priests, to market women, to traditional healers, and the media.

As a result of Jalloh's strategy, the number of new cases fell from more than 500 cases per week in December 2014 to less than 400 per week in early January. By the end of January, there were fewer than 100 new cases each week, and the number kept dropping: from March 2015 onward, there were fewer than 20 per week. And because officials convinced patients to seek early treatment (and as a result of the vigilance and clinical skills of Sierra Leone's doctors and care teams), the country's Ebola fatality rate of 28 percent was the lowest among the three most affected countries. It was dramatically less than Guinea's rate of 67 percent.[48] President Koroma later reflected, "One abiding lesson from this epidemic is that reinforcing trust relationships among leaders and citizens is key, as are community participation, ownership, and buy-in for any initiative to achieve its desired outcomes."[49]

How Mainstream Media Can Help

Working on behalf of the president's National Ebola Response Centre, SMAC also systematically engaged the local radio stations and dozens of local media houses to disseminate accurate information about prevention. By contrast, in the U.S., the spread of "Ebolanoia" at the hands of the press did nothing to end the Ebola epidemic, but it did inspire unnecessary fear.

The questions for those in the media are these: When the next epidemic hits, how can reporters be more helpful in stopping the spread of disease? What can the news media do besides pay attention to bad actors and mayhem? How can journalists dispense public-health information that engages readers in ways that appeal to their emotions without playing to their biases? How can the media best dispel rumors and distribute facts?

The worst thing the news media can do is to chase sensationalist, fear-mongering stories and pretend that its role is detached from health outcomes. In the case of an epidemic, combining compelling storytelling with objective science and avoiding sensationalism is a true journalistic calling. In a dire emergency, people need reporters to supply them with a flow of consistent, factually correct, and locally appropriate information that also engages readers. Research has shown that intensive, "how to protect yourself" media coverage of the kind Sierra Leone deployed can alter the course of an epidemic, from guiding people to seek appropriate care at the right moment to decreasing infection and death rates.[50, 51] Reporters and editors should bear this awesome responsibility in mind when choosing between a hyperbolic or balanced story and tone, and between chasing the gruesome story or informing people with reliable and actionable science. People need reporting that provides meaningful details that help them gauge their personal risk in a rational way.

Here's a positive example. During the SARS outbreak, Singapore's authoritarian government media communicated with the public through every conceivable channel and medium. National TV and radio channels constantly broadcasted SARS information—there was even a special SARS TV channel. The government printed educational ads in local newspapers and mailed pamphlets on SARS to every household. Some TV stations reported in a range of local dialects (a rare practice) and hosted live call-in SARS forums.[52] In addition, news and articles largely supported the state's official guidance and called on the public to comply with recommended action. As a result, SARS was quickly brought under control with the public's full trust and cooperation.

In any epidemic, journalists can provide facts, contribute to a climate of compassion, editorialize expressions of empathy for victims, examine unfounded fears and rumors, spotlight inspiring community projects, profile the vulnerable (children, the elderly), and—most importantly—hold leaders accountable. And they can do all this without generating panic. Such reporting earned Sheri Fink and her *New York Times* colleagues the 2015 Pulitzer Prize in International Reporting. The Pulitzer board cited the *Times* "for courageous front-line reporting and vivid human stories on Ebola in Africa, engaging the public with the scope and details of the outbreak while holding authorities accountable."[53, 54]

In poor nations, local media operations are often threadbare, yet journalists on the front lines are closest to the people and have their attention. Local journalists understand the all-important cultural context—language, religion, hot-button issues—but may lack experience in science-based reporting. They have limited access to evidence and are generally unskilled in the ability to appraise, translate, and communicate that evidence. One of the most important things we can all do is to better meet local journalists' needs for training and infrastructure so that they can be outbreak ready.[55, 56]

The Double-Edged Sword of Social Media

The nineteenth-century American writer and world traveler Mark Twain once said, "A lie can travel halfway around the world while the truth is putting on its shoes."[57] In the uncontrollable world of social media, everyone with an opinion can circulate his or her notions. Unlike professional news sources, Twitter, Facebook, and the rest don't benefit from fact-checkers. Everywhere around the world, the internet is both a wonderful supplier of misinformation and the most efficient rumor-spreader ever known.[58]

For example, more than 50 million of Nigeria's 180 million citizens reported Ebola cases on social media before the country's ministry of health had even made a public announcement. Nearly half the world's population tweeted about Ebola in one week near the height of the epidemic.[59] Researchers who reviewed all tweets in English with the terms "Ebola" and "prevention" or "cure" from Guinea, Liberia, and Nigeria during a seven-day period in 2014 found that most tweets and retweets contained misinformation, rumors, and false reports. "Death is inevitable once you catch Ebola" was one such report. "Drinking large quantities of salt water will protect you" was one Ebola-centric tweet. (Doing this actually killed a few people and sent many more to hospitals.)[60]

Like traditional media, social media can fuel or quell the spread of illness. In West Africa, where even the poorest people had access to cell phones that could send and receive texts and tweets, a war between fact and rumor raged on WhatsApp, Twitter, Facebook, Instagram, and elsewhere. Fortunately, for every gripping, false tweet, text, or posting about cures and conspiracies, someone else posted or shared facts. Young people particularly find user-generated digital content (status updates, tweets, peer reviews, blog posts, and so on) 50 percent more trustworthy and 35 percent more memorable than traditional media sources like newspapers or TV.[61]

Craig Manning, a CDC health communications specialist, told *Fast Company* that you have two choices: "You can refute the rumors one at a time or you can change the information environment with new, accurate scientific information. When we have gotten the messages out there, it prevents the ability of rumors to thrive."[62] In Sierra Leone, Manning had the good sense to record a presentation given by an expert on Ebola at the U.S. Embassy about mitigating transmission risks. He then edited 30-second snippets and had them translated into ten local languages and broadcast over local radio stations, television, and the web. Finally, he teamed up with BBC Media Action to bring together radio station managers from across the country to help spread the word.[63]

In the midst of the Ebola outbreak, Lawal Bakare, a Nigerian dentist, created the Twitter campaign @EbolaAlert, which shared legitimate information validated by links to original authoritative sources. Within a few weeks, Bakare had 76,000 followers receiving advice about prompt reporting and good environmental and personal hygiene. (The campaign also debunked Ebola myths.[64]) One link, "How to Conduct Safe and Dignified Burial of a Patient Who Died from Suspected or Confirmed Ebola (EVD)," connected to guidance from WHO.[65] On Facebook and Twitter, a popular campaign called KickEbolaOut—a joint program created by medical student associations in Sierra Leone and Guinea—shared regular information from WHO. So did another campaign called @EbolaFacts. West Africans posted infographics on Ebola prevention and shared information about local rallies and fundraisers. In Cameroon, the cellular service Orange partnered with the ministry of health to launch a preventive health texting system called MyHealthline.[66] On YouTube, a Liberian rapper named Shadow created a music video that warned against kissing and shaking hands. It garnered nearly 100,000 views.[67]

In addition to spreading timely truth and battling misinformation, social media can also provide researchers with crucial information about where outbreaks are occurring, as I described in chapter 8. Likewise, when public-health officials keep track of Twitter data, they can see trends that indicate sources of anger, anxiety, or other negative emotions. This information can help officials focus communications efforts and messages in ways that reduce fear and improve understanding of the risk associated with Ebola or any other disease outbreak.[68]

When two medical workers returned to the U.S. for treatment after being infected with Ebola, worried citizens flooded the CDC with questions. The CDC was ready with a global health Twitter account, one of many it manages. It hosted public events on Twitter (#cdcchat) that answered questions and dispelled misconceptions. And it used visual information strategically, posting photos and infographics to help make its messages memorable. "We can't just tell people things, we have to show them," said the CDC's Barbara Reynolds. "When people are using the more primitive part of their brain, visuals are more powerful than our higher order tools, including language."[69]

The Power of Broadcast Drama

Let's say you were living in Sierra Leone in 2014, right before Ebola struck. Back then, AIDS was the beastliest disease around, sickening and killing thousands in your country. The mainstream news on the radio was devastating. So you switched channels to listen to your favorite program, a long-running soap opera called *Saliwansai* ("Puppet on a String"). One of your favorite characters was a college student named Hingah, who has unprotected sex with a woman. He learned that she had several other lovers. When Hingah got sick, his friend advised him to get tested for AIDS. He learned the dangers of having sex without using a condom. The show ended on a cliffhanger: Would Hingah test positive for HIV?

Saliwansai ran for 208 episodes, from April 1, 2012, through April 2014. It was produced in Krio, a language that up to 95 percent of Sierra Leone's population can either speak or understand. It was one of more than 35 dramas—some broadcast on television, some via the web, but most via radio—that Population Media Center (PMC) develops and broadcasts in more than 20 unique languages, helping people to live healthier lives in 50 countries around the world. The idea behind PMC is clever: if you want to change people's behavior, you have to reach them through their emotions. The goal is to change people's behavior through entertainment-based education and role-modeling. PMC dramatizes situations in the lives of real people who need to make tough decisions, appealing to audiences in their own languages and cultures while delivering information that can protect their health, too.[70]

The organization's methodology is based on an idea by Miguel Sabido, who was vice president for research at the Mexican broadcasting company Televisa during the 1970s. Sabido figured out that social learning theory could be applied to develop shows that promote literacy, family planning, and other social-development goals. Sabido understood that, emotionally speaking, adult humans' brains are not that much different from children's, although ours are more calcified and less adaptable. So if you want to promote good behaviors and show the consequences of bad ones, give people something interesting to observe, discuss, and think about. Give them colorful, interesting, realistic, nuanced characters in complex situations.

Because PMC's 3 million loyal listeners and watchers can talk with their friends about the difficult and even dangerous topics aired on the programs, there's a level of safety and intimacy that sterile government and public-health communications advisories can't achieve. And the results have been stunning. In PMC's markets around the world, 67 percent of new health clinic clients say that they came to seek services because they've heard or seen its dramas.[71] (A few have even been nominated for Emmys.)

Vaccine Rejection: A Massive Public-Health Communications Challenge

Eva Avital is an infant struggling with whooping cough. In a YouTube video posted in April 2016, her mother, Cormit Avital—a healthy but anxious Australian woman—holds the tiny newborn on her shoulder, stroking the baby's back. "We've been in hospital for the past three weeks. It's been a nightmare," she explains.[72]

Proud of her fitness, Avital had enjoyed a near-perfect pregnancy and a natural childbirth. But in the last two weeks of her pregnancy Avital had developed a cough. Soon after delivery she learned that she had passed a highly contagious, sometimes deadly bacterial disease called pertussis (also known as whooping cough) to Eva. Eva's cough turned into a "pretty scary horror movie," Avital says; the baby was so out of breath that she was "flopping in my hands." Eva even stopped breathing for three minutes, "going from red to blue to black." There were a few near-death scares. "It's a lot of suffering for a tiny little cute thing you love so much," Avital observes ruefully. But when her doctor had offered to immunize her, she had refused it, thinking, "I don't need that crap." At that time, Avital had been one of a growing number of vaccine skeptics (a.k.a. "vaccine deniers"): people who have access to recommended vaccines but choose not to have themselves or their children immunized. But reflecting on Eva's near-death experience, Avital concluded, "If I could turn back time, I would have protected myself."[73]

*　　　*　　　*

Of all the lifesaving medical science and public-health advancements, immunization stands at the absolute pinnacle. As I noted in chapter 8, vaccines eradicated smallpox and have put us on the verge of polio eradication. The impact of immunization for measles, which killed 200 million children in the last century alone, is a stunning example of vaccine success. Before 1963, when measles vaccine was introduced in the U.S., there were typically more than 500,000 cases and 500 deaths from the disease per year. By 2000, measles had been eliminated through widespread access to measles vaccine, public education, and required immunization for school entry. Between 2000 and 2015, measles deaths around the world dropped by nearly 80 percent, preventing an estimated 20.3 million deaths and making measles a public-health best buy.[74]

Vaccines continue to save 2 to 3 million children each year. Deaths from cervical and liver cancer can be dramatically reduced by immunizing against the virus that causes them. Tens of thousands of lives are saved each year by vaccines for seasonal influenza.[75] In the event of a large-scale global pandemic with a highly deadly influenza strain, mass immunization would save millions of lives and dramatically reduce the political, social, and economic disruption of such a catastrophic event.

Despite the protective power of vaccines, some parents, like Avital, are scared away from vaccinating their children by exaggerated claims of vaccine risk. A 2016 global survey of vaccine confidence found that in one in five countries surveyed, at least 20 percent of the population believe that vaccines are unsafe.[76] While some are suspicious of vaccines, others are lulled into complacency because they (fortunately) have never experienced a measles epidemic. The result: between 2005 and 2015, there were nearly 2,000 cases of measles in the U.S.[77] In 2011 alone, 33 European countries suffered more than 30,000 cases of measles.[78] Data from early 2017 reveal that measles outbreaks were sharply spiking throughout Europe, correlating with a dip in measles vaccinations below the critical 95 percent threshold.[79] After decades of decline, whooping cough came blistering back from just 1,248 cases in 1981 to 20,762 cases in 2015 in the U.S. alone.[80] The vast majority of cases are occurring in the unvaccinated.

These are worrisome trends. Consider measles: spread through the air like influenza and many other viruses, measles is one of the most infectious viruses we doctors know. Each infected child spreads it to at least 12 others. In

January 2015, a *single* (presumably) unvaccinated person brought measles into Disneyland in Anaheim, California, and passed it to 35 people, including 14 children.[81] From there, it spread to 147 people in the U.S. and about 159 in Canada and Mexico.

And it's not only parents and children we should worry about. Immunization rates are also low for adults of all ages who are at risk for seasonal influenza, resulting in thousands of preventable deaths worldwide each year. Millennials are particularly wary of vaccines. Quoting from a Pew Research Center study, *Forbes* writer Maureen Henderson reported that one in five millennials believe the disproven theory that vaccines cause autism.[82] During the 2009 H1N1 swine flu epidemic, fewer than 20 percent of millennials were immunized.[83]

Where Vaccine Skepticism Comes From

The vaccine-refusal damage has been extensive, largely because of the distrust-in-authority issues I discussed earlier. Unfounded rumors that the tetanus toxoid contained a sterilizing agent or caused miscarriages have at times gained traction in the Philippines, Kenya, and several countries in Latin America—in some cases leading to a resurgence of neonatal tetanus. The most dangerous instance of vaccine rejection was the 2003 boycott of polio vaccination by five states in northern Nigeria, which quadrupled the number of polio cases, spread the disease to 17 countries on three continents, resulted in over 1,000 polio cases, stalled global polio eradication efforts for nearly a decade, and cost more than $500 million to reverse.[84]

What's behind the trend in vaccine rejection? Factors vary across countries, cultures, and times. They include fear of autism and other developmental disabilities, skepticism of modern medicine, presumed toxins, religious beliefs, local politics, perceived business motives, and various conspiracy theories (such as one belief that a vaccine contains birth control). Some people have refused vaccines because they are unwilling to accept the risks associated with each vaccine. Others reject vaccines based on the concept of individual exceptionalism, i.e., "I don't need to vaccinate my child because everyone else has vaccinated theirs."[85, 86] This dangerous misconception denies the reality that it takes only one unvaccinated child to infect many.

In the U.S. and Western Europe, the most provocative lightning rods for vaccine rejection have been the widely publicized claims that the mercury-containing preservative thimerosal and the measles vaccine each can cause autism in children. Hundreds of scientific studies have failed to show a link between autism and either thimerosal or the measles vaccine. Out of an abundance of caution, thimerosal has been removed from virtually all commonly used childhood vaccines.[87]

*   *   *

The unfounded link between autism and the measles vaccine dates to a 1998 article by former British doctor Andrew Wakefield that appeared in the *Lancet*, the most widely respected international medical journal. The article generated wall-to-wall coverage, followed by aggressive follow-up pieces. Measles immunization rates plummeted in the U.K.

The deception all came apart in 2004, when investigative journalist Brian Deer from the *Sunday Times* exposed Wakefield's *Lancet* paper not only as woefully lacking scientific basis, but also as influenced by substantial payments from lawyers who stood to gain from autism-related claims.[88] These revelations set off a chain reaction: Wakefield's coauthors issued a retraction and *Lancet* editor Dr. Richard Horton acknowledged the journal had been deceived in publishing the "utterly false" paper.[89] Described as having perpetuated "perhaps, the most damaging medical hoax of the last 100 years,"[90] Wakefield was delicensed for medical fraud. The British *Guardian* newspaper opined that "many journalists should be hanging their heads in shame. . . . They helped to create the climate of fear about the MMR [measles mumps rubella] vaccine, which caused immunization rates to plummet and allowed a childhood illness that had pretty much been consigned to the dustbin of diseases to return once more."[91]

After vaccine uptake bottomed out in 2004 at 80 percent,[92] Britain was able to make a comeback from the Wakefield debacle. Reporters in the U.K. widely publicized the discrediting of Wakefield's article. The government worked hard to rebuild vaccine confidence. Sadly, however, after having reached 92 percent coverage in 1996, it was not until 2015—17 years after Wakefield's fraudulent publication—that the U.K. reached the goal of 95 percent of children vaccinated, a percentage determined by WHO scientists to be the level needed to halt measles outbreaks. The U.K. had finally reversed the impact of the anti-MMR vaccine movement, but not before U.K. parents and children had experienced more than 12,000 cases of measles; hundreds of hospitalizations, many with serious complications like pneumonia and meningitis; and at least three deaths.[93] Precious time and money had been diverted from other pressing public-health needs.

Unfortunately, that fateful article has had a long life, despite the facts. Antivaccine advocates still point to it to support their arguments. Here's the sad irony: even as children are being put at risk by Wakefield's deceit, WHO reported that between 2000 and 2015 measles immunization saved 17.1 million lives worldwide.[94]

Protecting Us All from Epidemic Threats

Dr. Heidi Larson is a leading anthropologist and researcher who once led global immunization communications for UNICEF and now directs the Vaccine Confidence Project, supported by the Bill and Melinda Gates Foundation. In these leadership roles, Larson has studied attitudes toward vaccines around the world. She has found that "shouting louder" by peppering deniers with evidence doesn't work. It turns out that when people with a strong belief are confronted with opposing evidence, they actually become even more convinced of their belief and less likely to change their behavior.

Economist Brendan Nyhan calls this the "backfire effect."[95] Nyhan first observed this dynamic in politics as a campaign worker in the 2000 election. He then became interested in whether the same dynamic applied to personal health choices like immunization. Nyhan and colleagues tried four different messages to get antivaccination parents to accept the measles vaccine. It turned out that the messages not only failed to change parents' minds about the risk of autism but actually *decreased* the percentage of parents who said that they would be likely to vaccinate their children. The same thing happened when he tried to increase acceptance of influenza vaccine among adults who believed the myth (held by a whopping 43 percent of the American public) that flu vaccine can give you the flu. Those most worried about vaccine side effects actually became significantly *less likely* to get vaccinated when provided with evidence that flu vaccine does not cause the flu.[96]

These findings are troubling. "We found that people react in a defensive manner when challenged," says Nyhan. It seems that once false information linked to fear morphs into belief, as occurred following the publication of the Wakefield article, it can be very hard to turn such thinking around. "When people are skeptical of information they don't want to hear, they will double down on the myth in question," says Nyhan. Countering misinformation with rational explanations isn't likely to be the most effective strategy.[97, 98] So if evidence-based, authoritative information does not convince the skeptics, what does?

Turns out, the answer has surprisingly little to do with facts and more to do with trust based on personal relationships. Nyhan and his team studied influenza vaccine acceptance among college students, and found that self-reported immunization rates nearly doubled (and safety concerns were reduced) when students' social networks (parents, spouses, friends) supported vaccination.[99]

It All Comes Down to Trust

Speaking as a family doctor, I believe the human touch works best in persuading individuals to protect their own and their loved ones' health. When we sit down and listen deeply to a parent's fears in an empathetic way, from *their* point of view, as Julienne Anoko did with the Guinean villagers, we recognize that people's concerns warrant a serious response.

We can start by acknowledging the reality of a concerned parent's fears. It's true that some vaccines have had problems, including early formulations of the smallpox and polio vaccines, as well as the vaccine against swine flu (although enhancements to development, production, quality control, and regulation have since reduced the risk).[100]

We can also dig deeper to discover what parents are really afraid of, because in some cases the core fear may be different from what is openly stated. In India, for example, rumor had it that the polio vaccine caused sterilization. Researchers probed deeper and found that the people's objections had nothing to do with sterilization. Some people wished that a woman, rather than a man, give the shots to their children; others wanted the vaccinator to be a known person from the local community, not some stranger. Health officials acceded to the requests, and in so doing they lowered people's fears—and more children were vaccinated.[101]

Dr. Larson believes that conversations about vaccines should avoid "patronizing 'expert' tones, and instead build confidence from a human, personal perspective."[102] These are not easy conversations. Physicians and parents alike need support to have a frank and honest exchange based on the facts. Larson is particularly concerned about parents who blame vaccines for autism. While she understands that these parents only wish to safeguard their kids, she worries that posters like the one she happened on at the Nairobi airport ("Are vaccines making your child mentally ill?") discourage lifesaving immunizations. Larson cites the U.K. experience as one rare instance in which a country was able to reverse widespread vaccine skepticism. She credits the U.K.'s success in rebuilding acceptance of the MMR vaccine for laying the groundwork for achieving the world's highest rates of human papilloma virus (HPV) vaccination, which is given to young people to prevent cancer.[103]

Larson's advice to health leaders for dealing with vaccine rejection is straightforward: "Get your radar out there. Listen for emerging concerns, be open to dialogue. The priority is to make sure the expressed concerns are not a signal of a safety or delivery issue, in which case it needs to be addressed. If there are other reasons for rejection, find out what they are. Never, never assume what is in the minds of people. And never forget that they can change. We need to move into real-time listening and response. This issue is moving very fast."[104]

Once again, trust is critical—in both the ability and competence of the healthcare provider and trust in the provider's motivation, she says. Most importantly, she believes, "[c]onfidence in vaccines is a reflection of confidence in government." That confidence includes trust that the government is making scientifically informed vaccine recommendations as well as ensuring the quality and safety of vaccines.

The example of the northern Nigeria polio vaccine boycott I mentioned earlier is a case in point. The predominantly Muslim north was suspicious of the predominantly Christian south, which was promoting polio vaccination. It took 11 months for a combination of local, regional, and global interventions to finally end the boycott. Most crucially, both sides entered into an open two-way dialogue with trusted local leaders, and they received support from the Organization of Islamic States, an influential imam from Egypt, and Muslim vaccine producers from Indonesia.

Fortunately, beyond ongoing communication efforts by WHO, CDC, and national health authorities, there are all kinds of pro-vaccine efforts that are engaged to persuade the public. A few of these are large-scale—including the Vaccine Confidence Project,[105] which monitors public confidence in immunization programs, and the Immunization Action Coalition (IAC), which creates and distributes information about vaccines to health professionals and the public.[106] On the grassroots end, some mothers have taken matters into their own hands on a blog called "Moms Who Vax," posting informative articles, links, and counterarguments to vaccine skeptics.[107] A Facebook page called "Crunchy Moms for Vaccines" asks others "who breastfeed, co-sleep, eat organic fruits and veg, and believe in science and vaccines" to join in.

It's also important to educate children about the importance of getting immunized, beginning with primary school health programs. By the time they are teenagers, many kids can't distinguish real from fake news, so it's crucial for parents and teachers to show kids how to think critically and look at hard evidence from an early age.[108]

What happens if the words of personal healthcare providers, public-health authorities, and the instructions of trusted local leaders all fail to convince people of the need for vaccination? Supporters and opponents will continue to vigorously debate the necessity, effectiveness, and ethics of compulsory vaccination policies in schools, the military, healthcare institutions, and elsewhere.[109] Countries, government agencies, and health institutions have established compulsory immunization requirements to combat local outbreaks like yellow fever, to prevent deadly childhood illnesses like measles, and to protect healthcare workers, patients, and members of the military. Whether one agrees or disagrees with mandatory vaccination, such programs have been responsible for eradicating smallpox and polio and for historically high childhood immunization rates in the U.S.[110, 111] "I'm not a big fan of coercion, but I don't know who would put on seatbelts without laws. For highly infectious pathogens, it's sometimes acceptable," says Larson.[112] Indeed, in the event of a deadly epidemic, many experts agree that it may become necessary to make immunization mandatory.

Saving Lives and Preventing Panic with Public-Health Communications

Promoting healthy behaviors for prevention and response cannot wait until outbreaks occur; it has to be a continuous process before, during, and after outbreaks (see sidebar). Leaders of government agencies, as well as major institutions and those in the private sector, need to work in lockstep with public-health partners and deploy capable spokespeople who can clearly explain what is happening and how people can protect themselves.

Success depends on three critical factors.

First, public-health leaders at all levels—local, national, and global— have to make communication a central part of their job. Crisis communication is not an afterthought, something you make up on the fly. As we heard from the CDC's Barbara Reynolds, there is a playbook—proven principles and practices from experience.

Second, trust is the essential ingredient in effective communication—especially in the face of unexpected or unknown threats like Ebola or SARS. As the example of the murder of health workers in Guinea illustrated, lack of trust can be fatal.

Third, it's crucial to actively involve the community in the response. As Julienne Anoko and Mohammad Jalloh clearly demonstrated, the most effective communication strategies and messages come from systematic listening and learning throughout the course of an epidemic.

*   *   *

In the beginning of this chapter, I talked about trust. Trust builds by talking neighbor-to-neighbor and working day by day. Establishing trust also means that scientists, international agencies, governments, and the media must join together to prevent fear from squelching evidence and logic. In addition to quickly dispelling rumors, political leaders, public-health personnel, and the media must engage in widespread, unified communications campaigns to help people understand how to protect themselves and each other. If we do a better job of dispelling rumors and falsehoods, rely on science, and build trust, then we can go a long way toward preventing social upheaval in the face of an outbreak or an epidemic.

Health Behaviors for Epidemic Prevention and Preparedness[113]

Before Outbreaks

- Include infectious-disease prevention (personal hygiene, hand-washing, sanitation, safe water) in health education from primary school onward.

- Include epidemic prevention and preparedness in continuing education for health professionals, risk managers, and business continuity professionals.

- Promote vaccination through national policies, ensure access to immunization, and provide ongoing public education.

During Outbreaks

- Educate people about how the disease is spread.

- Work to reduce fear and panic by presenting clear, factual information.

- Gather volunteers and health workers to detect cases.

- Provide outbreak-specific immunization and medicines to prevent or cure disease.

- Encourage/mandate social distancing by closing schools and workplaces.

- Practice self-quarantine in the face of potentially serious infections, including seasonal influenza.

After Outbreaks

- Provide support and avoid stigmatizing those who are recovering.

CHAPTER 10

DISRUPTIVE INNOVATION, COLLABORATIVE TRANSFORMATION

Breakthrough innovations bring new tools for preventing, controlling, and eliminating infectious-disease threats.

We can stop epidemics by surrendering conventional wisdom and looking at each unmet challenge afresh. For example, some pioneering companies are using blood sampling and digital technology to look for microbes that could jump from animals to humans. We could soon employ these techniques to predict outbreaks. We can also use technologies like multilingual web crawlers to rapidly identify new disease outbreaks from online reports. We can use drones to bring diagnostics and vaccines to hard-to-reach places. And most promising is a novel approach for a vaccine to protect us from pandemic influenza, the greatest known viral threat.

The Fourth of July, 1916, was not a day of celebration for many New Yorkers. Instead of going to a ballgame or attending one of the many celebrations in the city, they sat locked in their homes. They feared that health officials would take away their sick babies in an effort to quell the polio epidemic that had attacked children and gripped the city. By the end of that summer, an estimated 9,300 New York City children would be paralyzed and at least 2,200 would die.

Polio had many famous victims as well, like Franklin D. Roosevelt, who wore braces that he tried to disguise from the public, and the singer/songwriter Joni Mitchell, who survived it as a child in Canada and suffered from a recurrence in adulthood.

Polio is caused by an intestinal virus that moves from the gut to the lymph nodes. At first, it produces fevers and an upset stomach. Then it spreads into the neurons of the brain stem, making it difficult to breathe and swallow, which is how many patients ended up encased on their backs in a medical ventilator called an "iron lung." Polio also attacks the spinal cord and muscles of the arms, legs, and abdomen, leading to crippling. The virus spreads fast through clothing, bathing sites, and drinking water. It can live up to 60 days outside the body.[1]

Polio would have crippled more people and claimed far more lives than it did had it not been for the innovative work of Dr. Jonas Salk and Dr. Albert Sabin, the scientists who discovered and delivered the inactivated polio vaccine in 1955, followed by the oral vaccine in 1961. The polio vaccine has since been distributed so widely that the disease was completely eliminated in the Western Hemisphere in 1994 and has been virtually eradicated worldwide. Since WHO launched the Global Polio Eradication Initiative in 1988, the incidence of polio has dropped 99 percent, to just 37 reported cases worldwide in 2016.

It's taking longer than hoped to wipe out the last remnants of the disease, largely because the remaining cases are in war-torn areas like Pakistan and Afghanistan that are difficult for health workers to access.[2] But the world is well on its way to ridding itself of another ancient scourge, and that is something to celebrate. Innovation in vaccines and so much more has saved an infinite number of lives, which is why it's yet another element in The Power of Seven.

A Proud History of Innovation

As the saying goes, necessity is the mother of invention. In the campaign to eradicate smallpox, Mother Nature compelled a breakthrough innovation in vaccine development.

Following Edward Jenner's development of the smallpox vaccine in 1798, use of the vaccine spread in Europe and the United States despite initial safety problems. As early as 1803, Dr. Francisco Javier de Balmis set out to vaccinate millions of people in what is now Central and South America. In the world's first international vaccine campaign, de Balmis successfully delivered the vaccine to thousands of people in present-day Colombia, Ecuador, Peru, Bolivia, and Chilean Patagonia. But the liquid vaccine had to be kept cool, which required mules hauling kerosene refrigerators on their backs, making immunization impossible for hot, remote villages in South America or Africa.

Four decades later, Dr. Leslie Collier, an English virologist and bacteriologist, would devise a way to freeze-dry the vaccine so that it could be carried into remote tropical areas without refrigeration. A vaccinator could now carry a simple kit containing enough of the mass-produced powder that could be reconstituted and delivered on-site, enough to inoculate 200 people in a village.[3] The result was a much-improved vaccination "take rate" in tropical settings.[4]

Another early problem in battling smallpox had to do with the shots themselves. The standard method was to dip needles into a vaccine vial and then stick them in the patient's arm multiple times, making the process both painful and time-consuming. An American microbiologist named Dr. Benjamin Rubin figured out a better method in 1961. He ground off the end of a sewing machine needle and opened the thread hole (the eyelet) to produce a fork-like, two-branched (bifurcated) needle. The new needle could hold enough vaccine in the space between the two sections to completely vaccinate a person with a few pokes. The bifurcated needle also used less vaccine, which meant that more people could be vaccinated.[5]

Another innovator in the fight against smallpox was a creative thinker named Dr. Bill Foege, an epidemiologist who worked on the eradication campaign. Foege solved a crucial problem by finding a way around conventional wisdom, which held that 80 percent of a target population must be vaccinated to prevent outbreaks from spreading. But what happens when you are faced with a potentially large outbreak in a remote area and don't have enough vaccine for the whole population?

Foege attacked this problem by applying an idea he learned as a young firefighter in the Pacific Northwest. Since a fire can't live without fuel, firefighters create a fuel-free ring around the fire area. Using the same systematic approach, Foege surmised that if you built a ring of immunity around smallpox cases, you could wipe out the disease more quickly. He tested the theory in Nigeria beginning in 1968. First, he mapped the existing cases. Then, using two-way radios, he contacted the susceptible population in surrounding villages within 24 hours. By strategically using the limited number of vaccines, he created a human shield of immunity that encircled the epidemic's epicenter. The smallpox outbreak was stopped, and Foege's innovative "surveillance and containment" (also known as "ring vaccination") strategy became a guiding principle in smallpox eradication.[6] "The whole emphasis is not on protecting people en masse. It's on being so intelligent that you can out-think the virus . . . and look at who is at risk and where the virus is," Foege told the *Washington Post*.[7]

Years later, Foege's approach worked again, this time in a test of an Ebola vaccine. In March 2015, researchers evaluated a single dose of the newly developed vaccine in contacts of nearly 100 Ebola patients. About 4,000 close contacts of those patients participated in the trial, and the vaccine was also given to 1,200 of Guinea's frontline Ebola response workers. None of the people who were vaccinated got sick with Ebola, and it showed 100 percent protection.[8]

Five Disruptive Innovations

Much has changed since the development of polio vaccine and the eradication of smallpox. Today we have the scientific know-how and the technology to beat back remaining and potentially new epidemic diseases, if we only apply the expertise, the willpower, the leadership, and the investment dollars to do so. The landmark polio vaccine changed the fates of millions. We now have highly effective vaccines for many common microbes, including the major childhood killers, several forms of influenza, more than a dozen tropical diseases, most causes of meningitis, and the viruses that lead to cervical and liver cancer. As of this writing, scientists are closing in on a vaccine against the Zika virus and, astonishingly, one that might even protect us from every kind of flu.[9]

In applying innovation to fighting epidemics, it's helpful to think about what we mean by effective innovation in the first place. "Disruptive innovation"—a term coined by Harvard Business School professor Clayton Christensen—is a new approach that utterly displaces a standard one, in the same way that the iPod and streaming music "disrupted" record stores and Netflix disrupted video rental stores.[10] Just as Sabin and Salk used new approaches to bring the polio vaccine to the world, scientists and health professionals around the world are applying fresh thinking to create novel technologies, systems, and approaches to vaccine development that flaunt conventional wisdom. To win the fight against epidemics, they look at each unmet challenge afresh, and they are beginning to outwit possible outbreaks with new approaches in vector control, surveillance, logistics, and other avenues.

I believe we need disruptive innovations in five areas: (1) new vaccines for some of the wiliest pathogens; (2) truly effective mosquito control; (3) low-cost, rapid tests for a wide range of pathogens with pandemic potential; (4) a global early warning system akin to that used to warn against hurricanes; and (5) mapping the genes of half a million potential viral enemies through the Global Virome Project. These five areas offer openings for entrepreneurs and investors and hope for everyone else.

Vaccines for the Wiliest Pathogens

Nothing can stop an epidemic in its tracks as effectively as a vaccine, which is fundamentally an immunological trick on the body. Inserting an inactive virus, a weakened live virus, or a viral protein into a person's bloodstream stimulates the immune system to build antibodies against the virus without causing disease. The body's finely tuned immune system remembers the invader so that if the same virus reappears later, the immune system knows how to fight it off.

Salk's polio vaccine, made from killed poliovirus and introduced in 1955, was given to 440,000 children. This inactivated (dead) vaccine was the first to be proven safe and effective in the largest clinical trial in history. But the injection was painful, and many, including yours truly, were reluctant to submit themselves to it. Five years later, Sabin introduced a different delivery method for a live oral vaccine. Instead of a painful shot, the live vaccine could be delivered straight into a child's mouth or via a drop on a sugar cube, proving Mary Poppins correct in that a spoonful of sugar does help the medicine go down. Not only were children and parents much more comfortable (even delighted, in the children's case) with this form of immunization, but the live virus actually produced a mild contagion that spread immunity to others. Sabin's breakthrough oral vaccine in the 1950s paved the way for today's polio eradication effort.

Although we have effective vaccines for more than two dozen common infections today, we still lack effective vaccines for a number of major viral killers.[11] Developing a new vaccine is still an unpredictable trial-and-error process that can take decades, which is why scientists are aggressively looking for new vaccine development strategies. A look at two high-priority targets that have bedeviled scientists—the human immunodeficiency virus (HIV) that causes

AIDS and the influenza virus—will give you a window into a few promising approaches.

*   *   *

Dr. Dan Barouch is a man who exudes patience, but when it comes to fighting viruses like HIV and Zika, he's a man on a mission. After earning his PhD in immunology at the age of 26, he managed to earn an MD in just four years. (He's also an accomplished violinist.) During his medical school residency as an infectious-disease specialist, he began publishing research papers. At the age of 29, he started his own research lab and began attacking the tricky problem of developing an effective vaccine against HIV. Now in his mid-forties, he is usually one of the youngest people in professional conference rooms.

In developing vaccines, Barouch's lab first adopted the traditional course: growing the whole virus and then using a chemical to kill it. But the lab developed two other completely novel approaches. With "naked DNA vaccination," researchers use a purified piece of DNA that contains a single gene of the HIV virus. Cells near the injection site take up the DNA and begin to synthesize proteins associated with the virus; the immune system then mounts a response. Another "viral vector" approach uses a common cold virus to help bring a single gene of the HIV virus into cells. "With these novel approaches, one can control exactly what genes are put in," says Barouch. "We can be very precise about which parts of the HIV virus to put in, which strains, so it gives us complete flexibility."[12]

These new methods could considerably speed up vaccine development time, in large part because the technologies allow for a lot of flexibility. A DNA vaccine for West Nile virus has been shown effective in horses, and a team of scientists from Brazil and Boston are using this technique to work on a vaccine for Zika. If the naked DNA approach works in humans as well as it does in horses, it would revolutionize vaccine development.[13] "The DNA and viral vector vaccines have been explored for many pathogens, for everything from flu to HIV to malaria to tuberculosis," says Barouch.

Another breakthrough in vaccine development called "retrovaccinology" is being used to outsmart HIV. In this approach, scientists work backward to create a vaccine. Instead of trying to create antibodies by injecting a weakened virus into someone, they deploy antibodies from someone who already has HIV to create the vaccine. According to Dr. Seth Berkeley, founder of the New York–based International Aids Vaccine Initiative (IAVI) and current head of Gavi, the Vaccine Alliance, such a thing had never been done before.

Here's how it works. AIDS, as we have already seen in chapter 2, is a very slippery, fast-changing virus. Getting the body to make the right antibodies to protect against AIDS has defied scientists' attempts so far. But in the retrovaccinology case, researchers were able to isolate several so-called "broadly neutralizing" antibodies from the blood of a person with HIV, and those antibodies provided full protection from HIV in monkeys. They had discovered a new, relatively unchanging site on the HIV virus that the antibodies could cling to, like a rock climber who finds a sudden solid ledge on a sheer, daunting face. "It's like, as many times as the virus changes its clothes, it's still wearing the same socks. Now our job is to make sure we get the body to really hate those socks," Berkeley told a TED audience in 2010.[14] The researchers hope to prompt the immune system into making matching, broadly neutralizing antibodies. Though the vaccine has not been developed as of this writing, scientists believe they are getting tantalizingly close.[15]

Like the AIDS virus, flu virus is very slippery, and it presents different challenges for vaccine developers. Jonas Salk and a colleague, Dr. Thomas Francis Jr., developed the first flu vaccine in 1938.[16] But it's never been a great vaccine. Today's flu vaccines use either attenuated influenza virus given by injection or a nasal spray with a weakened live virus that cannot cause influenza. Both vaccines attack the flu virus's two proteins, hemagglutinin and neuraminidase, which give the influenza viruses their H and N designations (e.g., H1N1). The problem is that these proteins, which sit on the outer surface of the mushroom-shaped virus's head, are constantly mutating. The flu shot is effective when the vaccine strain closely matches the circulating virus, because our immune system creates antibodies to fight these specific antigens. Unfortunately, it's not so effective when the virus's head mutates, because the virus in the vaccine no longer matches the head.

The holy grail for vaccine researchers is a universal vaccine that protects against all types of flu. Encouragingly, after years of hopeful but unfruitful research, clinical trials are now underway to test a universal vaccine, and genetic mapping is helping. Peter Palese, PhD, chair of the department of microbiology at New York's Icahn School of Medicine, worked to build the first genetic maps for influenza A, B, and C viruses. His team's new strategy redirected the immune response away from the proteins in the head toward the protein in the stalk, which remains more constant over time. Once again, it's as if they have found a stable shelf on a slippery rock face.[17] "We all have been infected with influenza A subtype H1 viruses, so we all have antibodies," says Palese. "Although most of our antibodies are against the head, we have some against the stalk."[18] When given to animals, including mice, ferrets, and monkeys, the new vaccine protected against flu strains like H5N1 avian flu and H1N1 swine flu. Best of all, this new vaccine could be created only once and could protect for many years, or even an entire lifetime, against all flu viruses. If the vaccine proves successful in humans, it would go a long way toward combating the nightmare scenarios that worry every epidemic professional.

Michael Osterholm, PhD, MPH, author of *Deadliest Enemy* and founder of the highly respected Center for Infectious Disease Research and Policy, feels so strongly about the development of a universal flu vaccine that he has called for a "Manhattan-like project" to develop a "game-changing influenza vaccine." He estimates that such an effort would take seven to ten years at a cost of $1 billion per year. In his view, one I wholeheartedly share, such an innovation would be "[t]he single most consequential action that we can take to limit, and possibly even prevent, a catastrophic global influenza pandemic."[19]

Conquering Mosquitoes

Mosquitoes have plagued humankind forever with diseases like malaria, dengue, West Nile virus, chikungunya, yellow fever, all kinds of encephalitis, and, of course, Zika. The tiny disease-spreaders are prolific; a single female *Aedes aegypti* mosquito, the kind that transmits Zika, can produce up to a billion progeny. Barbara Han, PhD, a disease ecologist from the Cary Institute of Ecosystems in New York, and her colleagues have identified three dozen species of mosquitoes (out of 3,000 known) that have Zika-transmitting potential, seven of which are found in the U.S.[20]

Aside from swatting them, we can battle mosquitoes by getting rid of standing water, cleaning out potential breeding sites, ensuring window screens are intact, using mosquito traps, spraying indoors and outdoors, hanging insecticide-treated nets, using mosquito repellent, and treating our clothes with insecticide.[21, 22] But what innovations could better control these pests?[23]

Today, some scientists are applying the CRISPR gene-modification technology, described in chapter 4, to block virus transmission or reduce the mosquito population. A biotechnology company called Oxitec has developed genetically modified male mosquitoes that could wipe out the Zika-carrying *Aedes aegypti* bugs. The female mosquito's eggs are injected with genetically modified DNA, and the males born from those eggs mate with the wild females (only female mosquitoes bite). The eggs produced from their connubial bliss carry the altered DNA, and the offspring don't live to maturity. According to Oxitec, field tests in Piracicaba, Brazil, resulted in an 82 percent decline in the mosquito population over an eight-month period.[24] But nobody yet knows how scalable the gene-modification approach is, and the public is generally apprehensive about messing with Mother Nature.

While acknowledging this issue, Nina Fedoroff, PhD, a molecular geneticist, and John Block, former U.S. secretary of agriculture, argued in the *New York Times* that genetically modified mosquitoes "may be our best hope for controlling the mosquito-borne Zika virus."[25] They cited the greatest insect-control success story known: the eradication of the screwworm, an insect that killed livestock by laying eggs in open wounds of animals. Edward Knipling, the top entomologist at the U.S. Department of Agriculture, had found that high doses of X-rays made screwworms sterile. After a large-scale test was conducted in 1951, millions of irradiated screwworm flies were packed in boxes and released from small planes. At the program's peak, more than 300 million sterile flies were released weekly. The program worked. By 1982, screwworm cases had disappeared in the U.S., followed by Mexico, Guatemala, and Belize.

Rapid Tests for Early Detection and Surveillance

On the evening of June 23, 2014, a middle-aged woman suffering from a fever was admitted to the common area of Phebe Hospital in Bong County, Liberia, one of the country's most respected rural healthcare centers. The workers there suspected malaria. But within a week, the hospital's first Ebola patient had died, and within a few more weeks, six of the nurses who cared for her also perished.

Phebe is just a few hours' drive from a busy border crossing with Guinea, where Ebola had been raging for months, but a diagnosis of Ebola was never considered for the woman. Even if it had been, it would have taken more than a week to send off a sample and get the results back from Conakry, Guinea, the nearest city with a lab capable of detecting Ebola.

In past outbreaks, Ebola was initially misdiagnosed as malaria, dengue fever, yellow fever, or one of nearly two dozen other diseases. On average misdiagnosis nearly doubles the time until a correct diagnosis is made and, therefore, doubles the time before control measures appropriate to the specific disease are taken. The difference can be a matter of days or weeks—long enough to allow epidemics to start spiraling out of control.[26]

A solution to this kind of problem would have been a rapid diagnostic test for Ebola. Rapid tests, or point-of-care diagnostics, are typically small, portable devices capable of detecting the presence or absence of infection within minutes or a few hours. Such tests offer a highly mobile alternative to large, complex, costly machines that have to be maintained and operated by skilled staff. Examples of rapid tests include home pregnancy tests, point-of-care diagnostic tests that can identify the presence of HIV/AIDS and influenza, and others that can measure blood levels of glucose and proteins released during a heart attack. Many such tests are no bigger than a USB drive, and sometimes as small as a one-inch-diameter piece of paper.[27]

Rapid tests can help in disease surveillance, traveler screening, and early outbreak detection.[28] According to infectious-disease experts at Imperial College London, the number of Ebola victims in Sierra Leone might have been reduced by over a third had a fast, accurate diagnostic testing been available in 2014.[29] If the same were true in Guinea and Liberia, nearly 4,000 people who perished might still be alive today. But such a test didn't exist until March 2015, a year into the outbreak.[30]

When rapid testing became available to Phebe Hospital, the waiting time for results shrank from a week to less than an hour. Phebe's ebullient medical director, Dr. Jefferson Sibley, proudly showed me a screening unit at the hospital entrance. Anyone coming to the hospital with suspected Ebola was tested before entering the hospital grounds. Those who tested positive were immediately isolated; others were directed to the outpatient and emergency departments for further evaluation.

We know the difference rapid diagnostics can make.[31] In Tanzania, where 93 percent of the population is exposed to malaria, a simple chemical-coated card can detect the virus from a patient's drop of blood in only 15 minutes.[32] It's estimated that early diagnosis with a rapid test can save over 100,000 lives per year from malaria alone.[33] Rapid tests are also helping to loosen HIV's stranglehold in impoverished and HIV-ravaged regions across Africa. In as little as five to 40 minutes, rapid HIV tests performed in community clinics or in the privacy of one's home are helping to increase the number of people on ARVs.[34, 35]

Rapid tests to detect multiple pathogens (multiplexed point-of-care diagnostics) are now in development to improve disease surveillance. With their potential to quickly sort infected people from everyone else, rapid tests can prevent overcrowding in healthcare settings and lower the opportunity for pathogens to leapfrog to new hosts. During an influenza pandemic, low-cost home tests would enable people to reduce the spread of the disease both at home and in clinics, lower the number of people quarantined, and help target resources to the sick.

Unfortunately, the development of rapid tests is not keeping up with the need. Despite their long history and proven value, it took months before rapid tests became widely available for SARS, the H5N1 bird flu, and Ebola.[36] As of this writing, rapid tests are still not available for Zika, dengue, or several other pathogens of regional or global pandemic potential. Some critics warn that rapid point-of-care tests for malaria and other diseases are less reliably accurate than conventional and expensive microscopy and other lab-based tests to examine blood. Nevertheless, our approach to innovation should be governed by the "need for speed" and for approaches that can succeed outside conventional settings.[37] With strong public-private collaboration, we could build systems to quickly scale up production. We can do this, and we should.

Fighting Our Viral Enemies with Their Own Genes[38]

New epidemics, from AIDS to Ebola, have reminded us that the faster we identify and genetically map a new pathogen, the faster we can develop a rapid test, a treatment, or a vaccine, and the more lives we will save. There are an estimated 500,000 viruses with the potential to cause a new form of human epidemic. And hundreds of new viruses get added to the list each year. They are lurking in or on animal "hosts": chickens, wild birds, pigs, bats, monkeys, camels, domestic dogs, or rodents.

A trifling 1 percent of these global viral threats have been genetically mapped, and there are far fewer for which vaccines, medicines, or rapid tests are available. If scientists already had the genetic code and could immediately match it to the virus causing the new human epidemic, however, it would save precious time that could save thousands of lives.

Launched in 2016 following a conference at the Rockefeller Foundation Center in Bellagio, Italy, the Global Virome Project has been described as a "moonshot" intended to do the job of mapping all these viruses within a decade. The projected ten-year cost of the effort is $3.4 billion. This is a fraction of the annual cost of fighting epidemics and would be one of the best investments the U.S. and the world could make in protecting us from pandemic spillover from the bush or the barn.

Global Early Warning and the Promise of Data Analytics

Over the last 50 years, weather forecasting and monitoring systems have seen dramatic improvements. Combined with national and local preparedness and response, these innovations have reduced deaths tenfold from storms, floods, bushfires, and other natural hazards, from nearly 3 million deaths between 1956 and 1965 to fewer than 250,000 deaths between 1996 and 2005.[39] Could the same thing happen in the field of pandemic prevention?

For Nathan Wolfe, whom you met in chapter 2, hope lies in digital technology and data analytics, which can make predictive sense of the virus information gathered from the field. Thanks to this fascinating, paradigm-shifting work, Wolfe and his colleagues are detecting new diseases as they jump from animals to humans and are discovering how to stop epidemics before they start.

Wolfe spent years hunting for viruses brewing in the blood of animals native to the hot, impassable jungles of Africa. Wolfe and his teams pioneered ways to investigate biological threats in Africa, Asia, and southern China, working in places where people come into close contact with wild animals. They collected blood samples from bushmeat hunters and their wild prey in hopes of discovering a new virus that hopped from beast to human. To this end, they distributed a special filter paper to villages in the countries where they worked. When hunters killed a wild animal, the researchers squeezed a few drops of the creature's blood onto the paper, recording what kind of animal was butchered and where. The teams collected the papers, which could preserve blood samples for months. "It's amazing the amount of information you can get from a single drop of blood," Wolfe said. Over more than a decade of work, Wolfe and his teams collected and analyzed more than 20,000 blood samples. They discovered several viruses, including one related to adult T-cell leukemia, that have spread from animals to humans. "In infectious disease, we're where cardiology was in the 1950s," Wolfe told *Time* magazine in 2011. "We're finally beginning to understand why pandemics happen instead of just reacting to them."[40]

Wolfe and his colleagues have since developed a data-management system called the Emerging Infectious Disease Information Technology Hub (EIDITH). EIDITH tracks wildlife specimens and associated metadata for USAID's Emerging Pandemic Threats (EPT) and PREDICT programs, which work with partners in 31 countries to build platforms for disease surveillance.[41] PREDICT analyzes the data for emerging diseases and releases the information through a public data-sharing and visualization platform hosted by HealthMap, an expansive globe-spanning project that processes an average of 133 disease alerts a day. This kind of multilayered risk modeling makes it easier to detect emerging zoonotic diseases.[42, 43]

Scientists are also getting better at predicting precisely where and whom the next epidemic will strike. EcoHealth Alliance, a New York–based organization, uses data analytics to discover what causes viruses to emerge, how to find them, and what pathways they will follow. "It's getting to be like predicting an earthquake," says Peter Daszak, a dark-eyed, shaven-headed, and quick-witted Englishman who is the organization's president. "The science is better. We know where the riskiest places are. Once it emerges and starts spreading you can predict accurately where and whom it will hit."[44]

As an example, Daszak points to the West Nile virus, a mosquito-borne illness that first struck New York in 1999, then spread across the U.S. To determine when and how the disease would reach Hawaii, EcoHealth Alliance picked apart the data on likely carriers (pets, migratory birds, poultry, and airplanes) and discovered that the disease would reach the islands only by hitchhiking on planes.[45]

In fact, EcoHealth Alliance has already used climate patterns, travel patterns, and socioeconomic factors to accurately predict where Zika would strike in the U.S. The prevalence of the Zika virus in the southern U.S. in the summer of 2016 had to do not only with the number of *Aedes aegypti* mosquitoes carrying it and the fact that 2016 was the hottest year on record but also with the intensity of airline travel from Zika-affected countries like Puerto Rico to Florida and New York.[46]

Dr. Barbara Han of the environmental research organization the Cary

Local to Global Early Warning System

Local data, monitored and analyzed at the national and global levels, will lead to more rapid, more effective community, national, and international action to prevent, detect, and respond to epidemics.

Local Data

Humans
- Population growth and movement
- Social factors—culture, poverty
- Travel data—air, land, sea
- Business data

Animals
- Wildlife surveillance
- Distribution of animal reservoirs
- Migratory patterns—esp. birds
- Livestock/food animal surveillance

Health System
- Healthcare systems
- International health regulation capacity

Viral and Other Pathogens
- Changing distribution
- Antimicrobial resistance

Environmental Drivers
- Climate change
- Seasonal weather patterns

Mosquitoes, Ticks, Other Vectors
- Changing distribution
- Susceptibility to control measures

National Monitoring & Analytics
- Local disease risk mapping
- Local transmission patterns
- National forecasting
- Local scenario analysis

Global Forecasting & Analytics
- Disease risk mapping
- Transmission modeling
- International forecasting
- Global scenario analysis

National & Community Action
- Risk-specific communication
- Preparedness for first responders
- Local travel alerts
- Targeted surveillance
- Stockpile review

International Action
- Outbreak alerts
- Vaccine development
- Research on new threats
- International travel alerts
- Surge capacity review

SOURCE: Adapted from Alexander K, Sanderson C, Marathe M et al. What factors might have led to the emergence of Ebola in West Africa? *PLOS Neglected Tropical Diseases* 2015; 9: e0003652. Han B, Drake J. Future directions in analytics for infectious disease intelligence. *EMBO Reports* 2016; 17: 785–89. About ProMED-mail. International Society for Infectious Diseases. 2010. http://www.promedmail.org/aboutus/ (accessed 7 July 2017).

Institute believes that a combination of data on human populations, animals, and environmental factors can guide prevention and preparedness. "For far too long our main strategy for tackling infectious disease has been defense after emergence, when a lot of people are already suffering," Han told *Science Daily*. "We are at an exciting point in time where technology and big data present us with another option, one that is anticipatory and has real potential to improve global health security."[47]

Disrupting the Last Mile

Innovation isn't just about the development of new products and technologies. It's also about finding new ways of delivering existing resources. In countries where public access to medical care is a crucial issue, innovation in procurement, supply chain, and delivery systems is making a huge difference.

In Rwanda, for example, a country of 11 million people riven by disease and emerging from a dark history of genocide, another approach to the "last mile" delivery problem is taking shape. Landlocked in east-central Africa, Rwanda is called the "land of a thousand hills" after its rough terrain. If you were lying in a hospital bed in Rwanda in desperate need of a blood transfusion during the rainy season, you might easily die because the unpaved roads are washed out and it's been impossible for medical supplies to get to the clinic for many weeks.

But a solution is on the way, courtesy of drones. When we think of drones, we might think of warfare or the nosy neighbor trying to get a better look at you. But drones are also being used for good. In the context of infectious-disease outbreaks, drones have the potential to maintain disrupted supply channels, transport blood samples for testing, or identify factors underlying an outbreak. Drones are now being used to make deliveries to medical stations and to improve contraceptive access for women in hard-to-reach villages in Ghana and parts of Eastern Europe. A Silicon Valley firm called Matternet has demonstrated the value of drones for transporting blood samples from isolated areas in Bhutan and Malawi. And in remote parts of Malaysia, drones are surveying changes in ground cover to better understand an unusual form of malaria and to monitor disease-carrying macaque monkeys.[48]

Elsewhere on the African continent, a Silicon Valley company called Zipline is working with United Parcel Service (UPS) and another public-private partnership, Gavi, to deploy a fleet of specialized drones in Rwanda. The company's founder and chief executive officer, Keller Rinaudo, thinks Zipline can deliver supplies in much less time than a motorbike messenger could.

Here's how it works. A doctor sends a text message to a medical warehouse. Within minutes, the supplies are dispatched from the facility to a nearby hub, where a drone operator inserts them into a padded cardboard box. He then places the box into the cargo holder of a specially designed drone—a small, fixed-wing craft built to withstand the rainy season—which can carry up to a little over three pounds of medical supplies. After putting a fresh battery on the drone's nose, the operator uploads the flight plan from an iPad and launches the device, which flies off at a speed of around 60 miles per hour at an altitude of between 300 and 400 feet. Following the flight plan up to a distance of around 74 miles, the drone drops the cargo (which is tethered to a parachute) at the destination and then returns.

Zipline's drone delivery program is an example of an adventurous partnership of creative people and organizations dedicated to solving a problem. UPS, one of those partners, provided $800,000 and its logistics expertise to get things started. The Rwandan government, which is very forward-looking and anxious to try out new solutions to address problems, is interested, says Rinaudo: "Rwanda is kind of a startup country. It is still one of the poorest countries of the world, but it is run by an incredibly innovative and technology-focused government that is willing to make big bets on the future."[49, 50]

*   *   *

Walk down a long, hot, dusty, red-clay road in the Ruvuma region of southern Tanzania, and you see village houses roofed with tin or thatch, people selling fruit laid out on cloth on the roadside or clothing from carts, the occasional bicyclist, and women in colorful garb and headdresses, babies slung from their backs. As in many developing countries, when someone from Ruvuma gets sick, their first stop is not a clinic or a pharmacist. Instead, it's the local medicines seller—typically a nearby shop that sells soap, aspirin, and other over-the-counter pharmaceuticals. In the past, such shops, called *duka la dawa baridi* (cold medicines shop) also sold prescription drugs illegally, usually a small quantity and at a high price. Because the shopkeepers were untrained, they often gave people the wrong drug, with the result that their customers often got sicker or even died.

If you went looking for treatment today in Ruvuma, you would meet a smiling, uniformed woman named Frieda Kamba, looking jaunty in a white cap and shirt and welcoming you into her small but tidy *duka la dawa muhimu* (essential medicines shop). Frieda would ply you with reliable health information for preventing or addressing your illness, whether it be a cold or a serious condition like AIDS.[51]

Frieda is a new kind of health worker; she operates a scalable social enterprise called an Accredited Drug Dispensing Outlet (ADDO). The ADDO program was created by the Tanzanian government, MSH, the Gates Foundation, and Tanzania's private sector. Today Frieda is a specially trained, licensed health dispenser who improves health and saves lives in her own community while enjoying the financial security of running her own business.[52] By 2015 there were more than 15,000 "Friedas" in Tanzania and more like her in Uganda and Liberia, which together provide health information, prevention, and treatment for common illnesses to more than 36 million customers in Africa.[53]

Inspired by the ADDO program, and also with the support of the Gates Foundation and MSH, Uganda launched the Accredited Drug Shops program in 2009. Because local dispensers were very often the first source of care, and because Ebola and other infectious diseases were still lurking in monkeys and other forest animals in Uganda, trainees were taught how to prevent, identify, report, and respond to hemorrhagic fevers like Ebola and Marburg, dengue and chikungunya fevers, meningitis, yellow fever, and other contagious diseases.[54]

In 2012, Liberian Medicines and Health Products Regulatory Authority, the Gates Foundation, and MSH teamed up to create the Accredited Medicines Stores program, also patterned after the Tanzania experience. When Ebola struck in 2014, nearly 500 dispensers had been trained in Montserrado County, where Liberia's capital, Monrovia, is located. Most of the 600-plus medicines stores and 112 pharmacies continued to provide prevention services and treatment for common illnesses such as malaria and pneumonia. Pharmacy students were mobilized to provide these outlets with Ebola-awareness training, advice on counseling customers, and guidance in referring suspected Ebola cases. While health facilities throughout Monrovia closed due to fears among staff and patients, the medicines stores and pharmacies not only stayed open but more than doubled the number of clients they saw.[55]

In 2016, I met with a group of 50 or more medicine-shop owners and operators and visited several in their stores in Monrovia. All were proud to have been able to reduce the burden on Liberia's crippled health system. They stayed open throughout the crisis, despite the risk to their own health. They protected themselves carefully and required customers to wash their hands in chlorinated water in buckets outside their shops. From behind the counter, wearing gloves, they used a noncontact infrared thermometer to check customers' temperatures and wiped down their shop repeatedly with bleach. Morkoi Kolleh, one of the store owners whom I visited, told me that after a very ill-looking woman vomited blood in the small shop bathroom, Kolleh disinfected her shop, then quarantined herself and closed the shop for the incubation period of 21 days. Sadly, at least 11 shop owners were known to have died from the disease despite their precautionary measures.

The ADDO programs in Tanzania, Uganda, and Liberia provide inspiring examples of public-private partnerships in which the government provides the training, accreditation, and monitoring; the Gates Foundation provides the resources and oversight; nonprofit organizations like MSH provide the know-how; and the local private sector becomes a sustainable social enterprise. ADDOs are now distributing mosquito-repellent nets, antimalarial medicines, and condoms; following HIV patients; and doing referrals.

If we are to address epidemics at the vital grassroots community level, then trusted local programs like ADDO will make all the difference.

Collaboration for the Innovations We Need

By now it should be evident that there are huge opportunities to dramatically reduce the threat to humanity from infectious-disease outbreaks. Given the compelling reasons to move forward, what will it take to aggressively pursue these opportunities?

Until now, the critical missing ingredient has been visionary and strategic leadership. No organization has had the responsibility and comprehensive mechanism to track the pandemic threats and coordinate the innovation agenda. The question of leadership was addressed in late 2015 and early 2016 when international leaders, government policymakers, public-health officials, and researchers were catalyzed into action by the 2014 Ebola epidemic.[56] In a series of high-level commissions, the international experts concluded that the role of the World Health Organization is "to galvanize acceleration of research and development, define priorities, and mobilize and allocate resources."[57] In response, in May 2016, WHO began work on a research and development "Blueprint for Action to Prevent Epidemics."[58]

I would agree with the group's conclusion that despite some missteps in recent epidemics, WHO stands as the only organization with the international mandate, access to needed technical expertise, and convening power to carry out such a task. However, I believe that leadership in such a broad and rapidly moving field requires a collaborative, not a command-and-control, dynamic. The 2017 launch of the Coalition for Epidemic Preparedness Innovations (CEPI) is a prime example of an effective collaborative dynamic. Created by the governments of Germany, Japan, Norway, and India; the Wellcome Trust; the Gates Foundation; and the World Economic Forum, CEPI is a partnership among international, government, corporate, philanthropic, and civil-society organizations. Its aim is to catalyze the development of vaccines for priority pathogens and to accelerate research and development.[59]

Collaborative work among scientists produced the world's first Ebola vaccine. When Ebola struck West Africa in 2014, the Public Health Agency of Canada (PHAC), whose researchers had developed an experimental Ebola vaccine in 2003, and the U.S. biopharmaceutical firm NewLink Genetics (to whom PHAC had licensed the vaccine) immediately went into overdrive. Working with the U.S. National Institutes of Health (NIH) and WHO, they moved the vaccine into clinical trials to test the effectiveness and safety in humans.[60] In November 2014, NewLink exclusively licensed rights to Merck to manufacture the trial vaccine. At the same time, Gavi, the Vaccine Alliance, committed up to $390 million for 12 million doses of an Ebola vaccine.[61]

Next came the field tests. In 2015, WHO—together with the Guinean health ministry, Médecins Sans Frontières, the Epicentre Research Center, the Norwegian Institute of Public Health, and other partners—conducted a study of the vaccine in Guinea. Not one of the nearly 6,000 people who received it contracted the Ebola virus.[62] In just ten months, the vaccine was proven to be 100 percent effective and safe.[63, 64]

In another set of initiatives, Grand Challenges (a partnership of USAID and the Gates Foundation), and governments around the world are partnering with private donors to provide millions in funding to grow a pipeline of technologies that can be administered in community settings. For example, USAID's Grand Challenges Initiative supports global innovators in fighting

Zika through the rapid development of innovations like diagnostic tests.[65] In April 2016, USAID asked innovators around the world to submit cutting-edge technologies and approaches to prevent, detect, and respond to Zika in the short and long term. While the U.S. Congress was busy debating how to fund resources to fight Zika, 900 entrepreneurs competed in a *Shark Tank*–like challenge to present their ideas. In August 2016, USAID awarded $15 million in grants to 21 innovators for inventions, including an electronic force field that repels mosquitoes, a mobile app that detects whether mosquitoes are carrying the virus, and low-cost treated sandals to prevent bites.[66]

*   *   *

As we've seen, innovations in science and technology have made our world safer from epidemic diseases. But the pace of innovations is not even close to keeping up with the accelerating risk of infectious-disease outbreaks. I've described five breakthrough innovations that I believe could dramatically reduce the risk of devastating pandemics: new vaccines, more effective mosquito control, proactive development of rapid tests, global early warning systems, and genetic mapping of viral threats. Our scientists, engineers, technology gurus, and field researchers have the capacity to develop far stronger tools to prevent, predict, detect, and respond to emerging pathogens. What's needed now is an aggressive investment plan—the subject of the next chapter.

CHAPTER 11

INVEST WISELY, SAVE LIVES

The equivalent of just $1 per year for every person
on the planet ($7.5 billion annually) will save lives
and pay for itself in lower emergency costs and
reduced economic disruption.

Epidemics are bad for people, they are bad for governments, and they are bad business. An ounce of prevention, in terms of dollars, is truly worth a pound of cure when it comes to stopping epidemics. By investing an extra $1 per year for every person on the planet ($7.5 billion annually) in the right prevention and preparedness measures at the right times, we can substantially reduce the chance of epidemics and more than repay ourselves in savings.

Dr. Jim Yong Kim—a physician, anthropologist, and cofounder of the nonprofit Partners in Health with global health legend Dr. Paul Farmer—was a surprise candidate when President Barack Obama nominated him as president of the World Bank in 2012.[1, 2] In his 2000 book, *Dying for Growth*, he had argued that an unfettered quest for growth had "worsened the lives of millions of women and men."[3] Today, he leads the World Bank with a vision of ending extreme poverty and creating opportunity for everyone.

Jim has been a friend and colleague since we worked together in the early 2000s on access to treatment for AIDS and tuberculosis. He's an inspiring visionary, activist, scientist, and humanitarian. Slightly balding with minimalist wire-rim glasses and a wry sense of humor, Jim applies to his work the same agility that he deployed as a high school quarterback and point guard.

Telling Jim something can't be done is like waving a red flag in front of a bull. Together with Paul Farmer, he has doggedly tackled one seemingly insurmountable health problem after another. While the world debated whether it was possible to treat AIDS in developing countries, these two men were on the ground proving treatment was quite feasible in places like Haiti. When WHO said treatment for highly drug-resistant tuberculosis was unrealistic, they mounted a successful program in Peru.

So when the West Africa Ebola epidemic exploded in August 2014 and the world seemed immobilized, it was no surprise that Jim's World Bank took the first responsive step in the international community. The bank made an unprecedented emergency commitment of $200 million to fight the disease.[4] "Responding to short-term emergencies . . . is not what the World Bank does," he told his board, "but we are not seeing the massive response that's needed. If we don't send a message, no one's going to do anything."[5] He pushed the bank to work at record speed. The money started flowing to West Africa within nine days. By 2015, the bank had mobilized more than $1.6 billion out of a total of $7 billion raised for Ebola response and recovery efforts.[6]

Making funds available fast, before a disease has a chance to spread, is crucial. Money to fight Ebola in West Africa did not begin to flow until three months later after the devastation began, during which time the number of cases increased tenfold. The poorest and most marginalized people have far less chance of receiving health care, despite their greater need for it. Had there been a mechanism to provide an initial $100 million in July 2014 when Ebola was erupting in West Africa, the money could have been used to hire health workers, purchase equipment, mount communications and containment campaigns, and much more that would have significantly limited the spread and severity of the epidemic.[7]

Investment is one of the most obvious and critical anchors of The Powers of Seven for a very simple reason. While trillions could be lost in a global pandemic (as I explained in chapter 5), investing a tiny fraction of what we spend in cleaning up after an epidemic would save billions. Just $1 per year for every person on the planet spent on epidemic preparedness and public health would save untold lives and dollars. When governments, NGOs, and the private sector work to invest the proverbial penny to strengthen health systems, the pound of cure proves the penny investment's worth.

The Politics of "Now"

As a public-health leader who has seen the impact of prevention and as a family physician who has cared for the sick, I ask myself: Why wasn't even a fraction of the money committed to emergency response and recovery used to maintain WHO's global response capacity? Why didn't we invest in building the three lines of defense in vulnerable countries before the Ebola epidemic came along?

The answer is: it's all about the economics and politics of now. "The response to pandemics is cycle of panic, neglect, panic, neglect," Jim Kim says. "It happens every time."[8] Typically, commitment and compassion, fear and self-interest only come together once an epidemic threatens to go worldwide. It's only then that the money flows, and typically too slowly.

National and international leaders have been fatally slow to put public-health knowledge into action. Epidemic preparedness is a highly vulnerable area of public spending because funding flows when there is obvious danger and ebbs when there isn't. There was a big boost of investment for funding pandemic prevention following the SARS epidemic and again when the 2009 H1N1 swine flu captured worldwide attention. In both cases, funding was short-lived. As always happens, the inflow of resources quickly dwindled to a trickle without another epidemic in the news. The disheartening fact is that countries that haven't experienced a recent epidemic don't spend money that should go into strengthening their health systems, preferring to spend it on other things.

When the 2008 global financial crisis hit, the World Health Organization was forced to cut nearly $1 billion from its proposed two-year budget, only about 20 percent of which comes from dues paid by member nations.[9] Facing difficult choices, WHO member countries chose to protect spending against chronic ailments like heart disease and less on outbreak and emergency response (which was not particularly well funded in the first place). The emergency-response department at WHO was so decimated that it looked "like a ghost town," according to one consultant. The epidemic- and pandemic-response department was also dissolved.[10] These cuts slowed WHO's ability to respond to Ebola, an avoidable epidemic that ended up costing the three most affected countries of Sierra Leone, Liberia, and Guinea $2.2 billion in lost GDP.[11] (As I noted in chapter 5, even a mild disease outbreak can have enormous financial consequences.[12])

In the U.S., biodefense and public-health emergency budgets increased after 9/11 and the anthrax attacks in Washington, D.C. But later, from 2006 to 2013, with budget pressures and no countervailing public concern, the U.S. Congress cut CDC public-health preparedness budgets by more than 50 percent. State and local health departments lost more than 45,000 jobs—demonstrating how the politics and economics of "now" repeatedly leave us vulnerable to major epidemics.[13]

During the summer of 2016, the U.S. Congress was embroiled in a row that prevented people in the U.S. Virgin Islands, Puerto Rico, Florida, and many U.S. states from getting the protection they needed from the increasingly rampant Zika virus. As Zika was turning into a public-health emergency, everyone understood that funding to fight Zika needed to happen. The problem was politics. Republicans wanted certain agendas dear to their hearts, such as defunding of Planned Parenthood, to be attached to the approval of money; Democrats vociferously disagreed.[14] The standoff prevented funding for Zika. Congressional members took a summer recess while more and more people were exposed to the disease. This shameful kind of political football while people are at risk of sickness and death is far too common.

Spending money on an epidemic when it's in the headlines doesn't prevent a crisis from occurring in the first place. Worse, far too much money goes to the wrong place at the wrong time. Once cases of an infectious disease are confirmed in a lab, various organizations, including the U.S. CDC and WHO, send in specialists to begin containing the disease. This strategy is both too slow and too late. Failing to fund prevention is like closing the fire department and canceling the fire insurance when cash is short and there hasn't been a conflagration in town for a few years. It's nothing short of idiotic.

How "Recency Bias" Trips Us Up: Will Short Memories Be Our Downfall?

To err is human, and we humans suffer from many psychological foibles. One is called "recency bias." Basically, we humans, like most animals, are creatures of habit who adhere to established behavioral patterns; our recent experience becomes the baseline for our future decisions. Instead of taking the long view and considering all the possibilities, we fall into a behavioral rut.

When it comes to investing money in things like keeping humankind safe from bad things like AIDS, SARS, and Zika, recency bias can trip us up. After the headlines fade and the tweets-per-day count plummets, we all forget about

Funding Rises and Falls with Public Attention

Pandemic-prevention funding commitments for developing countries rise during epidemic threats, like the avian influenza in 2006 and H1N1 swine flu in 2009, but fall when public interest declines ($millions).

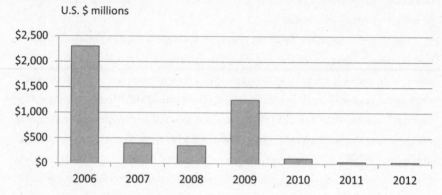

SOURCE: Jonas O. Pandemic risk. *Finance & Development.* 2014, pp. 16–17, based on United Nations and World Bank (2010) and World Bank (2012).

U.S. CDC Public Health Emergency Preparedness Funding has been reduced since 9/11, but the 2006 avian flu caught public attention.

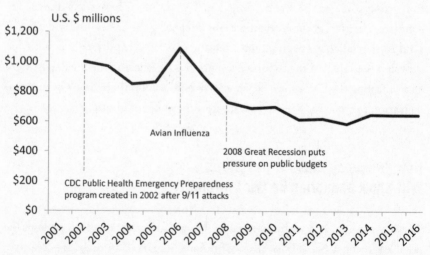

SOURCE: Centers for Disease Control and Prevention. The 2013–2014 National Snapshot of Public Health Preparedness. Cdc.gov. 2014. https://www.cdc.gov/phpr/pubs-links/2013/ (accessed 1 May 2017). Trust for America's Health. Public Health Emergency Preparedness Cooperative Agreement (CDC) Hospital Preparedness Program (ASPR-PHSSEF). TFAH. 2017. http://healthyamericans.org/health-issues/wp-content/uploads/2016/02/FY17-PHEP-HPP.pdf (accessed 1 May 2017).

the threat. As far as recent memory tells us, we're still okay. We go back to our patterns. We let our guards down. We don't consider the possibility, despite all the warnings, that we might be felled by some weird disease from the jungle or the barnyard. "Every time an event like an epidemic happens, we think it's unique," the behavioral economist Dan Ariely told me. "We simply don't understand the nature of epidemics."[15]

Recency bias is vividly illustrated in the World Economic Forum Global Risks Report, an annual survey of several hundred respondents from all regions of the world with diverse expertise in business, academia, and NGOs. In 2007, following widely publicized worries about avian influenza, pandemics ranked fourth out of two dozen economic, environmental, geopolitical, societal, and technological risks to countries and industries. By 2013, in the absence of a headline-grabbing infectious-disease outbreak, pandemics had dropped to twentieth place. In 2015, after Ebola struck, it shot back up to second place. And what was the ranking for perceived risk just two years later, after Ebola was out of the headlines? Down to eleventh place.[16]

Yet most informed experts would agree that the risk of pandemics has, if anything, steadily increased during this period.

The Political Case for Action

On September 11, 2001, the attacks on the World Trade Center and the Pentagon shook Americans to their core. The 9/11 Commission concluded that the attacks, which killed 3,000, "should not have come as a surprise." The U.S. had received clear warnings for several years. The commission argued that officials should have thwarted the plot, stating, "Across the government, there were failures of imagination, policy, capabilities, and management."[17]

In 2008, the collapse of several large financial institutions precipitated a global financial crisis and widespread recession, with devastating effects for millions of people around the globe. It seemed like a sudden event. But the 2011 U.S. Financial Crisis Inquiry Commission was unequivocal: the crisis had been avoidable, it said—"the result of human action and inaction."[18] Serious lapses in regulation, corporate governance, and risk management were compounded by a lack of transparency and accountability, and a sense of duty to protect the public.

A global pandemic on the scale of the Spanish flu would kill far, far more people than the 9/11 attack and wreak at least as much financial havoc as the

2008 crisis. And it could happen again if leaders fail to grapple with incipient problems before they become full-blown disasters.

Nothing shines a light on the quality of a country's leadership more than a public-health crisis. No president, prime minister, state or regional governor, or other leader wants to be condemned by his or her constituency for allowing a preventable disaster to happen. And when epidemics and pandemics do occur, leaders can either look like heroes or like they should not have been put in the job in the first place. There isn't a lot of room in between. When the government's response stutters, devastation and financial losses pile up, and so does the public criticism. Every time an infectious disease strikes and leaders show themselves to be ineffective in their response, they pay a political price. Consider:

+   The SARS epidemic turned into a major political crisis in China after authorities covered up the extent of the problem. They then scrambled to demonstrate that they had the situation under control, as I described in chapter 6. To make political matters worse, China's top leadership changed in the midst of the SARS outbreak. On April 19, 2003, Zhang Wenkang, the health minister and a protégé of the outgoing president of China, Jiang Zemin, was fired for lying to the press that China was "a perfectly safe place." And in what appeared to be political payback, Beijing mayor Meng Xuenong, a supporter of incoming president Hu Jintao, was also dismissed for dishonesty. Beijing party secretary Liu Qi, believed to be connected to Jiang, was forced to make a public "self-criticism" for covering up.[19]

+   In Mexico, the swine flu epidemic of 2009 brought criticism down on the head of President Calderon for being too slow to respond and too invisible. "In Mexico's flu crisis, where is Calderon?" the Reuters news agency asked. "The world's eyes are on Mexico and its deadly swine flu outbreak, but [the president] has gone to ground, barely showing his face since the crisis broke five days ago."[20] The absence of leadership during the crisis took a political toll: Calderon's party took a severe beating in the subsequent elections.[21]

+   In the U.S., Ebola turned into an explosive political issue after CDC director Tom Frieden declared that "we know how to stop Ebola." The Obama administration came under scorching attack by Republican presidential candidates who declared that the government wasn't doing enough to fight the disease. A 2014 Pew poll found that 41 percent of Americans said they had "not too much confidence" or "no confidence at all" that the government could prevent a serious Ebola outbreak in the United States.[22]

By contrast, when a government invests in public health, it saves the lives and money not only of its own people but also the world's. When national governments respond quickly, visibly, and responsibly, the public reacts with support and admiration.

An excellent example is Hong Kong. After the 2003 SARS outbreak killed nearly 300 of its citizens, Hong Kong learned its lessons and became a model for public health care. "If there is anywhere in the world that took a beating by SARS, it was Hong Kong," said Peter Cordingley, spokesman for WHO in Manila, to *Time* magazine in 2009. "The lesson was learned."[23]

Whenever a potential epidemic shows up on Hong Kong's shores, the country issues travel advisories. It increases scanning of travelers, taking their temperatures and detaining those who are sick with flu-like symptoms. It has tough infection-control policies in and out of hospitals. When a wild bird drops out of the sky, it gets dissected in a lab for traces of diseases. The public is disease-conscious: if residents of Hong Kong get sick or fear contracting an illness, they don surgical masks and wash their hands as a matter of social courtesy.[24] Would that all countries could be so adept.

Hong Kong is a small place whose government does the right thing for its own citizens and visitors. By contrast, when big, rich, developed countries like the U.S. decide to tackle disease, they can literally change the world. A shining model is PEPFAR, the U.S. President's Emergency Plan for AIDS Relief, a program George W. Bush announced in his State of the Union address in 2003—the same year the misbegotten "shock and awe" bombing of Iraq happened. Bush isn't beloved by many people around the world for starting a war that has riven the Middle East and brought about the deaths of millions. But he did do one thing really well as a self-described "compassionate conservative," and that was to wholeheartedly engage in the global battle against AIDS.

Spending money on AIDS treatment and prevention in Africa hasn't just boosted America's image among Africans; it has protected social institutions in these countries from degradation and collapse, thus contributing to security and effective governance. In effect, it not only helped shore up the legacy of George W. Bush but also helped governments in Africa do better, too.

The Business Case for Investment

An unexpected hero of the Ebola outbreak in Africa was not a doctor, nurse, or frontline worker. He was a broad-browed, professorial-looking fellow named Bernard Gustin, and he was the CEO of an airline. For a brief time, Brussels Air was the only one to provide services to the three stricken nations of Liberia, Sierra Leone, and Guinea. "We're not a humanitarian organization," Gustin pointedly told *Bloomberg News*, but "disconnecting completely from the rest of the planet would make the problem even bigger."[25]

Gustin was one of the very few people who connected the dots between human lives, economic well-being, investment, and private-sector engagement. By analyzing the facts and using cold reason, Gustin actively demonstrated how panicking would just make things worse. "Ebola is a very bad sickness but a very weak virus," Gustin said. "While the cases we see are shocking, we know very well how it is transmitted. I hope we keep reason, analyze the facts and get out of the panic mode. The hysteria must be overcome."

Gustin understood something that many corporate leaders have not: the typical human response to epidemics—fear, panic, and self-interest—is usually very bad for businesses and economies. And he was absolutely right. While the human cost of major epidemics is obvious and horrific, too many business leaders and government policymakers fail to adequately consider the staggering financial impact.

What Can Business Leaders Do?[26]

- **Encourage** governments in countries of operation to comply with the International Health Regulations (IHRs) to reduce risks to business.

- **Collaborate** with governments and NGOs to develop epidemic surveillance, preparedness, response, and other strategies.

- **Share** experiences and resources to assist governments and partners with a coordinated, multisector response to epidemics, so that their workforces and communities in vulnerable areas are protected.

- **Factor** outbreaks of infectious diseases and epidemics into business risk assessments and continuity planning.

As I noted in chapter 5, more than three-quarters of companies are not prepared for a public-health emergency. Pandemics are not "normal" business continuity risks—they are typically far more sudden, have a universal, disruptive impact on business and the economy, and affect larger numbers of people. Given that business is about making a profit, maximizing shareholder value, and getting a good return on investment, companies simply can't afford to operate in places that are uprooted by disease. Employees who are sick can't work; consumers who are sick can't shop. Epidemics can threaten market positions as well.

So what can companies do in the face of an epidemic? They don't just have to write checks to NGOs. They can also lend their expertise in logistics and supply chains, health, technology, data collection, mobile communications, management, and more to fill the gaps in often fragile and fractured health systems. Firms can offer specialized capabilities like communications technology, biopharma R&D, data analysis, and financial services, such as financing and mobile payments. Many companies have local personnel and equipment in outbreak areas, and their on-the-ground knowledge about communities and cultures can inform relevant and effective emergency efforts.

During the Ebola epidemic, the mining company ArcelorMittal conducted community awareness and screening programs and built treatment centers in Liberia. Coca-Cola used its distribution network to deliver medicine and medical supplies in the affected countries. Logistics companies transported goods and health workers. Pharmaceutical and diagnostic companies used their teams, labs, and capabilities to develop and test Ebola vaccines. Johnson & Johnson (with Bavarian Nordic), GlaxoSmithKline (with the U.S. National Institute of Allergy and Infectious Diseases), Merck and NewLink Genetics (jointly with the Public Health Agency of Canada), and Novavax all invested in an Ebola vaccine.[27]

Many other firms provided in-kind goods and financial donations such as medical supplies, personal protective equipment, and vehicles. For example, the medical supplier Becton, Dickinson and Company donated protected needle devices that allowed health workers to perform blood sampling and intravenous therapy procedures safely. Unilever, in addition to its donation of millions of bars of soap to aid the response effort, used its expertise in consumer behavior to develop a workshop for the U.K. Department for International Development that helped them create a better strategy for working with the community.[28]

The Best Dollar We'll Ever Spend: Three Areas of Investment

Clearly, the maxim "an ounce of prevention is worth a pound of cure" is absolutely true in the case of infectious diseases. Consider, for example, the savings that an aggressive vaccine program for childhood illnesses in the world's poorest countries could generate. Researchers have found that the increased use of just six vaccines (for pneumonia, meningitis, rotavirus, pertussis, measles, and malaria) in 72 of the world's poorest countries could save 6.4 million lives, prevent 426 million cases of illness, and save 63,000 children from being disabled due to meningitis in less than a decade. Just keeping people out of acute care for these diseases would save $7.4 billion; another $145 billion would be recouped in productivity, because people could continue to work instead of staying home sick or caring for their families. Individual countries would save approximately $8.6 million in treatment costs alone, or about $7 per surviving infant, and highly populated places where these diseases are common—India, Nigeria, Indonesia, and Pakistan—would save the most money.[29]

So what if, instead of playing whack-a-mole with epidemics as they spread and spending billions to clean up after them (not to mention the enormous and ongoing costs of caring for the chronically sick or orphaned children afterward), we had the will and imagination to avert epidemics in the first place?

In 2014, researchers from EcoHealth Alliance, the University of Wyoming, the National Institutes of Health, and Princeton University showed that if we invested in strengthening prevention strategies such as disease surveillance and tracking, improving public-health systems, reducing deforestation, and enhancing farm biosecurity, we could reduce infectious-disease outbreaks by as much as 50 percent. This would require total expenditures of $344 billion over a 27-year period—an average cost of $12.74 billion a year, at least half of which is already covered by current spending. The research showed that prevention programs—as opposed to the business-as-usual strategy of addressing epidemics when they happen—would save between $344 billion and $360 billion over the next 100 years if implementation began today.[30]

Early in 2016, the U.S. National Academy of Sciences (NAS) convened a global commission of clinicians, scientists, social researchers, policy experts, industry leaders, financiers, and community leaders from 12 countries on five continents. They asked: What would it take to implement the WHO International Health Regulations along with the necessary Food and Agriculture Organization (FAO) standards in every country? They found that investments to upgrade public-health systems in developing countries would run $4.5 billion per year.[31] In addition, the commission report suggested enhancing WHO's pandemic prevention and response capabilities and financing WHO and World Bank contingency funds ($130 million to $155 million per year) as well as saving an additional $1 billion for research and development. The estimated total for all of that came to just 65 cents per person on the planet per year.

Add to the National Academy of Science the World Bank's Pandemic Emergency Financing program, described below, and the estimated research

The Cost of Making the World Safer

By investing an extra $1 per year for every person on the planet ($7.5 billion annually), we can make the world substantially safer from pandemic threats.

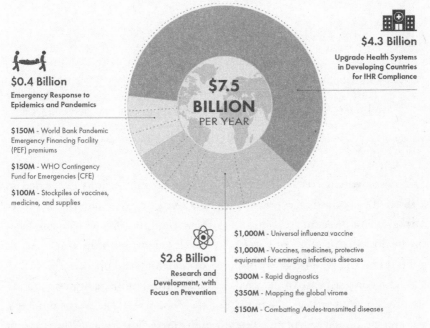

$4.3 Billion
Upgrade Health Systems in Developing Countries for IHR Compliance

$0.4 Billion
Emergency Response to Epidemics and Pandemics

$150M - World Bank Pandemic Emergency Financing Facility (PEF) premiums

$150M - WHO Contingency Fund for Emergencies (CFE)

$100M - Stockpiles of vaccines, medicine, and supplies

$7.5 BILLION PER YEAR

$2.8 Billion
Research and Development, with Focus on Prevention

$1,000M - Universal influenza vaccine

$1,000M - Vaccines, medicines, protective equipment for emerging infectious diseases

$300M - Rapid diagnostics

$350M - Mapping the global virome

$150M - Combatting Aedes-transmitted diseases

SOURCE: The neglected dimensions of global security. National Academy of Medicine. 2016. https://www .nap.edu/catalog/21891/the-neglected-dimension-of-global-security-a-framework-to-counter (accessed 1 May 2017). Osterholm M, Olshaker M. *Deadliest enemy: Our war against killer germs.* Boston: Little, Brown and Company, 2017. Sands P, Mundaca-Shah C, Dzau V. The neglected dimension of global security—A framework for countering infectious-disease crises. *New England Journal of Medicine* 2016; 374: 1281–1287. Røttingen J, Regmi S, Eide M et al. Mapping of available health research and development data: What's there, what's missing, and what role is there for a global observatory? *The Lancet* 2013; 382: 1286–307. Brende B, Farrar J, Gashumba D, Moedas C, Mundel T, Shiozaki Y, Vardhan H, Wanka J, Røttingen J. CEPI-a new global R&D organisation for epidemic preparedness and response. *The Lancet.* 21 Jan 2017; 389(10066): 233–35. Wilder-Smith A, Gubler D, Weaver S, Monath T, Heymann D, Scott T. Epidemic arboviral diseases: priorities for research and public health. *The Lancet Infectious Diseases* 2017; 17: e101–e106. Author estimate for diagnostics.

Savings-to-Cost Ratio for Four Pandemic Scenarios

To estimate the money savings alone, consider the following four scenarios, based on different severities (measured by GDP declines and frequencies over the next 100 years).

Annual Savings/Annual Cost Ratio

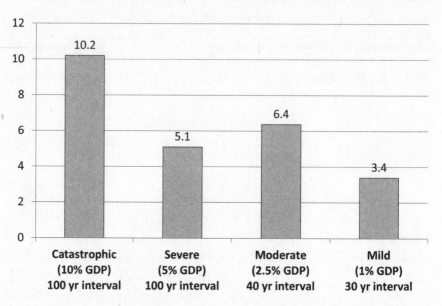

	Catastrophic (10% GDP) 100 yr interval	Severe (5% GDP) 100 yr interval	Moderate (2.5% GDP) 40 yr interval	Mild (1% GDP) 30 yr interval
	10.2	5.1	6.4	3.4

SOURCE: Author calculations based on 2016 Global GDP of US $75 trillion and pandemic cost data presented in chapter 5.

and development costs for the game-changing innovations described in chapter 10, and the total comes to an annual average of $7.5 billion for the three vital areas for investment: (1) health systems strengthening, with an emphasis on health security; (2) research and development, with an emphasis on prevention; and (3) emergency response to epidemics and pandemics.

These investments would save millions of lives, millions of jobs, and billions of dollars across global and national economies. If you do the numbers, the average annual cost of investment would average just under $1 per year for every person on the planet. Across four scenarios, every dollar spent returns between $3 and $10 in savings.

The projections above fit with evidence from other fields. Researchers from Stanford and Loyola Marymount University estimate that every $1 spent in the U.S. on preparedness for disasters such as floods, wildfires, and drought results in $15 saved in future damage mitigation. A 2014 study by UNICEF, the World Food Program, and the U.K. Department of International Development found preparedness interventions for humanitarian emergencies returned at least $2 for every $1 spent.[32]

Making the world safer from epidemic and pandemic threats amounts to less than $8 billion per year. That's an investment that pales against the $1.57 trillion the world spent on military defense in 2016.[33] And it's a fraction of the $91 billion spent on video games the same year.[34]

Where Should We Invest?

At essentially $1 per person per year to end epidemics, spending on epidemic prevention would obviously be the best investment we could ever make. Where should this funding come from?

1. Strengthening Public-Health Systems

As minister of health for Mexico, Dr. Julio Frenk (a friend and colleague from WHO, now president of the University of Miami and former dean of the Harvard School of Public Health) had a remarkably strong record in convincing the Mexican president and ministry of finance to invest in public health and universal health coverage. Realizing that finance people think and decide differently than health people, he told me, "To lead my new Economic Analysis Unit, I recruited a first-rate economist, with a PhD from the same top university as the minister of Finance, tasked him with producing the most solid economic analysis on each of our key policy proposals, and always took him with me when we met with the Treasury."[35]

National, state, provincial, and local governments bear the lion's share of the responsibility for building public-health systems capable of preventing, detecting, responding to, and recovering from epidemics. A whole-of-society response is needed, but governments must take the lead. High- and middle-income countries should cover these costs as part of their own government budgeting process, though this is often easier said than done. (In most countries, the head of state and the treasury department or the ministry of finance take the lead on the government budget. Health is often seen as an expense to be managed and contained, and health officials are not always adept at making the stronger case for investment.)

There is broad agreement that the Ebola crisis was not quickly contained, reversed, or mitigated because national health systems in West Africa were woefully underresourced, understaffed, and poorly equipped. In 2012, for example, the Liberian government spent $20 per person per year on health. Sierra Leone spent $16 per person per year, and Guinea $9 per person per year, far below the WHO recommendation of $86 per person to provide the minimum package of essential health services. By comparison, Norway spent $7,704 on health for each citizen. Health care in the poorest countries is so underresourced that the 40 poorest countries are collectively spending only $52 per capita on health care.[36]

Human resources are also woefully inadequate. The 40 poorest countries in the world have only an average of ten health workers per 10,000 people. (As a minimum, WHO recommends 23 health workers per 10,000 people.) There is a direct relationship between spending on health and the number of doctors, nurses, clinics, hospitals, equipment and medicines, and surveillance facilities that were available for emergency response when Ebola struck. Liberia had only 51 doctors in the whole country. Sierra Leone had 1,017 nurses and midwives. While the U.K. has one health worker for every 88 people, Liberia had one health worker for every 3,472 inhabitants and Sierra Leone one for every 5,319.[37] This means that most of the poorest countries do not have sufficient health workers to deal with routine health issues, let alone capacity to detect, prepare for, and respond to an epidemic.

One of the most important lessons from the Ebola crisis is the need to build comprehensive health systems with sufficient funding, staff, and equipment to deal with everyday health problems as well as infectious-disease outbreaks. All countries could make progress toward spending $86 of public funds per person on health. They could do this by collecting 20 percent of gross domestic product as tax revenue and allocating 15 percent of their budgets to health. Bringing an end to illicit financial flows and tackling tax avoidance, as well as putting innovative taxes in place, would close the gap too.[38]

2. Research and Development, with an Emphasis on Prevention

Each year, the world spends more than $250 billion on research and development for health, with most of it coming from high-income countries. Of this amount, 60 percent comes from the private sector, 30 percent from the public sector, and 10 percent from universities, foundations, and other sources. R&D for so-called "neglected diseases" like malaria, predominantly found only in low-income and some middle-income countries, accounted for only 1 percent of all health R&D.[39, 40] The U.S. government (National Institutes of Health, Department of Defense, USAID), European Commission, the U.K., and France top the list of public funders for health R&D. U.K.'s Wellcome Trust, the Gates Foundation, and France's Institut Pasteur lead R&D funding by the philanthropic sector.[41]

The private sector excels in developing and widely distributing health products when there is a large and proven market, as with seasonal influenza, the H1N1 swine flu vaccine, and antiviral medicines. Public and philanthropic funding can be catalytic, especially in new and basic areas of research such as universal influenza vaccine and the Global Virome Project. Public-private partnerships have proven successful in filling gaps that no one sector can fill, as in the case of Gavi, the Vaccine Alliance, and the Medicines for Malaria Venture.

We could dramatically reduce the pandemic threat if the world's major health R&D funders were to mobilize just 1 percent of the current $250 billion annual spending on a decade-long, collaborative program of innovation. A universal pandemic influenza vaccine would be the first priority. Michael Osterholm reckons that an investment of $1 billion per year, over seven to ten years, would probably get us there.[42] As of 2017, there were in fact nearly a dozen research teams working on such a vaccine, but they have only a fraction of the funding needed to maximize the chance of success.[43]

The Coalition for Epidemic Preparedness Innovation has actually been more successful, having in its first year generated $460 million of the $1 billion it needs to catalyze the development of vaccines for three viruses with pandemic potential. Commitments have come from the governments of Germany, Japan, and Norway, as well as from the Gates Foundation and the Wellcome Trust.

3. Emergency Response

Within weeks of mounting the emergency response to Ebola, Jim Yong Kim reached out to Unilever CEO Paul Polman and Nikolaus von Bomhard, the chairman of the insurance giant Munich Re. "Can't we do this better?" he asked them. "Isn't there a way of building a fail-safe instrument so that when the minute [epidemics] get bad it automatically releases emergency funds?"

The answer was an innovative $500 million Pandemic Emergency Financing (PEF) insurance policy for the 88 poorest countries. "Pandemic insurance uses the tools that rich people use every day to make themselves richer on be-half of the poorest people in the world," Jim told the audience at the Skoll World Forum 2017.[44] If this new form of insurance policy had existed and $100 million had been mobilized earlier in the Ebola outbreak, the number of cases could have been one-tenth of what they were, according to the World Bank.[45]

The PEF represents the first time in history that pandemic risk will be covered by insurance, making it easier for poor countries to protect their citizens and the world against outbreaks of infectious diseases. Instead of waiting for months or even years for money to arrive when an epidemic takes hold, poor countries can receive sufficient funding to mount a full-scale response. The insurance covers up to $500 million for a poor country for an initial period of up to three years.

It works like this: G7 donor countries and the World Bank purchase pandemic insurance coverage and pay insurance premiums on behalf of the 88 countries currently eligible for World Bank International Development Assistance. The coverage combines funding from the reinsurance markets (that is, companies like Munich Re that sell insurance to insurance companies) with the proceeds of World Bank–issued pandemic (catastrophe, or cat) bonds. Such bonds offer higher yields to investors in return for taking risks that are not correlated with the normal risks of business-cycle downturns.

"This has the potential to be a win-win-win," says the economist and former U.S. treasury secretary Larry Summers. "The World Bank is using financial innovation to mitigate a major threat to the world, and especially the world's poor. The vast resources of the global capital market are being tapped to provide vitally important insurance—and bring much-needed financial discipline to pandemic preparedness and response. And investors who, at this time of zero rates, are desperate for return are getting a new vehicle in which to invest."[46]

In the event of an outbreak, the PEF will release funds quickly to countries and qualified international agencies. In addition to helping poor countries contain infectious disease, the money can be used to shore up national health systems. A cash reserve, in the $100 million range and made up of long-term pledges from development partners, will provide additional funding to low-income countries to address outbreaks covered by insurance but that need larger and earlier payouts. That $100 million can also go toward responding to new or unknown pathogens not covered by the PEF insurance (like Zika) and toward surge funding for development partners to channel resources in the event of a crisis.

The PEF is expected to create a new market for pandemic insurance by incentivizing investments that can be used to respond better and quicker than ever before. The PEF can potentially save thousands of lives and keep the cost of response in the millions rather than the billions.

Invest Now or Pay Later

There are a million (or 7.5 billion, the current size of the world's population, and growing) reasons why it makes sense to invest in public health, not the least of which is to skirt the danger to ourselves, our families, and our societies. When outbreaks are not tackled early on and become epidemics, it takes far longer to control them, the death toll is much higher, and the secondary impacts on businesses, governments, and national and world economies much greater.

There are only two choices when it comes to epidemics: invest now in prevention and preparedness or pay later in lost lives, closed businesses, and social upheaval. Most health systems and businesses are not prepared for pandemics. They should be. As Jeremy Farrar, a prolific researcher and now director of the U.K.'s Wellcome Trust, observes, "We spend gazillions to defend ourselves from military attack, but from the beginning of the twentieth century far more people have died from infection. We are hugely vulnerable from a public health perspective."[47]

Of course, not every area of investment will be successful. There are uncertainties about the exact magnitude and frequency of epidemics. But the reality is that the more we spend up front, the more lives and money we save today and down the road. And the wonderful thing about this Power of Seven action is this: even if we overinvest, we will have made the world much safer and more prosperous in any case. It's a win-win all the way around. It's a huge benefit for so modest an investment.

CHAPTER 12

RING THE ALARM,
ROUSE THE LEADERS

Citizen activists and social movements must
mobilize the public and hold leaders' feet to the fire.

The AIDS activist Zackie Achmat, who spent years fighting to bring AIDS treatment to Africa, showed that combating an epidemic is ultimately about social justice, human rights, and accountability. Health workers like Kaci Hickox, an experienced American nurse who cared for Ebola patients, fought against stigmatization of both caregivers and those who had been infected. Citizen activists, gathered together by organizations like Global Citizen and the ONE Campaign, are crucial for mobilizing the public and holding leaders accountable to fight against denial, dithering, and self-interest. Making the world safe from pandemic threats will require a social movement of a magnitude equal to providing universal AIDS treatment or eradicating polio.

The history of public health—and indeed social development in many spheres—is replete with social movements that have made the case for a healthier, better, fairer community, country, or world. Thanks to a panoply of efforts, from nineteenth-century attempts to improve the health of the urban poor[1] to more recent movements to reduce tobacco-related deaths, control drug abuse, protect women's reproductive rights, end female genital mutilation, eradicate polio, achieve an AIDS-free generation, and end preventable child and maternal deaths, public health has come a very long way indeed.[2, 3, 4]

Looking at social progress in the twentieth century, political scientist, author, and self-described activist Peter Dreier observes, "The radical ideas of one generation have become the common sense of the next. Social movements transformed these (and many other) radical ideas from the margin to the mainstream, and from polemic to policy." The story of public health in the twentieth century, Dreier says, is a remarkable demonstration of progressive accomplishments against overwhelming odds.[5]

Activism is a Power of Seven element because without it, governments can remain stuck in the same recency bias, denial, and avoidance that put citizens at risk of suffering and dying. Sustained activism is not for the faint of heart, but when a leader provides the flint and a few followers set a spark going, others can join in the fight to get the health justice they need and deserve.

Fighting Ignorance at the Top

We couldn't believe our ears. On Sunday evening, July 9, 2000, Thabo Mbeki, the president of South Africa who had fought so hard to bring down apartheid, stood in front of 12,000 attendees at the International AIDS Conference in Durban and boldly insisted that the AIDS epidemic ravaging his country was a CIA conspiracy. The CIA had hatched HIV, he declared, to promote "poisonous" antiretroviral drugs that Western pharmaceutical companies hoped to foist on 4 million infected South Africans.[6]

Though Mbeki was intelligent, he had bought into bad science and false beliefs. Convinced that antiretroviral AIDS medicines (ARVs) were "biological warfare of the apartheid era," Mbeki believed that the directors of drug companies were white racists determined to treat his people like guinea pigs.[7] In his mind, only Africans should try to cure Africans; he held out hope for what turned out to be a highly toxic, ineffective, cheap drug called Virodene (the main ingredient of which was an industrial solvent) solely on the basis that it was developed in his country.

It was as if Mbeki had suddenly decided that the world was flat. His statements not only flew in the face of the overwhelming scientific consensus, but they displayed the most stunning denial in the face of a virulent epidemic that any of the experts in the audience had ever witnessed. The horrifying results of his intransigence had already spoken for themselves: 160,000 people had already died of AIDS in South Africa, leaving behind whole villages of orphaned children.

Though Mbeki proved to be tragically wrong about proper AIDS treatment, he was correct about one thing: poor people are always the first to succumb in an epidemic, and those in developing countries always suffer more when disease strikes. Just four years prior to the Durban conference, at the 1996 International AIDS Conference in Vancouver, Canada, the world heard the stunning news that ARV therapy was emptying hospitals in Europe and North America of patients suffering from AIDS and dramatically reducing death rates. People living with HIV/AIDS could even enjoy close to normal life expectancy. By 2000, while AIDS was fast becoming a manageable chronic disease in the global north, it remained a death sentence in the global south. In Africa, fewer than one in 20 of those infected knew they had the virus, and fewer than one in 100 of those in need of treatment were receiving it.[8]

Zackie Achmat, AIDS Denialism, and the Battle for HIV Treatment

The AIDS pandemic had ravaged many countries around the world for a generation before a combination of health education, preventive care, and the drugs that Mbeki decried finally brought the disease under a semblance of control in the global north. But the story of AIDS in South Africa is a particularly telling one. The struggle to get ARV drugs to the African poor was extremely difficult and dishearteningly long.

One of the great heroes of the fight for AIDS treatment in South Africa was Zackie Achmat. Graced with a warm, brotherly smile, Zackie led the biggest protest movement in that country since Nelson Mandela fought apartheid. I first saw Zackie in action during the 2000 Durban conference at which Mbeki made his stunning announcement. Zackie was direct, matter-of-fact, and unwavering in his condemnation of both Big Pharma prices and Mbeki's denialism.

Zackie was a determined fighter for poor South Africans all his life. Growing up in a mixed-race Muslim neighborhood on the Western Cape in the 1960s, he was part Malaysian, with honey-colored skin and a round, boyish face framed by curly, now-graying dark hair. In his "HIV Positive" T-shirt, he looked a lot more like a kindly high school teacher and soccer coach than the street fighter he's always been. Zackie was classified as "colored" under apartheid, so he was denied the privileges of whites. He detested the whites' treatment of the black friends and neighbors who worked in the same factories as his mother. In 1976, at age 14, he set fire to his school in protest.

Having developed a distinct taste for struggling against injustice, Zackie then organized for the African National Congress against apartheid. He wound up spending 15 years in jail, enduring beatings and hunger strikes.[9] Zackie also had a secret. Before going to jail, he had worked as a male prostitute. When he was 27—a few years after his release from jail and before the end of apartheid—he learned that he had contracted HIV and that AIDS was coming to kill him. In South Africa, the "gay disease" brought with it all the stigma that its sufferers had felt in America, and more.[10, 11]

In the late 1990s, he became a gay-rights and AIDS activist. When the HIV virus living in his blood finally gave him full-blown AIDS, he started a campaign to make expensive ARV drugs affordable for poor South Africans. Big Pharma was the target; brand-name drugs cost $10,000 per person per year.[12] Poor South Africans could not afford the medicine and groups like Médecins Sans Frontières and others could not raise enough money to treat patients.

Zackie founded what he called the Treatment Action Campaign, or TAC. TAC quickly caught hold, attracting dozens, then hundreds and thousands of activists. People with HIV and their supporters alike began wearing T-shirts announcing their HIV-positive status—something that previously might have gotten them beaten or killed. (The clever T-shirt tactic also made it impossible to distinguish the infected from the uninfected.) The campaign took up the cause of the 40,000 South African HIV-positive babies whose mothers could not afford the ARV drug nevirapine. Not wanting to be accused of killing babies, the country's health minister finally acquiesced and rewrote the Medicines Act to allow the government to import generic versions of the ARV drugs.

But the generics were not soon to be had. Thirty-nine of the largest drug companies sued the South African government to prevent implementation of the new legislation. And the Clinton administration, bowing to the drug industry lobbyists, initially threatened trade sanctions on South Africa. However, increasing public pressure by groups like TAC and ACT UP, and a strong legal defense provided through the WHO essential medicines program I was leading at the time, forced the industry to drop their suit in April 2001.

After three years the court battle had been won, but much work remained to make low-cost generics available.

Meanwhile, Zackie had decided to put his own life on the line. Until the government committed to extending access to AIDS treatment to all South Africans, he refused any expensive treatment for himself. In 1999, he told reporters, "That probably means I will die a horrible death . . . even though medical science has made it unnecessary." He knew the risk inherent in his pledge, but felt he had to take it. "It's wrong to be able to buy life," he said.[13]

During his long struggle with the Mbeki government, one of Zackie's closest friends and allies was Justice Edwin Cameron, a judge on the Constitutional Court. Cameron deeply believed that the law should be more than an instrument of rebuke and correction. Openly gay since the 1980s, Cameron had created an advocacy group called the AIDS Law Project, for which Zackie worked in the 1990s.[14] Cameron himself was ill with AIDS when he worked as a high-court judge, but he was able to keep going thanks to the $10,000-per-year ARVs that he could afford, unlike most poor South Africans. He also benefited from a secure job and a loving family. "What saved me from poverty was that I was white," he wrote.[15]

After witnessing Zackie's courage, Cameron recalled, his own silence was becoming unbearable. So, in 1999, he announced his condition to the world, making him one of the first public figures in his country to do so. "Speaking publicly was an enormous relief," he said.[16] For Cameron, justice first meant fighting the racism and discrimination at the root of apartheid. On the public provision of ARV, he noted, "I was campaigning for more than just a public issue. I was campaigning also for myself."[17]

Though Cameron was reviled in some quarters, his position as a respected high-court judge and as a gay man with AIDS gave him enormous credibility as a speaker and writer. During the fight for drug access, Cameron walked a precarious judicial tightrope. Yet while he had to meticulously avoid crossing the legal and political divide, he felt morally compelled to speak out for what he knew to be right.

*   *   *

Organizers for the TAC campaign put great effort into spreading the word about how treatment could save lives. The afternoon before the Mbeki speech that shocked us all, thousands of people marched in the streets of Durban to demand affordable treatment.

The AIDS conference in 2000 proved to be a pivotal moment for TAC and, as it turned out, for the movement for global access to AIDS treatment. The morning after Mbeki's speech, the conference officially opened with a powerful, moving plea by Justice Cameron on the "deafening silence of AIDS."[18] He criticized Mbeki's ignorant stance and noted that each month, 5,000 South African babies were born with HIV. He called for equitable drug pricing.[19] "In my own country, a government that in its commitment to human rights and democracy has been a shining example to Africa and the world, has at almost every conceivable turn mismanaged the epidemic," he said. Three years later, Cameron would deliver a stinging speech at Harvard Law School in which he linked AIDS denialism in South Africa to Holocaust denial.[20, 21]

Even as government denial and dithering persisted, TAC fought back by sending teams to rural villages and crowded city townships to teach people how to use ARVs properly (with what limited supplies were available). TAC did this despite the Mbeki administration's insistence that the hospitals didn't have the infrastructure to deliver the drug treatment. All the while, people with HIV were getting sicker and dying; Zackie still refused to take expensive lifesaving drugs. Word of his drug strike spread and people around the world began paying more attention to the cause. Elton John made Zackie a guest of honor at his annual AIDS Foundation ball. *Time Europe* selected him as its annual "Hero."[22] Finally, after a long and disturbing silence, former president Nelson Mandela went on television to publicly embrace what TAC was doing. TAC's combination of mass protests, a widespread treatment-literacy campaign and AIDS education program, and media outreach was critical in changing hearts and minds. In addition to enlisting Nelson Mandela in the fight, TAC prompted other widely respected South African leaders to speak out for AIDS treatment.

Despite these efforts and the rising national and international outcry, President Mbeki remained intransigent. It was time to escalate the battle to the courts. Nathan Geffen, TAC's astute campaign strategist, cleverly advised TAC's leaders not to reach straight for the "golden ring" of universal access to AIDS treatment. The battle would be won instead through a step-by-step series of smaller legal wins. In 2002, TAC asked South Africa's highest court to make nevirapine available to HIV-positive pregnant women to prevent transmission of the virus to their children. "We showed that this program would save costs by keeping kids from getting infected," Geffen told me. "We weren't asking the court very much in terms of changing policy, other than to say that the current policy wasn't reasonable. Also, the rights in the constitution with regard to children were much more enforceable than they were for adults."[23] The South African courts had little choice but to hand over a victory. "We got criticized because we were asking for something so modest. But it didn't matter, because it was a plank on which the bigger program was built," Geffen said. South Africa's highest legal body, the Constitutional Court, agreed with TAC, and eventually women began receiving the drug.[24]

Geffen attributed the legal win to TAC's four-point strategy: (1) research—understand the disease, the medicines, and what it takes to deliver treatment; (2) mobilization—talking to people about how treatment saves lives, getting thousands of people marching and building a "crescendo of people calling for treatment"; (3) media outreach—taking the moral and practical case for treatment access to the public; and (4) legal strategy—using the courts to push the boundaries that could not otherwise be breached.[25]

When I asked Geffen whether ARVs for pregnant women would have come sooner if TAC had simply gone straight to court, without all the public protests, he was unequivocal: "Without the other three components, the legal strategy could not work." He explained that there had been many successful court cases against South African injustices. But even the greatest victory was empty without enforcement. With the nevirapine win, he explained, "the health minister made it clear she would not carry out the judgment."

In contrast to the case of SARS in China, public shaming of Mbeki and his cabinet ministers was not doing the trick. A bigger fight was necessary. So, in 2003, Zackie and TAC organized a massive campaign of civil disobedience. Activists put up "wanted" posters with the cabinet ministers' faces everywhere. Every day, hundreds of people crowded into police stations and government buildings all over the country. The public support was enormous.

By this time, Zackie was desperately ill and many people, including Mandela, argued that his drug strike had to stop because he was much more useful as a living leader than as a martyr. He gave in only when TAC demanded at its annual conference that Zackie stop his drug strike. Within two weeks of taking the ARV pills, his energy came flowing back.

Jim Yong Kim, then head of WHO's AIDS division and a vigorous champion of social justice, joined the battle. He was appalled that the same government that had fought so hard to end apartheid could be so stubbornly opposed to helping its people when it came to AIDS treatment. "To succeed, you've got to have political buy-in from the very top—you can't have the president and the health minister ambivalent about scaling-up care. The epidemic is fundamentally dropping the life expectancy of Thabo Mbeki's people," said Kim. "He has to get personally involved and hold people accountable. He has to say, 'Okay, how many did we get this week, why are we going so slowly?' If he did that, South Africa could get to treating 500,000 people in a matter of months—they have so much more capacity than any other country in Africa."[26]

Mbeki's government finally gave in to the pressure and slowly began rolling out AIDS treatment in 2004. However, it was not until 2008, when Mbeki was removed from power, that a new minister of health, Barbara Hogan, could officially declare that "[t]he era of denialism is over completely in South Africa."[27] Treatment access accelerated so much that a million people were on medication by 2010, making South Africa's program the biggest in the world.[28] There it remains today.[29]

Zackie's fight to bring AIDS treatment to Africa showed that fighting an epidemic is ultimately about far more than public health. Making the world safe from pandemic threats in the future will require that millions of us around the world stand up not just for public health but also for social justice, human rights, and political accountability.

From Local Campaigns to a Global Movement

Despite President Mbeki's paranoid rhetoric, the year 2000 proved to be a positive tipping point for people at risk of AIDS. That year, the Clinton administration, pressured by the HIV/AIDS patient advocacy organization ACT UP, said "no" to the Big Pharma–funded lobbyists who had refused, on patent (and greedy) grounds, to sanction the use of generic ARV drugs in South Africa. In September, combating AIDS became one of the eight Millennium Development Goals to which world leaders committed themselves. Led by UN secretary-general Kofi Annan, WHO director-general Gro Brundtland, UNAIDS executive director Peter Piot, Irish rock-star-turned-activist Bono, Bill and Melinda Gates, and committed governments on every continent, the multibillion-dollar Global Fund to Fight AIDS, Tuberculosis, and Malaria was launched in 2002. At his 2003 State of the Union address, George W. Bush announced the U.S. President's Emergency Plan for AIDS Relief

(PEPFAR). Together these programs created the largest public-health program to treat a single disease in global health history.[30]

What began as campaigns by ACT UP, TAC, MSF, and AIDS activists around the globe had become a highly successful social movement driven collectively by international agencies, national governments, universities, NGOs, and a host of other partners.[31, 32, 33] AIDS first showed up in the early 1980s; it took more than 15 years for an effective antiretroviral treatment to become available, and millions died in the interim.[34] Yet in the 15 years from 2000 to 2015, those with access to lifesaving AIDS medicines increased 25-fold, from 690,000 to 17 million people worldwide.[35, 36]

Enormous threats to life and health around the world remain, of course. But if we consider how much has changed in the world of HIV/AIDS alone, clearly the success spurred by activists has been stunning. "What the facts are telling us is that the long, slow journey—humanity's long, slow journey of equality—is actually speeding up," Bono told a TED audience in 2013. "Look at what's been achieved. . . . Since the year 2000, since the turn of the millennium, there are 8 million more AIDS patients getting life-saving antiretroviral drugs."[37]

Fighting Stigma and Politics

Regardless of their station in life, the people who get sick, as well as their caregivers, are also among the first to be suspect, thanks to the fear-driven and uninformed human desire to stigmatize anyone associated with disease. Sometimes, as ACT UP has so successfully demonstrated, the only way to fight back against stigma and political ignorance is with activism.

Consider the parallels between the AIDS epidemic, which first spread in the U.S. more than 30 years ago, and the West African Ebola virus, which resurfaced issues of scapegoating, political grandstanding, blame, and human rights. Public hysteria over AIDS drove people to stigmatize and harass gay men and heroin users. In her book *Betrayal of Trust: The Collapse of Global Public Health*, the journalist activist Laurie Garrett summarized the "othering" of HIV/AIDS victims this way: "[T]he homes of hemophiliacs were burned, masses of gay men died with little attention from the heterosexual communities around them, intravenous drug users were denied sterile syringes, female prostitutes were imprisoned or denied access to health care, and many medical and dental providers refused to allow HIV positive individuals access to care unrelated to their infections."[38]

The stigma suffered by Ebola patients and their caregivers was strikingly similar to the experiences of AIDS patients. After recovering from the near-death experience of an Ebola infection, survivors in Liberia reported facing hostility, exclusion, and unemployment. Many survivors came home to find their possessions destroyed.[39] Even those risking their lives to help patients with Ebola faced devastating stigma; some medical workers were murdered. "If we fall victim [to the disease]," a physician's assistant with MSF wondered, "will the [people in my hometown] rejoice and be happy we're dead and gone?"[40]

One of the victims of stigma was a 35-year-old nurse named Kaci Hickox who worked with MSF to treat Ebola patients in Sierra Leone; previously, she had responded to outbreaks of cholera, measles, and yellow fever. As was the case with all MSF medical volunteers, she had been extremely careful to follow the standard protocols to protect herself from contracting the virus. After spending four exhausting and emotionally draining weeks in Africa, she was looking forward to returning to her home in Maine when she arrived at Newark International Airport in October 2014. She'd been traveling for two days. She was hungry, tired, and jet-lagged when she arrived. She had no idea that she was about to undergo an even more trying ordeal, courtesy of New Jersey governor Chris Christie.

Along with the governors of New York, Illinois, and Florida, Christie had issued a mandatory 21-day quarantine on anyone returning from West Africa, against the recommendations of public-health and infectious-disease experts. Although she had tested negative for Ebola, Hickox was quarantined in a plastic tent inside an unheated parking garage at the University Hospital in Newark, New Jersey. Her quarantine was stricter than federal standards required. The tent was equipped with a bed, a port-a-potty, and no shower. She was not allowed visitors and could only communicate with her family by cell phone. "I felt like Governor Christie was trying to hide what he was doing to me," she recalled. "I felt scared and alone. It made no sense that I could not see and speak to my loved ones through the tent window."[41]

Quarantine is reasonable in certain medically justifiable circumstances, such as when people are suffering with active cases of Ebola and other highly contagious diseases. But policies based on fear rather than scientific evidence inflame hysteria because they lead the public to believe that those without symptoms are secretly infectious. Hickox turned out to be a convenient political tool. Christie, who was then head of the Republican Governors' Association and planning a run for the U.S. presidency, made a great show of uncalled-for decisiveness in this situation, despite the fact that Hickox posed no risk to anyone. He lied about her condition, saying she was "obviously ill."[42] "I don't believe when you're dealing with something as serious as this that we can count on a voluntary system," Christie told Fox News. "The government's job is to protect [the] safety and health of our citizens. And so we've taken this action, and I absolutely have no second thoughts about it."[43] In a perfect example of fearmongering, a Christie representative told *Newsweek* that the quarantine policy was meant to calm public hysteria "and to give people a sense of certainty that people who may have Ebola will not be traveling around their neighborhoods."[44] Such edicts only made people more afraid.

Governor Bobby Jindal of Louisiana, another failed 2016 presidential contender, similarly turned the Ebola epidemic into fodder for his campaign to halt immigration. Jindal suggested that the U.S. ought to close its borders to people coming from West Africa, a move that would have increased the isolation of devastated countries and made it harder to deliver essential aid there.[45] As WHO assistant director-general Bruce Aylward stated, such arbitrary travel bans make the world sicker, not safer. "The more difficulty you have with travel and trade, the harder it is to have an appropriate response," Aylward noted.[46] Indeed, drastic policies can backfire in other ways. As was the case with the Texas Ebola patient Thomas Duncan, patients returning from pandemic-affected countries may be disinclined to report their travel history. And what doctor or nurse would want to volunteer to work in the hot zone, only to return to stigma and the prospect of isolation in a cold, showerless plastic tent?

After she was released from quarantine, Hickox went home to Maine. There, her governor wanted to hold her under yet another quarantine, but a judge overruled that move.[47] The judge's decision set a legal precedent that may have dissuaded other government officials from isolating more returning Ebola workers. With support from the ACLU, Hickox filed a lawsuit against Christie and other state officials for $250,000, alleging false imprisonment, invasion of privacy, and violation of due process, among other claims. Once more, the AIDS activist group ACT UP helped, creating a Facebook profile called ACT UP Against EBOLA and calling for a "smart, science-based reaction" to the disease. ACT UP sent a letter cosigned by 114 AIDS researchers, activists, and public-health experts to New York governor Andrew

Cuomo, calling the quarantine order unscientific and shameful. Mark Harrington, an ACT UP member and executive director of TAC and ACT UP, told *Newsweek* that "[o]ne of the clearest lessons we learned from the AIDS epidemic is that politicians make bad scientists."[48]

Other activists helped to protect health workers against stigma and to ensure their protection. Human Rights Watch, Amnesty International, and other advocacy organizations demanded better protection for health workers. After two Texas nurses came down with Ebola, an 18,000-member professional organization called National Nurses United polled thousands of nurses at hospitals in 46 states. Of those who responded, 85 percent said their hospitals were not providing training during which nurses could ask questions. Taking these numbers to the press, the nurses spoke out loudly and clearly about the need for the very best protective suits and training and against attempts to blame them for the spread of the disease.[49]

"When we allow government officials to create policies that are not scientifically sound and fail to protect the health of the public, we allow the diseases we are fighting against to win," Hickox insists. "As a nurse, I was trained to be an advocate, yet I never thought I would need to be an advocate for myself and my colleagues in order to advocate for our patients. We need to learn from our mistakes in order to be better prepared for the next public-health crisis, and to protect people from government overreach during times of fear."[50]

Global Citizen and ONE: Strength in Numbers

All great civil rights struggles succeed when the number of people who participate in them is so overwhelmingly large that leaders have no choice but to meet their demands. Today, in an era of Twitter, Facebook, and other popular social media outlets, calling for change has never been easier; the trick is to get people to do more than click on a link, however.

One contemporary example of a mass online civil action movement is Global Citizen. The *New York Times* has called its founder, 33-year-old Hugh Evans, "a prodigy of philanthropy." When the Australian "philanthropreneur"[51] was 14, he spent time in a Manila slum where he became friends with Sonny Boy, a child who lived on a mountain of steaming garbage. "'Smoky Mountain' was what they called it," Evans says in his February 2016 TED talk.[52] "But don't let the romance of that name fool you, because it was nothing more than a rancid landfill that kids like Sonny Boy spent hours rummaging through every single day to find something, anything of value."

After that experience, Evans declared that he would spend his life ending extreme poverty. As cofounder of the advocacy organization Global Poverty Project and founder of Global Citizen, he's stuck with that vision ever since—cleverly using rock music to achieve it. "If we're to try to help kids like Sonny Boy, it wouldn't work just to try to send him a few dollars or to try to clean up the garbage dump where he lived, because the core of the problem lay elsewhere," Evans told the TED audience. "Although charity is necessary, it's not sufficient. We need to confront these challenges on a global scale and in a systemic way. And the best thing I could do is try to mobilize a large group of citizens back home to insist that our leaders engage in that systemic change."

Beginning with the premise that music is an irresistible lure, Evans organized the first of Global Citizen's massive benefit concerts on the Great Lawn of New York's Central Park in 2012. He persuaded city officials to grant the permit and got a concert promoter to produce the show gratis. Rock stars like Neil Young donated their time, along with well-known bands like Foo Fighters and the Black Keys. By 2015, Stevie Wonder, Kings of Leon, Alicia Keys, and John Mayer were headlining the late-September festival. True to his word, Evans wasn't just trying to raise money but to get people to take action. Concertgoers could not buy tickets; they had to earn them by signing up at globalcitizen.org, where they could gain points toward tickets by watching videos about extreme poverty and disease around the world, posting information on social media, signing digital petitions, and donating money to charities. The intent, Evans told the *New York Times*, was to "gamify the whole experience" and create a "sustainable movement."[53]

Evans claims that in 2015, Global Citizen signed up an astonishing 100,000 members every week. That's a lot of people committed to ending poverty, disease, environmental damage, and more. Working together, millions of Global Citizen members claim to have persuaded governments around the world to invest in education, sanitation, and health care. Pressure on world government leaders to step up has worked; from the stage of the Global Citizen concert, World Bank president Jim Yong Kim announced donations from various government entities worth $15 billion.

On the health front, one of Global Citizen's efforts is to generate support for Gavi, the Vaccine Alliance, which is dedicated to increasing access to vaccines. Since 2000, GAVI has helped to immunize more than half a billion children. Global Citizen directly asks world leaders to pledge the resources needed to vaccinate more children. For example, 46,000 members of the group signed a petition in partnership with the ONE Campaign and delivered it to USAID administrator Raj Shah in 2014. Pledges from around the world exceeded GAVI's fundraising goal of $7.5 billion to vaccinate 300 million more children in developing countries.[54]

Gavi leverages its strength by partnering with another advocacy organization, the aforementioned ONE Campaign. It's called "ONE" because it's about bringing its 7 million members around the world together to have one voice to end poverty and disease, particularly in Africa. ONE's tagline is "We're not asking for your money, we're asking for your voice." ONE hires PhDs to prepare policy papers, conduct research, and lobby governments in an effort to raise awareness about health and poverty issues and to shine a light on governmental secrecy and corruption that prevents people in poverty from getting the help they need.

Like Global Citizen, ONE raises public awareness and puts pressure on political leaders, but unlike Global Citizen, it doesn't distribute money on the ground. Rather, it partners with organizations like World Vision, Oxfam, and the Bill and Melinda Gates Foundation to further their programs. ONE claims that its advocacy efforts have helped more than 10.7 million people living in sub-Saharan Africa today to have access to AIDS medication, up from only 52,000 in 2002. The organization says malaria deaths have been cut by 66 percent in sub-Saharan African countries since 2000, and 60 million more children across sub-Saharan Africa are now going to primary school compared to 2000, thanks to its campaigns.[55]

Like Global Citizen, ONE rouses members to action through the heavy use of online communities, social media, YouTube ads, and, of course, rock star power. Celebrity spokespeople such as U2 front man Bono (ONE's cofounder) talk to the media and take televised trips to areas suffering from poverty in order to illustrate the issues ONE is attempting to solve. Bono has proven an excellent spokesperson for ONE, not only because he is a celebrity but also because he loves data and has no compunction when asking people who otherwise might be strange bedfellows to help out. To persuade George W. Bush to continue funding for the PEPFAR program, he applied all the persuasive tools in his control. "Bono came in and floored me with his knowledge, his energy, and his faith," Bush said.[56] Bush persuaded Congress to buy in, and PEPFAR was refunded.

Thanks to the activists' work, we now know much more about how individuals and community-based organizations can fight back against dithering, denial, complacency, greed, and secrecy. We now understand how individuals can deploy scientific, legal, and media resources to fight for public health, and how mass civil actions and protests can bring those who can't or won't protect the poor and the ostracized to heel.

Building a Social Movement to End Epidemics

I'm always astonished at how a single powerful but misguided leader like Mbeki and his compliant minions—combined with public ignorance, fear, and inertia—can condemn thousands of innocent people to preventable deaths. But if there is one thing I've learned about stopping epidemics, it's that activism works. As Gandhi understood, civil action often involves terrible personal sacrifice and limitless patience to force systemic change. Zackie Achmat, Edwin Cameron, Nathan Geffen, and countless other TAC members and supporters changed the lives of people living with HIV/AIDS in South Africa. Like the incessant beating of waves upon rocks, the ongoing work of people like them—and every single one of us—can force change over time. We all win when thousands or millions of us join together to force ignorant leaders and complacent governments to do the right thing through loud and energetic protests; evidence-based, irrefutable science; strong alternative leadership; ongoing media attention; and legal action.

Campaigns like TAC, the ONE Campaign, and Global Citizen are examples of essential forces that can achieve local progress. But major social change requires a larger-scale social movement that is broader and messier than individual campaigns. TAC, for example, became part of the movement to provide universal access to AIDS treatment. The efforts of ONE and Global Citizen are part of the broader social movement to end extreme poverty. When individual campaigns combine, the forces of activism strengthen from gale-force winds to hurricanes.

What are the prospects for building such a social movement to end infectious-disease epidemics? I would say they're quite good. Combining

Building a Successful Social Movement

Large-scale social change and impact require the right people, a persuasive case, tangible goals, and strategies for action.

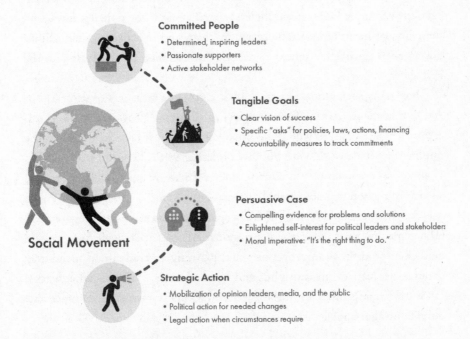

Committed People
- Determined, inspiring leaders
- Passionate supporters
- Active stakeholder networks

Tangible Goals
- Clear vision of success
- Specific "asks" for policies, laws, actions, financing
- Accountability measures to track commitments

Persuasive Case
- Compelling evidence for problems and solutions
- Enlightened self-interest for political leaders and stakeholders
- Moral imperative: "It's the right thing to do."

Social Movement

Strategic Action
- Mobilization of opinion leaders, media, and the public
- Political action for needed changes
- Legal action when circumstances require

SOURCE: Authors' synthesis formulation based on: Busby J. *Moral movements and foreign policy.* Cambridge: Cambridge University Press, 2010. Berridge V. Public health activism: lessons from history? *British Medical Journal* 2007; 335(7633): 1310–2. Dreier P. Social Movements: How People Make History. Mobilizing Ideas. 2012. https://mobilizingideas.wordpress.com/2012/08/01/socialmovementshowpeoplemakehistory/ (accessed 6 March 2017). Quick J. Smith F. 15 March 2017; by email. Fryer B. Coe J. 17 June 2016; by email.

Nathan Geffen's four-point strategy for the AIDS Treatment Action Campaign, described earlier, and the observations of researchers and effective advocates together suggest four critical factors for a building a high impact social movement: committed people, tangible goals, a persuasive case, and action strategies.

In reality, the movement to end epidemics has already started, as illustrated by the success stories and examples of leadership I have described in the preceding pages. The increasing pandemic threat has already attracted increased attention and action by world leaders, business leaders, WHO, the World Bank, scores of governments, and countless universities and citizen organizations, as I will describe in the epilogue.

Today, the success of the movement to end pandemic threats might be measured by the very high degree of consensus among public-health leaders and scientists about what must be done to contain them.[57, 58] There are exciting achievements in many critical areas, but, as I have pointed out, there are critical gaps yet to be filled. Nonetheless, specific "asks" for policies, laws, and financing commitments are increasingly clear, and there are accountability measures to track achievements against commitments, as I'll describe in the epilogue.

For many social movements, there are tangible measures of success. For AIDS treatment, that indicator is access to affordable drugs. For polio eradication, it's zero cases of wild poliovirus. For poverty, it's the reduction in the number of people worldwide who live on less than $1.25 per person per day. Even for issues as complex as climate change, there are quantifiable measures, such as reduction in global greenhouse gas emissions.[59]

Sustained, broad-based progress in epidemic prevention and preparedness takes time, just as it did in the fight against AIDS, the struggle for access to medicines, and the eradication of polio. Fighting an epidemic is ultimately about social justice, human rights, and accountability. We know what works. If we are to end epidemics in the twenty-first century, we must embrace and build upon that knowledge.

EPILOGUE

HEADLINES FROM THE FUTURE

The threat is imminent. The pathway is known.
The time for action is now.

At this point in my career, I have seen enough horror to know what's at stake for the world today and for our children and grandchildren. I have also seen epidemic diseases eradicated and global health challenges that just a few years ago seemed impossible to deal with come to an end. It's within our power to free the world from the risk of catastrophic epidemics.

It's unacceptable that a healthy 12-year-old child would develop a sudden fever one day and die just a few days later, as Eddie MacNeal did during the 1918 flu. It's intolerable that nurses caring for Ebola-stricken patients should be vulnerable to the disease themselves, as happened to Nina Pham and Amber Vinson, who fell ill while working in a Dallas, Texas, hospital. It's tragic that whole families and communities should be wiped out, as they were in the West Africa Ebola epidemic. And it's nonsensical that entire cities should be closed to travelers because of epidemics, as were Toronto and some Chinese cities during the 2003 SARS outbreak.

The Ebola epidemic put international, national, and local governments, as well as public-health officials, on immediate notice. It was a real-life test of national and international prevention and response capabilities, and the verdict was not good: we were caught flat-footed. The health systems of West Africa were not ready to deal with the crisis. And if they can be excused because of lack of resources, what about the World Health Organization, which was also unprepared? What about the CDC? And what about the people of countries outside West Africa, who were also unprepared?

The Good News

In part I of this book, I presented compelling evidence that the pandemic threat is real, potentially devastating, and growing. Bill Gates's nightmare of a global pandemic that kills millions is not science fiction. The threat has never been greater. Population growth, urbanization, international travel, food animal production practices, forest clearance, and a rapidly warming climate all increase our collective risk. The potential for international bioterror attacks or accidental laboratory bio-error events only adds to our worries.

Paradoxically, despite the magnitude of the danger, our potential to prevent and stop epidemics has never been greater either. For 50 years, we have made dramatic progress in controlling infectious diseases, beginning with the eradication of smallpox. Each year, highly trained public-health experts in countries around the globe successfully contain hundreds of outbreaks. While public-health systems in Liberia, Guinea, and Sierra Leone utterly failed during the first months of the West Africa Ebola epidemic, three neighboring countries (Nigeria, Mali, and Senegal) stopped Ebola in its tracks. And advances in vaccines, drugs, and twenty-first-century technologies such as web crawlers—combined with a better-informed public—put effective solutions within reach.

In part II, I described The Power of Seven—the critical areas for action. Together, these actions will save millions of lives. A very modest annual investment of $1 for each global inhabitant will return $3 to $10 in savings. Perhaps the strongest argument for collective action is the moral imperative: we cannot leave our families and our children with a world that is increasingly at risk for deadly epidemics and pandemics.

Since I began working on this book, much has changed in the world of epidemic prevention. There is much good news. Following the Ebola peak in 2015, international agencies, national governments, the business sector, civil society, academia, and other stakeholders became much more engaged in global health security. In chapter 6, I shared how courageous, decisive leaders stopped deadly viruses. In chapter 7, I described how more than 60 countries have committed to the WHO Joint External Evaluation initiative to bring their epidemic prevention and preparedness capabilities up to international standards. In chapter 8, I illustrated how vaccines, mosquito control, and other prevention efforts stop killer diseases before they spread. In chapter 9, I demonstrated the role that empathic listening, fact-based communication, and local engagement play in combating epidemics and preventing panic. In chapter 10, I showed how new programs such as the Coalition for Epidemic Preparedness Innovations are accelerating innovation in vaccines, medicines, diagnostics, and other essential areas. In chapter 11, I described how increased investment in global health security by governments, the World Bank, the private sector, and foundations can dramatically reduce the risk of disease outbreaks. And in chapter 12, I showed how citizen activists can force their governments to do the right thing.

Despite all the hard work that emerging-disease teams are doing, however, we're not yet close to where we need to be. Making the world safe from epidemic threats requires major commitments. It demands continuing political and financial support from all around the world—from Brasilia, to Brazzaville, to Berlin, to Beijing. It requires funding from foundations and the private sector. Such commitments cannot depend on which political party is in power. They can't be made and kept by some countries and not others, or held only when there is a disease outbreak. To get where we need to be, such commitments require sustained international support over the next 10 to 20 years.

I do not believe such commitments can be kept without a visible and vocal social movement. Consider the increasingly diverse demands on governments, corporations, and research institutions: humanitarian crises, refugee crises, natural disasters, cyber threats, global warming, hunger, and others. Each of these threats demands attention and resources. Given the pressure on leaders, it's unlikely that sufficient attention will be paid to the risk of a devastating epidemic or global pandemic without significant pressure from all of us.

What Can You Do?

I hope you will apply what you've learned from this book to your personal health habits, your family, your community, your political and civic engagement, and your work.

If you are a local or national political leader, you can make epidemic awareness one of your priorities. Be sure your public-health team is keeping you informed of the epidemic risks they are confronting. Ask them what actions they are taking to prevent, detect, and respond to threats. How are they assessing their own readiness? Do they have the resources they need to protect the people for whom you're responsible?

If you are a business leader, ask yourself and your executive team: Do we have the strategy we need to keep our business in business through a global pandemic? What is our plan to keep our staff safe? How can we apply our expertise and capacity to combat epidemics and support our stakeholders?

If you are a scientist, can you teach or study subjects having to do with epidemic prevention and response? Can you connect your work to the full landscape of knowledge, experience, and innovation that affects our epidemic and pandemic readiness?

If you are a healthcare professional, are you fully informed about epidemic threats like influenza, Zika, or new pathogens? Are you able to answer questions and talk about the benefits of childhood and adult immunizations with patients and families? Are you able to guide them to reliable sources of information and to thoughtfully separate false claims from real ones? Do you practice what you preach by getting an annual flu shot and being vigilant when traveling?

If you are someone interested in your own health, the health of your family and friends, or the health of future generations, do you know how to protect against infectious diseases with good personal hygiene, immunization, clean water, safe food, and a healthy local environment? Are you aware of the resources available in your community for epidemic prevention and preparedness? Do you know if your community and your nation are taking necessary action to keep you safe from infectious disease threats? Do you know where to turn if you're interested in supporting action to end epidemics?

Whoever you are, joining the movement to combat infectious-disease threats will put you in good company. The necessity and capacity to end epidemics have attracted many inspiring champions: Bill Gates, MSF president Dr. Joanne Liu, World Bank president Jim Yong Kim, Unilever CEO Paul Polman, and others, about whom you've read in the preceding chapters. You can join a rapidly expanding network of committed stakeholders from a wide range of organizations and sectors whose work crosses political, professional, geographic, generational, cultural, and social boundaries.

For example, my own nonprofit health group, Management Sciences for Health (www.msh.org), is working to build resilient, locally led health systems in more than two dozen countries in Africa, Asia, and Latin America. And we are advocating for increased support to combat pandemics from the U.S. government and the G7 and G20 countries. You can join with groups like Global Citizen (www.globalcitizen.org), which is mobilizing people of all ages around the world to fight the world's biggest challenges, including poverty and pandemics. You'll find more on these and other opportunities to help on *The End of Epidemics* website (www.endofepidemics.com).

Headlines from the Future

What will success look like after one to two decades of effective, persistent action? Here are examples of the sort of headlines I believe could one day be true:

"Near Perfect" Response Stopped SARS-M4

Bellagio, Italy, September 2, 2026 (AP)—"Rapid, decisive action" on the part of health officials and scientists prevented a deadly new virus, SARS-M4, from turning into a global pandemic. That was the conclusion the World Health Organization's (WHO) director-general Dr. David Collins shared with experts attending a three-day response-review conference at Italy's Rockefeller Foundation Bellagio Center.

Collins said that the 2025 outbreak of the highly infectious airborne SARS-M4 (a genetic cousin of the 2003 SARS virus) could easily have infected over 5 million people in scores of countries and lasted several months. Instead, SARS-M4 was contained in fewer than eight weeks. There were 5,065 cases and 570 deaths reported in 15 countries.

In March of last year, SARS-M4 was detected in bat populations in Asia and Latin America. In the first week of June, the first human cases were reported almost simultaneously in Brazil and China. By June 30, the new Global Outbreak Early Warning System (GOEWS) had identified SARS-M4 cases in the cities of Nairobi, Kenya; Dar es Salaam, Tanzania; Kampala, Uganda; and Rio de Janeiro, Brazil. A Chinese businessman who had traveled to Nairobi and two American tourists returning from Rio de Janeiro died of the disease.

On July 3, Collins declared a PHEIC (Public Health Emergency of International Concern) immediately following a conference call with the WHO public-health emergency committee. Within 24 hours, China, Brazil, and all three affected East African countries had activated emergency operation centers. On July 7, the UN Health Security Council convened a meeting of national and business leaders to address the threat of the virus and contain economic disruption.

By July 20, more than 500 cases of SARS-M4 had been reported from East Africa. Though hospitals were quickly overwhelmed by patients requiring the highest-level isolation, teams of expert volunteers, mobilized through the expanded Global Outbreak Alert and Response Network (GOARN), arrived in East Africa and Brazil from Britain, the U.S., Sweden, China, and Israel. Meanwhile, scientists quickly developed rapid tests, which streamlined patient and traveler assessments.

Erika Mitchell, an emergency-room nurse at Dallas Presbyterian Hospital, identified the first U.S. cases in the travelers from Brazil, who were quickly admitted and placed in isolation units. Mitchell, who also came down with the virus, was quickly treated and has fully recovered.

Collins, a veteran of the 2003 SARS pandemic, told the assembly at Bellagio that containment of SARS-M4 is a "near-perfect example of how the new global epidemic prevention and response strategy is working."

New Vaccine Highly Effective against Deadly Avian Flu

Atlanta, Georgia, April 15, 2028 (Reuters)—The CDC announced today that the Universal Influenza Vaccine (UIV) has proven highly effective against the deadly H7N9 avian flu that broke out last month in Guangdong, China. According to CDC director Dr. Barbara Frye, there were fewer than 6 million cases and 2 million deaths worldwide, compared to more than 150 million cases and 50 million deaths in the 2020 pandemic.

Introduced in September 2027, the UIV vaccine has been given to over 80 percent of the world's 8.3 billion people. More than 150 national pandemic-response teams working in every country distributed the vaccine.

The UIV was the product of the $12 billion NIH-led decade-long U.S. Presidential Pandemic Initiative. NIH director Dr. Ted Shuster credited "extraordinary collaboration among university research teams, regulatory agencies, and pharmaceutical companies worldwide" for both vaccine development and innovation that enabled rapid production of sufficient vaccine.

Measles Eradicated Worldwide

Geneva, Switzerland, May 25, 2038 (Deutsche Zeitung)—World Health Organization director-general Atul Panjabi announced to the World Health Assembly that measles, one of the greatest-known childhood killers, has been eradicated. The last reported measles cases occurred in the Central African Republic and a vaccine-skeptical community in the U.S. state of Minnesota in 2037. Since that time, no further cases have been reported.

Inspired by the 1977 eradication of smallpox, the measles campaign follows the elimination of Guinea-worm (dracunculiasis) in 2024, polio in 2028, sleeping sickness in 2034, and malaria in 2037.

The measles eradication battle was fought first in poor countries with weak governments and immunization programs. A concerted effort to strengthen health systems and a decade-long public-health education program resulted in immunization rates of 95 percent.

The second front in the eradication fight took place in Europe and North America, where discredited theories of vaccine harm drove down immunization rates. Following measles outbreaks that sickened and killed thousands of children in Italy, Romania, and the U.S. states of Minnesota and California, a grassroots campaign led by Morgan McCulloch, who lost her only child to measles, became a global movement. "Mothers for Vaccines" turned the antivaccine tide through thousands of local community gatherings.

"Today, thanks to vaccine acceptance, we celebrate the end of yet another disease that has killed and maimed children for centuries," Panjabi told the assembly.

*   *   *

I truly believe that courageous leadership, resilient health systems, active prevention, effective communication, breakthrough innovations, and very modest annual investment will put us on the right path before the next pandemic takes a terrible toll. It will take all of us to make these "headlines from the future" a reality. But we can do it. We know how to stop the next epidemic. There is no excuse for unpreparedness. If we are to save ourselves and our children, we must act decisively. The threat is real. The pathway is known. The time for action is now.

ACKNOWLEDGMENTS

Writing a book is always a journey of people, places, and ideas. I was really blessed to have had the right fellow travelers at each step in the creation of *The End of Epidemics*. At the start of the journey were Jim Stone, then chair of the MSH Board of Directors, and Mim Nelson, an MSH Board member and best-selling author. Jim grasped what was at stake from the beginning and urged me to write about preventing pandemics. I decided fairly quickly that I did not want to write another technical book or textbook, but instead one aimed at a much broader audience and impact. Mim Nelson mentored and encouraged me in navigating the publication process.

The blueprint for this book was developed during a four-month sabbatical from MSH in the fall of 2015, the central part of which was a resident fellowship at the Rockefeller Foundation Bellagio Center on Italy's Lake Como. Michael Myers and Robert Marten provided encouragement, and Julio Frenk, David Heymann, and Ariel Pablos-Mendez provided essential support for my fellowship application.

From our first conversation at the Chart House in Boston, my agent, Todd Shuster, grasped the urgency of the challenge of infectious-disease epidemics and my vision for the book. Through multiple drafts of the book proposal, he pushed me to distill the nature of epidemics threats and the plan for attacking them into compelling stories with convincing evidence.

Todd connected me with my collaborator, Bronwyn Fryer. She is a passionate writer who cares deeply about contributing to a fairer, better world. Bronwyn has a gift for separating the wheat from the chaff, and she continually challenged me to get the heart of the matter. Her probing questions and frank feedback always made for a better product. For me, writing a book has been a journey of hills and valleys each time. Bronwyn was always ready to celebrate the view from the hills and to help push me out of the valleys.

At St. Martin's Press, editor-in-chief George Witte and associate publisher Laura Clark identified the need to dramatically expand descriptions of the threats from the bush, the barn, and the bioterrorist. George's clear, steady, and matter-of-fact style—combined with the upbeat, supportive approach of assistant editor Sara Thwaite and production editor Donna Cherry—made for a very smooth publication process.

I was fortunate to have highly capable MSH staff and colleagues assisting in this effort. Jo Ellen Warner made invaluable contributions through her outstanding writing skills, experience in epidemic and crisis communications, wise advice, and organizational skills. Jon Rohde and Fred Hartman provided extremely helpful critiques of the full manuscript. Mia Roca Alcover, who developed the infographics, was a wonderfully insightful, creative, and responsive partner throughout the process. Christine Rogers, Niranjan Konduri, JoAnn Paradis, and Mackenzie Allen provided very helpful reviews of the draft infographics. My deep appreciation also goes to Chelsey Canavan for her thoughtful suggestions and in-depth research during the early phases of this work; Elaine Appleton Grant and Sherry Knecht for their superb manuscript editing and smart questions; Amanda Kirk for meticulous proofreading, fact-checking, and formatting of references; and Leah Perkinson for her excellent, speedy research.

Throughout the journey from concept to completion of this book, MSH colleagues past and present from the home office and the field were incredibly encouraging and supportive. I will be forever grateful to Larry Fish, chair, and the entire MSH Board of Directors; Marian Wentworth, current MSH president and CEO; MSH leaders Catharine Taylor, Douglas Keene, Pat Nicklin, Vickie Barrow-Klein, and Paul Auxila; the MSH communications team led by Barbara Ayotte, who was a vital, steady resource; and MSH No More Epidemics campaign staff Frank Smith and Ashley Arabasadi.

Above all, I would like to thank the Ebola response officials, healthcare workers, and survivors in Sierra Leone and Liberia who welcomed me into their offices, hospitals, and villages where they bared their souls about their experience of the devastating epidemic. They awakened the world to the need and the possibility for ending devastating epidemics once and for all, and kept the fire blazing in my heart to deliver this book. Sjoerd Postma, Murtada Sesay, Garfee Williams, and Arthur Loryoun from MSH Liberia and Sierra Leone made these visits possible.

Finally, with apologies to anyone I may have missed, I would like to express my profound gratitude to the following individuals whose vision, insights, and experience contributed to this book through their encouragement, interviews, personal conversions, or public presentations: Kesetebirhan Admasu, James Allen, Nancy Aossey, Dan Ariely, David Barash, Dan Barouch, Kenneth Bernard, Larry Brilliant, Barbara Brilliant, Gro Harlem Brundtland, Charlanne Burke, Edwin Cameron, Dennis Carroll, Robert Clark, Bernice Dahn, Peter Daszak, Nils Daulaire, Jose Esparza, Paul Farmer, Ron Fouchier, Donald Francis, Maria Freire, Julio Frenk, Stefanie Friedhoff, Laurie Garrett, Bill Gates, Nathan Geffen, Larry Gostin, Richard Greene, David Heymann, Kaci Hickox, Mohammad Jalloh, Jonathan Jay, Bonnie Jenkins, Ashish Jha, Bob Kadlec, Olivia Kasenge, Rebecca Katz, Ilona Kickbusch, Marie-Paule Kieny, Jim Kim, Ann Marie Kimball, David Kirby, Minister Klinge, Alan Knight, Irene Koek, Outi Kuivasniemi, Stephen Kunitz, Randy Larsen, Heidi Larson, Jon Lidan, Marc Lipsitch, Joanne Liu, Catherine Machalaba, Rebecca Marmot, Jonna Mazet, Carolyn Miles, Michael Myers, David Nabarro, Tolbert Nyenswah, Michael Osterholm, Ariel Pablos-Mendez, Raj Panjabi, Anibal Peru, Peter Piot, Sjoerd Postma, Mark Potok, Scott Ratzan, Barbara Reynolds, David Ropeik, Peter Sands, Geary Sikich, Mark Smolinski, Jeff Sturchio, Alan Tennenberg, Dick Thompson, Oyewale Tomori, Elioda Tumwesigye, Suwit Wibulpolprasert, Desmond Williams, Nathan Wolfe, and Prashant Yadav.

Financial support for *The End of Epidemics* was provided by Management Sciences for Health, Inc. and a generous contribution from the James M. and Cathleen D. Stone Foundation.

I am deeply indebted to Dr. Ron O'Connor, founder of Management Sciences for Health, who 40 years ago took a risk on a young medical student when he sent me around the world on an eight-country study of pioneering essential medicines programs. His "Go the People" philosophy of working shoulder to shoulder for the success of our colleagues on the front line of health care has inspired me throughout my career in global health.

The journey of hills and valleys was perhaps toughest on my wife and daughters, who endured vacations postponed and time stolen from holidays for me to meet book deadlines. Despite this, they remained thoroughly supportive throughout the project, for which I am most grateful. Our loved ones are the most precious fellow travelers in our passage through life. My most earnest hope is that *The End of Epidemics* will help make the world safer for my daughters, for their families, and for everyone's loved ones for generations to come.

NOTES

Prologue: A Fear I'd Never Felt Before

1. Brown M. Bill Gates' greatest fear for humanity is absolutely terrifying—and likely to happen. GeekWire. 2016. http://www.geekwire.com/2015/bill-gates-greatest-fear-for-humanity-is-absolutely-terrifying-and-likely-to-happen/ (accessed 18 November 2016).
2. Nahal S, Ma B. Be prepared! Global pandemics primer. Bank of America Merrill Lynch. 2014. http://www.actuaries.org/CTTEES_TFM/Documents/BankofAmericaPandemicArticle.pdf.
3. Henderson D, Klepac P. Lessons from the eradication of smallpox: An interview with D. A. Henderson. The Royal Society. 2013. http://rstb.royalsocietypublishing.org/content/368/1623/20130113.short (accessed 18 November 2016).
4. Sars: Mission impossible? News24. 2003. http://www.news24.com/SouthAfrica/News/Sars-Mission-impossible-20030425 (accessed 18 November 2016).

Chapter 1. Stop Epidemics with The Power of Seven

1. Worobey M, Han G, Rambaut A. Genesis and pathogenesis of the 1918 pandemic H1N1 influenza A virus. *Proceedings of the National Academy of Sciences* 2014; 111: 8107–12.
2. Influenza (flu) including seasonal, avian, swine, pandemic, and other. Centers for Disease Control and Prevention. 2016. http://www.flu.gov/pandemic/history/1918/the_pandemic/influenza/ (accessed 18 November 2016).
3. Lynch E. *Pennsylvania Gazette*: The flu of 1918. Upenn.edu. 1998. http://www.upenn.edu/gazette/1198/lynch.html (accessed 18 November 2016).
4. Shilts R. *And the band played on*. New York: St. Martin's Press, 1987.
5. Owen J. AIDS origin traced to chimp group in Cameroon. *National Geographic*. 2006. http://news.nationalgeographic.com/news/2006/05/060525-aids-chimps.html (accessed 18 November 2016).
6. Chin J. Global estimates of AIDS cases and HIV infections. *AIDS* 1990; 4: S277–83. See more at: http://www.avert.org/history-aids-1987-1992.htm#footnote94_0jqce8s.
7. Smith E, Yan H. Ebola: Patient zero was a toddler in Guinea. CNN. 2014. http://www.cnn.com/2014/10/28/health/ebola-patient-zero/ (accessed 18 November 2016).
8. Ebola: Mapping the outbreak. BBC News. 2016. http://www.bbc.com/news/world-africa-28755033 (accessed 18 November 2016).
9. Forbes Profile: Bill Gates. *Forbes*. 2014. http://www.forbes.com/profile/bill-gates/ (accessed 18 November 2016).
10. Nahal S, Ma B. Be prepared! Global pandemics primer. Bank of America Merrill Lynch. 2014. http://www.actuaries.org/CTTEES_TFM/Documents/BankofAmericaPandemicArticle.pdf.
11. Ibid.

12. Mutume G. In fact and fiction, U.S. officials play games with AIDS in Africa. Third World Network. 2001. http://www.twn.my/title/games.htm (accessed 18 November 2016).

Chapter 2. The Bush—Lessons from Ebola, AIDS, and Zika

1. Today, it's harder to find bushmeat delicacies in the markets of Guinea because the government authorities have attempted to ban the stuff in the wake of the Ebola outbreak. It's a little hard to enforce. Samb S, Toweh A. Beware of bats: Guinea issues bushmeat warning after Ebola outbreak. Reuters. 2014. http://www.reuters.com/article/us-ebola-bushmeat-idUSBREA2Q19N 20140327 (accessed 18 November 2016).
2. Roberts M. First Ebola boy likely infected by playing in bat tree. BBC News. 2014. http://www.bbc.com/news/health-30632453 (accessed 18 November 2016).
3. Stern J. Why a massive international effort has failed to contain the Ebola epidemic. The Hive. 2014. http://www.vanityfair.com/news/2014/10/ebola-virus-epidemic-containment (accessed 18 November 2016).
4. Dabbous W. Ebola outbreak. *Frontline*. PBS. 2014. http://www.pbs.org/wgbh/frontline/film /ebola-outbreak/ (accessed 18 November 2016).
5. Ebola is named for the Ebola River, where the disease was first identified.
6. MacDougall C, Suakoko L. In West Africa, medical workers risk becoming victims in Ebola fight. *Time*. 2014. http://time.com/3137012/liberia-west-africa/ (accessed 18 November 2016).
7. Achenbach J, Sun L, Dennis B, Bernstein L. How Ebola sped out of control. *Washington Post*. 2014. http://www.washingtonpost.com/sf/national/2014/10/04/how-ebola-sped-out-of-control/ (accessed 18 November 2016).
8. Quick J, Liu J. 7 June 2016; by phone.
9. Roland D. Experts criticize World Health Organization's "slow" Ebola outbreak response. *Wall Street Journal*. 2015. http://www.wsj.com/articles/experts-criticize-world-health-organizations -slow-ebola-outbreak-response-1431344306 (accessed 18 November 2016).
10. Elliott L. Ebola crisis: Global response has "failed miserably," says World Bank chief. *The Guardian*. 2014. http://www.theguardian.com/world/2014/oct/08/ebola-crisis-world-bank-president -jim-kim-failure (accessed 18 November 2016).
11. Dabbous. Ebola outbreak.
12. Stern. Why a massive international effort.
13. Botelho G. 2 Americans infected with Ebola in Liberia coming to Atlanta hospital. CNN. 2014. http://www.cnn.com/2014/08/01/health/ebola-outbreak/ (accessed 18 November 2016).
14. Winter M. Timeline details missteps with Ebola patient who died. *USA Today*. 2014. http:// www.usatoday.com/story/news/nation/2014/10/17/ebola-duncan-congress-timeline /17456825/ (accessed 18 November 2016).
15. Ibid.
16. Jacobson S. Rick Perry, health officials offer reassurances on Dallas Ebola case. *Dallas News*. 2014. http://www.dallasnews.com/news/metro/20141002-perry-health-officials-seek-to-reassure -public-about-ebola-case.ece (accessed 18 November 2016).
17. Schwartz I. Bill Maher: "I'm pissed off" about Ebola, "People are nervous and I don't blame them." Real Clear Politics. 2014. https://www.realclearpolitics.com/video/2014/10/17/bill_maher_im _pissed_off_about_ebola_people_are_nervous_and_i_dont_blame_them.html (accessed 12 November 2016).
18. Carmichael M. How it began: HIV before the age of AIDS. *Frontline*. PBS. 2006. http://www.pbs.org/wgbh/pages/frontline/aids/virus/origins.html (accessed 18 November 2016).
19. The size of an outbreak depends on the number of "primary" novel infections (species jumps) and the potential for transmission from one new host to another (e.g., human-to-human spread).
20. Hobbes M. Why was the AIDS crisis so much worse in the U.S. than Western Europe? *New Republic*. 2015. https://newrepublic.com/article/121270/aids-crisis-video-why-it-was-so-much -worse-us-w-europe (accessed 18 November 2016).
21. U.S. conservatives weren't exclusively at fault. Many liberals and gays opposed proven public-health practices such as testing and partner notification. In contrast to U.S. dynamics, Australia's conservative government quickly put sound, scientifically based health practices into place.
22. Engel J. *The epidemic: A global history of AIDS*. New York: Smithsonian Books/HarperCollins, 2006.
23. Ghiasi M. The origins of AIDS by Jacques Pepin—book review. Ghiasi. 2013. http://ghiasi.org /2013/03/the-origins-of-aids-jacques-pepin/ (accessed 18 November 2016).
24. HIV infected almost every hemophiliac born before 1985, when the virus was finally cleansed

from clotting factors. Who was Ryan White? HIV/AIDS Bureau. 2016. http://hab.hrsa.gov /abouthab/ryanwhite.html#how (accessed 18 November 2016).

25. Hobbes, M. Why did AIDS ravage the U.S. more than any other developed country? *New Republic.* 2014. https://newrepublic.com/article/117691/aids-hit-united-states-harder-other-developed -countries-why (accessed 18 November 2016).

26. Francis D. Interview. The Age of AIDS. *Frontline.* PBS. 2006. http://www.pbs.org/wgbh/pages /frontline/aids/interviews/francis.html (accessed 18 November 2016).

27. Ibid.

28. Romero S. After living Brazil's dream, family confronts microcephaly and economic crisis. *New York Times.* 2016. http://www.nytimes.com/2016/03/09/world/americas/after-living-brazils -dream-family-confronts-microcephaly-and-economic-crisis.html (accessed 18 November 2016).

29. Zika virus fact sheet. World Health Organization. 2016. http://www.who.int/mediacentre /factsheets/zika/en/ (accessed 18 November 2016).

30. Olivares P. Where did Zika virus come from and why is it a problem in Brazil? IFLScience. 2016. http://www.iflscience.com/health-and-medicine/where-did-zika-virus-come-and-why-it -problem-brazil (accessed 18 November 2016).

31. Ibid.

32. Zika cases and congenital syndrome associated with Zika virus reported by countries and territories in the Americas, 2015–2017: Cumulative cases. Pan American Health Organization/World Health Organization. 2017. http://www2.paho.org/hq/index.php?option=com _docman&task=doc_view&Itemid=270&gid=39692&lang=en (accessed 18 November 2016).

33. Cumming-Bruce N. Zika vaccine still years away, W.H.O. says. *New York Times.* 2016. http:// www.nytimes.com/2016/03/10/world/americas/zika-vaccine-still-years-away-who-says.html ?mabReward=R4&action=click&pgtype=Homepage&region=CColumn&module =Recommendation&src=rechp&WT.nav=RecEngine (accessed 18 November 2016).

34. Back then, abortion was illegal in Western countries, but some doctors began offering abortions to women who had had rubella during pregnancy. Löwy I. Zika and microcephaly: Can we learn from history? *Physis: Revista de Saúde Coletiva* 2016; 26: 11–21.

35. How scientists misread the threat of zika virus. NPR. 2016. http://www.npr.org/sections/health -shots/2016/02/19/467340791/how-scientists-misread-the-threat-of-zika-virus (accessed 18 November 2016).

36. de Vogel N. The facts on Brazilian income inequality. ICCO International. 2016. http://www .icco-international.com/int/news/blogs/nadine-de-vogel/the-facts-on-brazilian-income -inequality/ (accessed 18 November 2016).

37. The poor northeast is not the region with the highest incidence of dengue, yet it has the highest incidence of Zika. (As of this writing, researchers are trying to find out why dengue is particularly prevalent in Brazil's southeast and Zika most prevalent in the northeast.)

38. Romero. After living Brazil's dream.

39. Zika travel information. Centers for Disease Control and Prevention. 2016. http://wwwnc.cdc .gov/travel/page/zika-information (accessed 18 November 2016).

40. Zika epidemiological update. PAHO/WHO. 2017. http://www.paho.org/hq/index.php?option =com_docman&task=doc_view&Itemid=270&gid=39706&lang=en (accessed 7 July 2017).

41. Wolfe N. The jungle search for viruses. TED. 2009. https://www.ted.com/talks/nathan_wolfe _hunts_for_the_next_aids?language=en (accessed 18 November 2016).

42. Africa hunger and poverty facts. World Hunger. 2016. http://www.worldhunger.org/articles /Learn/africa_hunger_facts.htm (accessed 18 November 2016).

43. Friedman T. *Hot, flat, and crowded: Why we need a green revolution—and how it can renew America.* New York: Farrar, Straus and Giroux, 2008.

44. Mirkin B. World population trends signal dangers ahead. YaleGlobal Online. 2014. http:// yaleglobal.yale.edu/content/world-population-trends-signal-dangers-ahead (accessed 18 November 2016).

45. Baer, D. "The biggest change of our time" is happening right now in Africa. *Business Insider.* 2015. http://www.techinsider.io/africas-population-explosion-will-change-humanity-2015-8 (accessed 18 November 2016).

46. Global forest resources assessment 2010. FAO. 2010. http://www.fao.org/docrep/013/i1757e /i1757e.pdf (accessed 18 November 2016).

47. Muyembe-Tamfum J, Mulangu S, Masumu J, Kayembe J, Kemp A, Paweska J. Ebola virus outbreaks in Africa: Past and present. *Onderstepoort Journal of Veterinary Research* 2012; 79: 6–13.

48. Warming conditions allowed dengue virus in Texas, Lyme disease in Canada, and tick-borne encephalitis in Slovakia to spread. See Lukan M, Bullova E, Petko B. Climate warming and

tick-borne encephalitis, Slovakia. *Emerging Infectious Diseases* 2010; 16: 524–526. DOI: 10.3201/eid1603.081364.

49. Annual review 2015. International Air Transport Association. 2015. https://www.iata.org/about/Documents/iata-annual-review-2015.pdf (accessed 18 November 2016).

50. Factors that contributed to undetected spread of the Ebola virus and impeded rapid containment. World Health Organization. 2015. http://www.who.int/csr/disease/ebola/one-year-report/factors/en/ (accessed 18 November 2016).

51. Jones K, Patel N, Levy M et al. Global trends in emerging infectious diseases. *Nature* 2008; 451: 990–93.

Chapter 3. The Barn

1. Jones K, Patel N, Levy M et al. Global trends in emerging infectious diseases. *Nature* 2008; 451: 990–93.

2. Influenza (seasonal) fact sheet. World Health Organization. 2016. http://www.who.int/mediacentre/factsheets/fs211/en/ (accessed 18 November 2016).

3. No one knows for sure when or where the so-called "Spanish flu" got started, but Spain was neutral in World War I; the flu apparently was so named from news reports about outbreaks there. See: Appenzeller T. Tracking the next killer flu. *National Geographic Magazine*. 2005. http://ngm.nationalgeographic.com/features/world/asia/vietnam/killer-flu-text/2 (accessed 18 November 2016).

4. Byerly C. *Fever of war: The influenza epidemic in the U.S. Army during World War I*. New York: New York University Press, 2005.

5. Garrett, author of *The Coming Plague*, won the Pulitzer for her work on the Ebola virus for *New York Newsday*.

6. Appenzeller. Tracking the next killer flu.

7. Schmitz R. The Chinese lake that's ground zero for the bird flu. *Marketplace*. 2016. http://www.marketplace.org/2016/03/03/world/chinese-lake-has-become-ground-zero-bird-flu (accessed 18 November 2016).

8. As the demand for meat in the country goes up, so does the risk of more flu strains coming out of China. See: ibid.

9. Greger M. *Bird flu: A virus of our own hatching*. New York: Lantern Books, 2006. http://www.birdflubook.org/a.php?id=15.

10. And because Hong Kong is one of the most crowded cities in the world, the likelihood of catching an illness there is high, which is why the virus in the movie *Contagion* was transmitted there first.

11. Drexler M. *Secret agents: The menace of emerging infections*. Washington, DC: Joseph Henry Press, 2002: 174.

12. Types of influenza viruses. Centers for Disease Control and Prevention. 2016. https://www.cdc.gov/flu/about/viruses/types.htm.

13. Zitzow L, Rowe T, Morken T, Shieh W, Zaki S, Katz J. Pathogenesis of avian influenza A (H5N1) viruses in ferrets. *Journal of Virology* 2002; 76: 4420–29. Cited in Greger, *Bird flu*.

14. Evidence suggests that transmission of H1N1 to humans occurred through contact with infected poultry blood or bodily fluids through food preparation practices such as slaughtering, boiling, defeathering, cutting meat, cleaning meat, removing and/or cleaning internal organs of poultry; through consuming uncooked poultry products (e.g., raw duck blood); or through the care of poultry (either commercially or domestically). Van Kerkhove M, Mumford E, Mounts A et al. Highly pathogenic avian influenza (H5N1): Pathways of exposure at the animal-human interface, a systematic review. *PLOS ONE*. 2011: 6: e14582. http://journals.plos.org/plosone/article?id=10.1371/journal.pone.0014582#pone.0014582-Vong2 (accessed 18 November 2016).

15. Claas E, Osterhaus A, van Beek R et al. Human influenza A H5N1 virus related to a highly pathogenic avian influenza virus. *The Lancet* 1998; 351: 472–77.

16. Specter M. The deadliest virus. *New Yorker*. 2012. http://www.newyorker.com/magazine/2012/03/12/the-deadliest-virus (accessed 18 November 2016).

17. Appenzeller. Tracking the next killer flu.

18. Cumulative number of confirmed human cases of avian influenza A(H5N1) reported to WHO. World Health Organization. 2017. http://www.who.int/influenza/human_animal_interface/2017_04_20_tableH5N1.pdf?ua=1 (accessed 18 November 2016).

19. Specter. The deadliest virus.

20. Indonesia, Vietnam, and Egypt have reported the highest number of human cases to date. The

fact that it's endemic in poultry in parts of Asia and in Egypt provides continued opportunities for more instances of human infection and for more virus mutations that could lead to quicker and more effective spread among humans. Van Kerkhove et al. Pathways of exposure.

21. Sandoval E, Melago C. Queens educator felled by swine flu mourned by hundreds. *New York Daily News.* 2009. http://www.nydailynews.com/new-york/queens-assistant-principal-mitchell -wiener-swine-flu-city-victim-mourned-hundreds-article-1.410561 (accessed 18 November 2016).

22. The city of New York closed 15 schools over the course of about one month because of the large number of children coming down with flu-like symptoms like fever and coughing. See: Hartocollis A. Swine flu kills Queens school official; first in New York State. *New York Times.* 2009. http://www.nytimes.com/2009/05/18/nyregion/18swine.html (accessed 18 November 2016).

23. Taylor V. Family of woman who died from H1N1 urges flu shots. *New York Daily News.* 2014. http://www.nydailynews.com/life-style/health/family-woman-died-h1n1-urges-flu-shots -article-1.1598023 (accessed 18 November 2016).

24. Dawood F, Iuliano A, Reed C et al. Estimated global mortality associated with the first 12 months of 2009 pandemic influenza A H1N1 virus circulation: A modelling study. *The Lancet Infectious Diseases* 2012; 12: 687–95. DOI: 10.1016/S1473-3099 12, 70121–4.

25. Kirby D. *Animal factory.* New York: St. Martin's Press, 2010.

26. Facts on animal farming and the environment. *One Green Planet.* 2012. http://www.onegreen planet.org/animalsandnature/facts-on-animal-farming-and-the-environment/ (accessed 18 November 2016).

27. According to *Animal Factory* author David Kirby, U.S. CAFOs are well protected by agribusiness industry lobbyists and politicians who care more about lining their pockets than about public health. Fryer B, Kirby D. 16 March 2016; by phone. See: Paarlberg R. The changing politics of CAFOs. Farm Foundation Ag Challenge 2050. 2015. http://www.agchallenge2050.org/farm -and-food-policy/2013/02/the-changing-politics-of-cafos/ (accessed 18 November 2016).

28. As of this writing in 2016, Mexico's health ministry has reported 945 cases of H1N1 and 68 deaths, compared to only four cases and no deaths in the previous season. In 2015, an outbreak of swine flu in two southeastern provinces of Iran killed at least 33 people within three weeks. In Costa Rica, health officials reported that in 2015 the virus claimed 14 lives, including that of a three-year-old boy. And in February 2016, Fresno, California, reported two H1N1 deaths within a week of each other. See: H1N1 deaths reported in Fresno County. ABC News. 2016. http://abc30.com/news/2-h1n1-deaths-reported-in-fresno-county/1199290/ (accessed 18 November 2016).

29. Conditions in these feedlots are appalling. It's not the purpose of this book to plead the cause for the animals in them, though I sympathize with those who would like to get rid of the lots. The purpose of this book is, however, to focus squarely on the risk of pathogenic disease that these operations pose. CAFOs are enormously profitable and poorly regulated operations; they produce more than 50 percent of the meat products consumed in the United States alone.

Animals raised for meat are big eaters and big poopers; a single dairy cow discharges 20 times as much waste as a human per day, and a 1,000-cow CAFO will produce the same amount of waste as a city of 20,000 people. That poop attracts a lot of flies, which excel at carrying germs around. While most human waste is treated in sewer systems, no such thing exists on CAFOs. Farmers turn the manure into fertilizer; they also build lagoons to store the wastewater, some of which spills into irrigation ditches and river tributaries, poisoning the fish. CAFO employees also scrape waste from feeding sheds and run it through a series of settling ponds to separate solids. During the crop season, lagoon water is mixed with fresh water to irrigate crops. People who live anywhere near CAFOs suffer—not just from the stench, but from all kinds of health problems ranging from itchy skin and headaches to nausea and pulmonary problems. When thousands of animals are packed into feedlots full of manure, bacteria can get on their hides and feathers and then into the slaughterhouses. Contamination on even one animal can contaminate thousands of pounds of meat inside a slaughterhouse.

CAFOs originated in the United States, but CAFO operations are growing throughout the world, especially Eastern Europe. See: Rising number of farm animals poses environmental and public health risks. Worldwatch Institute. 2016. http://www.worldwatch.org/rising-number -farm-animals-poses-environmental-and-public-health-risks-0 (accessed 18 November 2016). See also: Kirby, *Animal Factory.*

30. Bittman M, Hermanns S, Weathers S. Health leaders must focus on the threats from factory farms. *New York Times.* 2017. https://nyti.ms/2qISgrc (accessed 7 July 2017).

31. Weathers S, Hermanns S. Open letter urges WHO to take action on industrial animal farming. *The Lancet* 2017; 389: e9. http://dx.doi.org/10.1016/ S0140-6736 17, 31358–2.

32. Grillo I. Inside Mexico's hospitals, a struggle to cope. Public Radio International. 2009. https://www.pri.org/stories/2009-04-30/inside-mexicos-hospitals-struggle-cope (accessed 7 July 2017).

33. Arkell H. "Find out who did this to me, mum": Mother reveals agony of watching. *Daily Mail.* 2013. http://www.dailymail.co.uk/news/article-2413564/Who-killed-son-Mothers-year-battle -truth-mad-cow-disease-24-year-olds-deathbed-plea-justice.html (accessed 18 November 2016).

34. In the United States, mad cow didn't take hold because cattle were fed soy protein. See Mad Cow Disease—Bovine Spongiform Encephalopathy (BSE). EHA. 2017. http://www.ehagroup.com /food-safety/bse-mad-cow/ (accessed 7 July 2017).

35. An official British inquiry noted that BSE developed into an epidemic as a consequence of what it calls "intensive farming practice—the recycling of animal protein in ruminant feed." Lord Justice Nicholas Phillips, who ran the inquiry, concluded that nothing could have prevented the emergence of BSE. See: BSE Inquiry: The Report, Executive Summary, Key Conclusions. Encyclopedia.com. 2017. http://www.encyclopedia.com/science/medical-magazines/bse-inquiry -report-executive-summary-key-conclusions (accessed 7 July 2017).

   The general response to the report was scalding. Richard Tyler, writing on the World Socialist website, had this to say: "Within the mass of data contained in the report can be found the economic considerations that encouraged cattle and dairy farmers to vastly increase the amount of MBM they gave their cows: 'The emphasis on increasing milk production led to the use of MBM in place of some of the cheaper vegetable proteins, which had been the main protein source up until then. From about 1982 the least cost formulation of rations manufactured for dairy cows recommended the inclusion of substantial amounts of MBM,' the report stated.

   "A single firm, Prosper De Mulder (PDM), which processed around 64 per cent of red meat waste in England and Wales and 80 per cent of poultry waste, dominates the U.K. rendering industry. In Scotland, William Forrest and Son (Paisley) Ltd had about 71 per cent of the red meat waste supply. The feed producers (where a near monopoly also operates) would mix the MBM with other ingredients to make the compound feeds sold to farmers. In this industry as well, the emphasis is on maximum profit for the lowest outlay." See: Tyler R. Britain's official inquiry into BSE/Mad Cow Disease finds no one to blame. World Socialist Web Site. 2000. https://www.wsws.org/en/articles/2000/10/bse-o31.html (accessed 7 July 2017).

36. Shortly after leaving office in 1998, Dr. Calman told a U.K. government BSE inquiry that he felt misled by the U.K. Ministry of Agriculture, Fisheries and Food (MAFF) that food safety rules were being enforced when they were not. BBC Health Background Briefings. Public "misled over BSE." BBC News. 1998. http://news.bbc.co.uk/2/hi/health/background_briefings/bse/191356 .stm (access 3 July 2017).

37. Ibid.

38. Tran M, Glover J. The threat to humans from BSE. *The Guardian.* 2000. http://www.theguardian .com/world/2000/oct/26/qanda.bse (accessed 18 November 2016).

39. Tyler R. Britain's official inquiry into BSE/mad cow disease finds no one to blame. World Socialist Web Site. 2000. https://www.wsws.org/en/articles/2000/10/bse-o31.html (accessed 18 November 2016).

40. Tagliabue J. Mad Cow Disease (and anxiety). *New York Times.* 2001. http://www.nytimes.com /2001/02/01/business/mad-cow-disease-and-anxiety.html (accessed 7 July 2017).

41. Houston C. Regulations for cattle and beef. Harvard Law School. 2004. https://dash.harvard .edu/bitstream/handle/1/8852126/regulationsbeef3.html?sequence=2 (accessed 7 July 2017).

42. Beef war turns bloody. CNN Money. 1999. http://money.cnn.com/1999/10/22/europe/beef/ (accessed 18 November 2016).

43. Presley J. Mad cow to cost firms almost $6 billion. *Spokane Review.* 2004. https://www .organicconsumers.org/old_articles/madcow/billion225-4.php (accessed 7 July 2017).

44. Nunez C. Mad cow disease still menaces U.K. blood supply. *National Geographic.* 2015. http:// news.nationalgeographic.com/news/2015/02/150215-mad-cow-disease-vcjd-blood-supply -health/ (accessed 18 November 2016).

45. See: Justice for Andy—Human BSE, VCJD, mad cow disease, who killed my son? Justice4andy. 2016. http://justice4andy.com/ (accessed 18 November 2016).

46. Fryer B, Kirby D. 16 March 2016; by phone.

47. Higgs S. "Manure flu" and other CAFO maladies. *Bloomington Alternative.* 2008. http://www .bloomingtonalternative.com/articles/2008/03/23/9196 (accessed 18 November 2016).

48. See: Kirby. *Animal factory.*

49. Food & Water Watch estimates that the livestock and poultry on the largest factory farms in 2012 "produced 369 million tons of manure—almost 13 times more than the 312 million people in the United States. This 13.8 billion cubic feet of manure is enough to fill the Dallas Cowboys' stadium 133 times. The household waste produced in most U.S. communities is treated

in municipal sewer systems. But factory farm manure is stored in lagoons and ultimately applied, untreated, to farm fields as fertilizer." What's Wrong With Factory Farms?—Factory Farm Map. Food and Water Watch. 2017. https://factoryfarmmap.org/problems/ (accessed 7 July 2017).

50. Mellon M, Benbrook C, Benbrook K. Hogging it! Estimates of antimicrobial abuse in livestock (2001). Union of Concerned Scientists. 2004. http://www.ucsusa.org/food_and_agriculture/our-failing-food-system/industrial-agriculture/hogging-it-estimates-of.html#.Vu6mlxIrKRs (accessed 18 November 2016).
51. McEachran A, Blackwell B, Delton Hanson J et al. Antibiotics, bacteria, and antibiotic resistance genes: Aerial transport from cattle feed yards via particulate matter. National Institutes of Health. 2015. http://ehp.niehs.nih.gov/wpcontent/uploads/advpub/2015/1/ehp.1408555.acco.pdf (accessed 18 November 2016).
52. Klein E, Smith D, Laxminarayan R. Hospitalizations and deaths caused by methicillin-resistant Staphylococcus aureus, United States, 1999–2005. *Emerging Infectious Diseases* 2007; 13(12): 1840–46.
53. Ibid.
54. McKenna M. Almost three times the risk of carrying MRSA from living near a mega-farm. *Wired*. 2014. http://www.wired.com/2014/01/mrsa-col-cafo/ (accessed 18 November 2016).
55. Human vs superbug: Too late to turn the tide? BBC Guides. 2014. http://www.bbc.co.uk/guides/z8kccdm (accessed 18 November 2016).
56. Baer D. Bill Gates just described his biggest fear—and it could kill 33 million people in less than a year. *Business Insider*. 2015. http://www.businessinsider.com/bill-gates-biggest-fear-is-a-killer-flu-2015-5 (accessed 18 November 2016).
57. Fryer B, Kirby D. 16 March 2016; by phone.
58. Barnett A. Feed banned in Britain dumped on Third World. *The Guardian*. 2000. http://www.theguardian.com/uk/2000/oct/29/bse.focus (accessed 18 November 2016).
59. Ungchusak K, Auewarakul P, Dowell S et al. Probable person-to-person transmission of avian influenza A (H5N1). *New England Journal of Medicine* 2005; 352(4): 333–40.
60. The best way to prevent the spread of H5N1 to humans is to eradicate it in poultry. But this takes infrastructure and resources, and access to public-health and personal-health services is uneven across the globe. In Hong Kong, it involved "vaccinating every chicken against H5N1; regularly testing chickens, pet birds, even wild birds; shutting down the hundreds of live-poultry stalls twice a month to disinfect them; and inspecting farms and markets obsessively." What works on an island with the resources to mount this type of offensive is not likely to be possible in places like Vietnam, where the government can afford to pay less than half of a bird's market value as compensation, creating a disincentive for farmers to report sick birds. See: Appenzeller. Tracking the next killer flu.

Chapter 4. The Triple Threat

1. For a riveting likely scenario from a respected bioterror expert, see: Osterholm M, Schwartz J. *Living terrors: What America needs to know to survive the coming bioterrorist catastrophe*. New York: Delacorte Press, 2000.
2. Snyder-Beattie A, Cotton-Barratt O, Farquhar S, Halstead J, Schubert S. Global catastrophic risks 2016. Global Priorities Project. 2016. http://globalprioritiesproject.org/2016/04/global-catastrophic-risks-2016/ (accessed 30 November 2016).
3. Anthrax is a bacterial disease of sheep and cattle, typically affecting the skin and lungs. It can be transmitted to humans, causing severe skin ulceration or a form of pneumonia (also called woolsorter's disease). Commonly found in herd animals, anthrax has surprised scientists by breaking out high above the Arctic Circle, thanks to melting permafrost that is exposing carcasses.
4. Immenkamp B. ISIL/Da'esh and "non-conventional" weapons of terror. European Parliamentary Research Service. 2015. http://www.europarl.europa.eu/RegData/etudes/BRIE/2015/572806/EPRS_BRI(2015)572806_EN.pdf (accessed 30 November 2016).
5. I've deliberately left chemical weapons off this list, as, horrific as they are, they don't propagate across time and continents to pose the same kind of pandemic threat as most biological weapons. See: Riedel S. Biological warfare and bioterrorism: A historical review. *Proceedings Baylor University Medical Center*. 2004. Oct; 17, 4: 400–6.
6. Wheelis M. Biological warfare at the 1346 siege of Caffa. Centers for Disease Control and Prevention. 2016. http://wwwnc.cdc.gov/eid/article/8/9/01-0536_article (accessed 30 November 2016).

7. Peck M. Don't forget, Japan used biological weapons on China. War Is Boring. 2013. https://warisboring.com/dont-forget-japan-used-biological-weapons-on-china-71ce4a8a303a (accessed 30 November 2016).

8. Garner M. 2 North Georgia men sentenced for terrorism plot. *Atlanta Journal-Constitution*. 2012. http://www.ajc.com/news/news/local/2-north-georgia-men-sentenced-for-terrorism-plot/nRMNj/ (accessed 10 May 2016).

9. Jury finds 2 Georgia men guilty in ricin plot. *USA Today*. 2014. http://www.usatoday.com/story/news/nation/2014/01/17/ricin-georgia-guilty/4592157/ (accessed 30 November 2016).

10. Fryer B, Potok M. 24 May 2016; by phone.

11. Mohr H. "The perfect poison": Ricin used in 3 recent cases. Yahoo! News. 2013. https://www.yahoo.com/news/perfect-poison-ricin-used-3-recent-cases-204805812.html?ref=gs (accessed 30 November 2016).

12. Bioterrorism overview. Centers for Disease Control and Prevention. 2007. http://emergency.cdc.gov/bioterrorism/overview.asp (accessed 30 November 2016).

13. Ibid.

14. Coleman K, Ishisoko N, Trounce M, Bernard K. Hitting a moving target: A strategic tool for analyzing terrorist threats. *Health Security* 2016; 14: 409–18. DOI:10.1089/hs.2016.0062.

15. His speech has been viewed more than 109,000 times. See: MEMRI TV. Kuwaiti Professor Anthrax. 2009. https://www.youtube.com/watch?v=M32M-2B2mz8 (accessed 30 November 2016).

16. Inglesby T. Plague as a biological weapon. The JAMA Network. 2000. http://jamanetwork.com/journals/jama/fullarticle/192665 (accessed 30 November 2016).

17. Plague is a bacterium, not a virus. But the intent is the same.

18. "The real difficulty in all of these weapons . . . [is] to actually have a workable distribution system that will kill a lot of people. . . . But to produce quite scary weapons is certainly within [the Islamic State's] capabilities," Magnus Ranstorp, research director of the Center for Asymmetric Threat Studies at the Swedish National Defence College, told *Foreign Affairs*. Doornbos H, Moussa J. Found: The Islamic State's terror laptop of doom. Foreign Policy. 2014. http://foreignpolicy.com/2014/08/28/found-the-islamic-states-terror-laptop-of-doom/ (accessed 30 November 2016).

19. Said-Moorhouse L. Iraq stops would-be child bomber for ISIS. CNN. 2016. http://www.cnn.com/2016/08/22/middleeast/would-be-child-suicide-bomber-iraq/ (accessed 30 November 2016).

20. Allen P, Webb S. Terrorist's backpack searched for bomb—but cops found something REVOLTING. *Mirror*. 2016. http://www.mirror.co.uk/news/world-news/isis-feared-planning-crude-biological-7715046 (accessed 30 November 2016).

21. Immenkamp. ISIL/Da'esh.

22. Colonel Randall Larsen, USAF (Retired). UPMC Center for Health Security. 2016. http://www.upmchealthsecurity.org/our-staff/profiles/larsen/ (accessed 30 November 2016).

23. Levine B. Chasing ground zero: Preparing for the unpredictable. North Carolina Biotech Center. 2016. http://www.ncbiotech.org/article/chasing-ground-zero-preparing-unpredictable/171511 (accessed 30 November 2016).

24. The *Bacillus globigii* germ is genetically identical to anthrax powder. The stuff is basically harmless, but anyone interested in weaponizing anthrax—which means reducing the molecules to the size of 3 microns, so that it would immediately reach the bloodstream—would experiment with *Bacillus globigii* first.

25. Quick J, Larsen R. 2 September 2016; by phone.

26. From 2009 to 2013, Dr. O'Toole served as undersecretary of science and technology (S&T) at the Department of Homeland Security. See http://www.upmchealthsecurity.org/our-staff/profiles/otoole/.

27. For more on this story, see: Hylton W. How ready are we for bioterrorism? *New York Times*. 2011. http://www.nytimes.com/2011/10/30/magazine/how-ready-are-we-for-bioterrorism.html?_r=0 (accessed 30 November 2016).

28. Garrett L. *Betrayal of trust: The collapse of global public health*. New York: Hyperion, 2000: 350.

29. Ibid, 358. For more on the Biopreparat program, see: Tucker J. Bioweapons from Russia: stemming the flow. *Issues in Science and Technology* 1999; 15 3. http://issues.org/15-3/p_tucker/.

30. On June 6, 2015, a North Korean scientist defected to Finland with 15 gigabytes of electronic evidence, claiming that it proves how the country is testing chemical and biological agents on its own citizens. North Korean dictator Kim Jong Un toured a factory that was ostensibly making pesticides. Analysis of the photos revealed that the Pyongyang Bio-Technical Institute can produce regular, military-sized batches of anthrax. That same day, a defector reportedly fled the coun-

try carrying human testing data. Hanham M. Kim Jong Un tours pesticide facility capable of producing biological weapons. 38 North: Informed Analysis of North Korea. 2016. http://38north.org/2015/07/mhanham070915/ (accessed 30 November 2016).

31. Russia, Iraq, and other potential sources of anthrax, smallpox and other bioterrorist weapons. Commdocs.house.gov. 2001. http://commdocs.house.gov/committees/intlrel/hfa76481.000 /hfa76481_0.htm (accessed 30 November 2016).

32. President Bush signs Project Bioshield Act of 2004. The White House. 2004. http://georgewbush -whitehouse.archives.gov/news/releases/2004/07/20040721-2.html (accessed 30 November 2016).

33. According to a July 2007 article in the *Los Angeles Times*, Alibekov had "won about $28 million in federal grants or contracts for himself or entities that hired him." Willman D. Selling the threat of bioterrorism. *Los Angeles Times*. 2007. http://articles.latimes.com/2007/jul/01/nation/na -alibek1 (accessed 30 November 2016).

34. Ibid.

35. Garrett. *Betrayal of trust.*

36. Scutti S. The cure could kill you. *Newsweek*. 2014. http://www.newsweek.com/2014/03/21/only -thing-scarier-bio-warfare-antidote-247993.html (accessed 30 November 2016).

37. Adapted from Biosafety in microbiological and biomedical laboratories. 5th edition. U.S. Department of Health and Human Services, 2009: 30–59. http://www.cdc.gov/biosafety /publications/bmbl5/BMBL.pdf.

38. It was all due to a software glitch, and some people at the CDC tried to avoid reporting the incident to federal regulators. *USA Today* learned about the incident through the Freedom of Information Act; it took the CDC more than three years to fulfill the newspaper's request. Young A. Newly disclosed CDC biolab failures "like a screenplay for a disaster movie." *USA Today*. 2016. http://www.usatoday.com/story/news/2016/06/02/newly-disclosed-cdc-lab-incidents -fuel-concerns-safety-transparency/84978860/ (accessed 30 November 2016).

39. Biolabs in your backyard. *USA Today*. 2015. http://www.usatoday.com/pages/interactives /biolabs/ (accessed 30 November 2016).

40. Christensen J. CDC: Smallpox found in NIH storage room is alive. CNN. 2014. http://www .cnn.com/2014/07/11/health/smallpox-found-nih-alive/ (accessed 30 November 2016).

41. Harris R. Feds tighten lab security after anthrax, bird flu blunders. NPR. 2014. http://www.npr .org/sections/health-shots/2014/07/11/330725773/feds-tighten-lab-security-after-anthrax -bird-flu-blunders (accessed 30 November 2016).

42. Neuman S. CDC says more workers potentially exposed to live anthrax. NPR. 2014. http://www .npr.org/sections/thetwo-way/2014/06/20/324077444/cdc-says-more-workers-potentially -exposed-to-live-anthrax (accessed 30 November 2016).

43. As *Newsweek* reported, "accidents also occur due to events beyond human control. A bird flew into a power transformer in the summer of 2008, knocking out power to the Centers for Disease Control and Prevention's (CDC) Emerging Infectious Diseases Laboratory in Atlanta for an hour. Primary as well as backup generators were temporarily down, and the negative air pressure system, which is essential for keeping dangerous agents from escaping the containment area, shut down. A building housing a BSL-3 lab—in which scientists are believed to have been studying a deadly strain of avian flu—was among those that lost power. It was dumb luck that no one became infected—an hour doesn't sound like much, but that's about 59 minutes more than a virus like the H5N1 flu needs to find a host and spread." See: Scutti. Cure could kill you.

44. 2015 annual report of the Federal Select Agent Program. Federal Select Agent Program. 2015. http://www.selectagents.gov/annualreport2015.html (accessed 30 November 2016).

45. Young A. GAO finds more gaps in oversight of bioterror germs studied in U.S. labs. *USA Today*. 2016. http://www.usatoday.com/story/news/2016/09/21/gao-inactivation-failures-high-contain ment-labs/90776218/ (accessed 30 November 2016).

46. Ibid.

47. European lab accidents raise biosecurity concerns. Reuters. 2009. http://www.reuters.com/article /health-biohazards-idUSLJ55693920090319 (accessed 10 August 2016).

48. Ibid.

49. Sample I. Revealed: 100 safety breaches at U.K. labs handling potentially deadly diseases. *The Guardian*. 2014. https://www.theguardian.com/science/2014/dec/04/-sp-100-safety-breaches-uk -labs-potentially-deadly-diseases (accessed 30 November 2016).

50. European lab accidents. Reuters.

51. Back in 1971, the Soviets tested weaponized smallpox and other horrors on an island not far from a research ship trawling for plankton samples. The smallpox powder exploded on the island, contaminating an area around 150 miles in radius. Thanks to the quick evacuation of about

50,000 residents of the Aral area, only ten people got sick and three died. A bug's life. *Economist*. 2011. http://www.economist.com/node/17849189/print (accessed 9 September 2016).

52. Young A. Deadly bacteria release sparks concern at Louisiana lab. *USA Today*. 2015. http://www.usatoday.com/story/news/2015/03/01/tulane-primate-bio-lab-bacteria-release/24137053/ (accessed 30 November 2016).

53. In the U.S. alone, there were 1,356 high-security bioweapons labs in 2009. By 2013, the U.S Government Accountability Office reported an increase in the number of labs but, as *Newsweek* reported in a 2014 article, it "also warned that because there is a lack of counting and registration standards, it can no longer provide an accurate estimate." Scutti. Cure could kill you.

54. Young A. Hundreds of safety incidents with bioterror germs reported by secretive labs. *USA Today*. 2016. https://www.usatoday.com/story/news/2016/06/30/lab-safety-transparency -report/86577070/ (accessed 30 November 2016).

55. Quick J. and Fryer B. Fouchier R. 31 August 2016; by phone.

56. For example, see: Specter M. The deadliest virus. *New Yorker*. 2012.

57. Enserik M. Fight over Dutch H5N1 paper enters endgame. *Science*. 2012. http://www.sciencemag .org/news/2012/04/fight-over-dutch-h5n1-paper-enters-endgame (accessed 12 September 2016).

58. Roos R. Experts call for alternatives to "gain-of-function" flu studies. Center for Infectious Disease Research and Policy. 2014. http://www.cidrap.umn.edu/news-perspective/2014/05/experts -call-alternatives-gain-function-flu-studies (accessed 30 November 2016).

59. In October 2014, the White House put a rare moratorium on funding these types of experiments— including some funding of Fouchier's lab—until advisors could think through the safety issues.

60. Fouchier interview.

61. Fryer B. Lipsitch M. 22 September 2016; by phone.

62. Greenfield-Boyce N. Biologists choose sides in safety debate over lab-made pathogens. NPR.org. 2014. http://www.npr.org/sections/health-shots/2014/08/13/339854400/biologists-choose-sides -in-safety-debate-over-lab-made-pathogens; National Academies of Sciences, Engineering, and Medicine. *Gain-of-function research: Summary of the second symposium, March 10–11, 2016.* Washington, DC: The National Academies Press, 2016. DOI: 10.17226/23484.

63. Shelley M. *Frankenstein, or, the modern Prometheus*. Revised edition. London: Penguin Books. 1992 (first published 1818): 29.

64. Garrett L. CRISPR: Transformative and troubling. Council on Foreign Relations. 2016. http:// www.cfr.org/biotechnology/crispr-transformative-troubling/p37768 (accessed 30 November 2016).

65. Venter C, Goetz T. Unlocking the mysteries of genetics with Dr. Craig Venter. City Arts & Lectures. 2012. http://www.cityarts.net/event/unlocking-the-mysteries-of-genetics/ (accessed 30 November 2016).

66. Dr. Venter became a controversial figure in the 1990s when he pitted his former company, Celera Genomics, against the publicly funded effort to sequence the human genome, the Human Genome Project. Venter had already applied for patents on more than 300 genes, raising concerns that the company might claim intellectual rights to the building blocks of life. See: Sample I. Craig Venter creates synthetic life form. *The Guardian*. 2010. https://www.theguardian.com /science/2010/may/20/craig-venter-synthetic-life-form (accessed 30 November 2016).

67. In the summer of 2016, a baby was born in New York who had three parents. See: Kolata G. Birth of baby with three parents' DNA marks success for banned technique. *New York Times*. 2016. http://www.nytimes.com/2016/09/28/health/birth-of-3-parent-baby-a-success-for -controversial-procedure.html (accessed 30 November 2016).

68. Garrett. CRISPR: Transformative and troubling.

69. Gronvall G. Hindsight not 20/20 for smallpox research. Start: National Consortium for the Study of Terrorism and Responses to Terrorism. 2015. http://www.start.umd.edu/news /hindsight-not-2020-smallpox-research (accessed 30 November 2016).

70. Bioterrorism, public health, superbug, biolabs, epidemics, biosurveillance, outbreaks, DNA sequencing. Homeland Security News Wire. 2015. http://www.homelandsecuritynewswire.com /dr20150224-dna-synthesis-creates-risk-of-resurrecting-deadly-viruses (accessed 30 November 2016).

71. Cotton-Barratt O, Farquhar S, Snyder-Beattie A. Beyond risk-benefit analysis: Pricing externalities for gain-of-function research of concern—working policy paper (revision 0.9). Global Priorities Project. 2016. http://globalprioritiesproject.org/wp-content/uploads/2016/03/GoFv9-3 .pdf (accessed 30 November 2016).

72. Church G. Synthetic biohazard non-proliferation. Arep.med.harvard.edu. 2005. http://arep.med .harvard.edu/SBP/Church_Biohazard04c.htm (accessed 30 November 2016).

73. Chyba C. Biotechnology and bioterrorism: An unprecedented world. *Survival* 2004; 46: 143–61.
74. Yuhas A, Kelkar K. "Rogue scientists" could exploit gene editing technology, experts warn. *The Guardian*. 2016. https://www.theguardian.com/science/2016/feb/12/rogue-scientists-could -exploit-gene-editing-technology-experts-warn (accessed 30 November 2016).
75. Ibid.
76. Araki M, Ishii T. International regulatory landscape and integration of corrective genome editing into in vitro fertilization. *Reproductive Biology and Endocrinology* 2014; 12: 108.
77. In 2015, the journal *Nature* surveyed 12 countries with well-funded biological research to identify the extent to which genome sequencing was regulated. In some countries, experimenting with human embryos at all would be a criminal offense, whereas in others, almost anything would be permissible. Japan, China, India, and Ireland have unenforceable guidelines that limit the modification of a human embryo's genome, while the U.K. may permit human genome editing for research but bans the practice in the clinic. Germany has strict laws on using embryos in assisted reproduction and limits research on human embryos—violations can result in criminal charges. Argentina, like Germany, bans reproductive cloning, but human genome editing is not clearly regulated. While the U.S. won't provide federal funding to modify human embryos, there are no genome-editing bans. See: Ledford H. Where in the world could the first CRISPR baby be born? *Nature*. 2015. http://www.nature.com/news/where-in-the-world-could-the-first-crispr -baby-be-born-1.18542 (accessed 30 November 2016).
78. National Academies of Sciences, Engineering, and Medicine. *Human genome editing: Science, ethics, and governance*. Washington, DC: The National Academies Press, 2017.
79. Quick J and Fryer B. Bernard K. 1 August 2016; in person.
80. Scientific advice and evidence in emergencies, third report of session 2010–11, volume II, additional written evidence. House of Commons. 2011. http://www.publications.parliament.uk/pa /cm201011/cmselect/cmsctech/498/498vw.pdf.
81. Quick J and Fryer B. Bernard K. 1 August 2016; in person.
82. Countering bioterrorism: Lessons from 2010 Israeli exercise, US perspectives, & international efforts. Center for Cyber & Homeland Security, George Washington University. 2010. https:// cchs.gwu.edu/countering-bioterrorism-lessons-2010-israeli-exercise-us-perspectives -international-efforts (accessed 30 November 2016). When I asked Kenneth Bernard if any other countries outside the U.S. have done a good job, he cited England for its superior work on apportioning risk—essentially, defining the risk of bioterror against other disasters, such as nuclear war, hurricanes, and earthquakes.
83. A national blueprint for biodefense: Leadership and major reform needed to optimize. Hudson Institute. 2015. http://www.hudson.org/research/11824-a-national-blueprint-for-biodefense -leadership-and-major-reform-needed-to-optimize-efforts (accessed 30 November 2016).
84. Mackler N, Wilkerson W, Cinti S. Will first-responders show up for work during a pandemic? Lessons from a smallpox vaccination survey of paramedics. *Disaster Management & Response* 2007; 5: 45–48.
85. A national blueprint for biodefense: Leadership and major reform needed to optimize. Hudson Institute. 2015. http://www.hudson.org/research/11824-a-national-blueprint-for-biodefense -leadership-and-major-reform-needed-to-optimize-efforts (accessed 30 November 2016).

Chapter 5. The Costs of Complacency

1. Homepage. Carlo Urbani Center. 2011. http://carlo-urbani-center.com/en/modules.php?name =Thongtin&go=page&pid=1 (accessed 9 June 2017).
2. McNeil D. Disease's pioneer is mourned as a victim. *New York Times*. 2003. http://www.nytimes .com/2003/04/08/science/disease-s-pioneer-is-mourned-as-a-victim.html (accessed 19 December 2015).
3. Korea Centers for Disease Control and Prevention. Middle East Respiratory Syndrome Coronavirus Outbreak in the Republic of Korea, 2015. *Osong Public Health and Research Perspectives* 2015; 6(4): 269–278.
4. Frangoul A. Counting the costs of a global epidemic. CNBC. 2014. http://www.cnbc.com/2014 /02/05/counting-the-costs-of-a-global-epidemic.html (accessed 15 March 2016).
5. SARS fallout to cost Toronto economy about $1 billion: Conference board. CBC News. 2003. http://www.cbc.ca/news/business/sars-fallout-to-cost-toronto-economy-about-1-billion -conference-board-1.363576 (accessed 19 December 2015).
6. Lee E. Ali Fedotowsky canceled her wedding in Mexico because of Zika: Details. The Knot News.

2016. http://www.theknotnews.com/ali-fedotowsky-canceled-her-wedding-in-mexico-because-of
-zika-it-was-such-a-huge-disappointment-10037 (accessed 12 March 2016).

7. Keogh-Brown M, Smith R. The economic impact of SARS: How does the reality match the predictions? *Health Policy* 2008; 88: 110–20.

8. Nahal S, Ma B. Be prepared! Global pandemics primer. Bank of America Merrill Lynch. 2014. http://www.actuaries.org/CTTEES_TFM/Documents/BankofAmericaPandemicArticle.pdf.

9. Ibid.

10. Much worse to come. *Economist*. 2014. http://www.economist.com/news/international /21625813-ebola-epidemic-west-africa-poses-catastrophic-threat-region-and-could-yet (accessed 19 December 2016).

11. Fox M. Cost to treat Ebola: $1 million for two patients. *NBC News*. 2014. http://www.nbcnews .com/storyline/ebola-virus-outbreak/cost-treat-ebola-1-million-two-patients-n250986 (accessed 19 December 2016).

12. Nahal and Ma. Be prepared!

13. Parpia AS, Ndeffo-Mbah ML, Wenzel NS, et al. Effects of Response to 2014–2015 Ebola Outbreak on Deaths from Malaria, HIV/AIDS, and Tuberculosis, West Africa. *Emerging Infectious Diseases* 2016;22(3): 433–441.

14. UNDP. 2014. "Assessing the socio-economic impacts of Ebola Virus Disease in Guinea, Liberia and Sierra Leone: The Road to Recovery." Accessed 22 March 2017. http://www.africa.undp .org/content/dam/rba/docs/Reports/EVD%20Synthesis%2023Dec2014.pdf.

15. Long H. Stock market scare as Dow drops 460 points. CNN Money. 2014. http://money.cnn .com/2014/10/14/investing/stocks-market-3-key-numbers-to-watch/index.html?iid=EL (accessed December 10 2016).

16. Nahal and Ma. Be prepared!, 41.

17. Ighobor K. Ebola threatens economic gains in affected countries. Africa Renewal Online. 2014. http://www.un.org/africarenewal/magazine/december-2014/ebola-threatens-economic-gains -affected-countries (accessed 4 January 2017).

18. News article: Ebola, food security and FAO's response. FAO. 2016. http://www.fao.org/news /story/en/item/270716/icode/ (accessed 24 October 2015).

19. Chavez D. The socio-economic impacts of Ebola in Sierra Leone. World Bank Group. 2015. http://www.worldbank.org/en/topic/poverty/publication/so-cio-economic-impacts-ebola -sierra-leone (accessed 20 October 2015).

20. Thomas A, Nkunzimana T, Hoyos A, Kayitakere F. Impact of West Africa Ebola outbreak on food security. European Commission. 2014. file:///C:/Users/npersaud/Downloads/JRC94257 _ebola_impact_on_food_securi-ty_jrc_h04_final_report.pdf (accessed 25 October 2015).

21. Fry E. Business in the hot zone: How one global corporation has managed the Ebola epidemic. *Fortune*. 2015. http://fortune.com/2014/10/30/arcelormittal-business-liberia-ebola-outbreak/ (accessed 2 November 2015).

22. Ibid.

23. HIV and AIDS cost $17 per employee for one Kenyan car manufacturer and $300 per employee for the Ugandan Railway Corporation. Dixon S, McDonald S, Roberts J. The impact of HIV and AIDS on Africa's economic development. *British Medical Journal* 2002; 324(7331): 232–34. http://www.ncbi.nlm.nih.gov/pmc/articles/PMC1122139/ (accessed 2 November 2015).

24. Fryer B. Ariely D. 7 September 2016; by phone. For an astute analysis of this psychological bias, see: Ariely D. *The upside of irrationality: The unexpected benefits of defying logic*. New York: Harper, 2010: chap. 9, "On Empathy and Emotion."

25. Kraft D. AIDS ravaging the teachers, education systems of Africa. *Los Angeles Times*. 2002. http://articles.latimes.com/2002/dec/01/news/adfg-nomore1 (accessed 20 December 2015).

26. United Nations. *The impact of AIDS*. New York: United Nations, 2004.

27. Think piece prepared for the Education for All Global Monitoring Report 2011. The hidden crisis: Armed conflict and education; The quantitative impact of conflict on education. UNESCO Institute for Statistics. 2010. http://www.uis.unesco.org/Library/Documents/QuantImp.pdf (accessed 20 December 2015).

28. An AIDS orphan's story. BBC. 2002. http://news.bbc.co.uk/2/hi/africa/2511829.stm (accessed 20 December 2015).

29. We have nothing: The human cost of Ebola. Sky News. 2014. http://news.sky.com/story/we-have -nothing-the-human-cost-of-ebola-10386164 (accessed 20 December 2015).

30. Bell C, Devarajan S, Gersbach H. The long-run economic costs of AIDS: Theory and an application to South Africa. SSRN. 2016. http://papers.ssrn.com/sol3/Papers.cfm?abstract_id=636571.

31. Epidemics and economics. *Economist*. 2003. http://www.economist.com/node/1698814 (accessed 15 December 2015).

32. Baker A. Liberian Ebola fighter, a TIME Person of the Year, dies in childbirth. TIME Health. 2017. http://time.com/4683873/ebola-fighter-time-person-of-the-year-salome-karwah/ (accessed 9 July 2017).

33. For an astute analysis of this psychological bias, see: Ariely. *The upside of irrationality.*

34. Slovic P. "If I look at the mass I will never act": Psychic numbing and genocide. *Judgment and Decision Making* 2007; 2: 79–95. http://journal.sjdm.org/7303a/jdm7303a.htm (accessed 20 December 2015).

35. WHO Global Malaria Programme. Guidance on temporary malaria control measures in Ebola-affected countries. World Health Organization. 2014. http://apps.who.int/iris/bitstream /10665/141493/1/WHO_HTM_GMP_2014.10_eng.pdf?ua=1 (accessed 31 March 2015).

36. Kieny M, Evans D, Schmets G, Kadandale S. Health-system resilience: Reflections on the Ebola crisis in western Africa. *Bulletin of the World Health Organization* 2014; 92: 850.

37. Walker P, White M, Griffin J, Reynolds A, Ferguson N, Ghani A. Malaria morbidity and mortality in Ebola-affected countries caused by decreased health-care capacity, and the potential effect of mitigation strategies: a modelling analysis. *The Lancet Infectious Diseases* 2015, 15: 825–32. http://dx.doi.org/10.1016/S1473-3099(15)70124-6.

38. The impact of HIV/AIDS on food security. June 2001. http://www.fao.org/docrep/meeting /003/Y0310E.htm (accessed 20 December 2015).

39. HIV Cost-effectiveness. Centers for Disease Control and Prevention. 2015. https://www.cdc.gov /hiv/programresources/guidance/costeffectiveness/index.html (accessed 31 March 2015).

40. Leefeldt E. The true cost of Zika in the U.S. could be staggering. CBS News. 2016. http:// www.cbsnews.com/news/the-true-cost-of-zika-in-the-u-s-could-be-staggering/ (accessed 31 March 2015).

41. Ubelacker S. SARS survivors struggle with symptoms years later. *Toronto Star.* 2010. https:// www.thestar.com/life/health_wellness/2010/09/02/sars_survivors_struggle_with _symptoms_years_later.html (accessed 31 March 2015).

42. Rettner R. What are the long-term effects of Ebola? Live Science. 2015. http://www.livescience .com/50039-ebola-survivors-health-problems.html (accessed 31 March 2015).

43. Discussion adapted from Nahal and Ma. Be prepared!

44. Cooper H. Liberian president pleads with Obama for assistance in combating Ebola. *New York Times.* 2014. https://www.nytimes.com/2014/09/13/world/africa/liberian-president-pleads -with-obama-for-assistance-in-combating-ebola.html?_r=0 (accessed 7 July 2017).

45. McNeil D. Starvation timetable in a pandemic. *New York Times.* 2015. http://www.nytimes.com /2015/06/23/health/starvation-timetable-in-a-pandemic.html (accessed 31 March 2015).

46. The twentieth century saw three of them, all of them influenzas (Spanish flu, Asian flu, and Hong Kong flu). Taubenberger J, Morens D. 1918 influenza: The mother of all pandemics. *Emerging Infectious Diseases* 2006. http://wwwnc.cdc.gov/eid/article/12/1/pdfs/05-0979.pdf (accessed 2 January 2017).

47. Most deaths from seasonal influenza are attributable not to the flu virus itself but to complications of bacterial pneumonia. Some medical experts believe that ensuring antibiotic treatment for such pneumonias would reduce pandemic influenza deaths. Seasonal flu is a different virus, however. Michael Osterholm, author of *Deadliest Enemy* and director of the Center for Infectious Disease Research and Policy based at the University of Minnesota, points out that with pandemic influenza viruses, the most common cause of death is an acute respiratory distress syndrome whose treatment requires respirators and intensive-care units. Such treatment is simply not available to most of the world's population and will not be available in adequate numbers even in the U.S., Europe, and other high-income countries if a big pandemic were to strike.

48. Pike J, Bogich T, Elwood S, Finnoff D, Daszak P. Economic optimization of a global strategy to address the pandemic threat. *Proceedings of the National Academy of Sciences* 2014; 111: 18519–23. http://www.pnas.org/content/111/52/18519.abstract.

49. Quick J. Marmot R. 27 October 2016; by phone.

Chapter 6. Lead Like the House Is on Fire

1. Neustadt R, Fineberg H. *The epidemic that never was: Policy-making and the swine flu scare.* New York: Random House, 1983.

2. Roan S. Swine flu "debacle" of 1976 is recalled. *Los Angeles Times.* 2009. http://articles.latimes .com/2009/apr/27/science/sci-swine-history27 (accessed 13 December 2016).

3. Hamburg, David A. in Neustadt and Fineberg. *The epidemic that never was.*

4. Troy T. *Shall we wake the president?: Two centuries of disaster management from the Oval Office.* Guilford: Lyons Press, 2016: p. 5 and appendix 3.

5. Barry J. *The great influenza: The story of the greatest pandemic in history.* New York: Penguin Books, 2005.

6. Dickens C. *Bleak House.* London: Bradbury & Evans, 1853: 344–45.

7. White M. Necrometrics: Estimated totals for the entire 20th century. Necrometrics. 2010. http://necrometrics.com/all20c.htm (accessed 9 June 2017).

8. Riedel S. Edward Jenner and the history of smallpox and vaccination. *PubMed Central (PMC).* 2005. https://www.ncbi.nlm.nih.gov/pmc/articles/PMC1200696/ (accessed 13 December 2016).

9. Langer E. D. A. Henderson, "disease detective" who eradicated smallpox, dies at 87. *Washington Post.* 2016. https://www.washingtonpost.com/local/obituaries/da-henderson-disease-detective -who-eradicated-smallpox-dies-at-87/2016/08/20/b270406e-63dd-11e6-96c0-37533479f3f5 _story.html (accessed 13 December 2016).

10. Ibid.

11. Ibid.

12. Quick J. Henderson D. 8 August 2015; by phone.

13. Langer. D. A. Henderson.

14. Ibid.

15. Quick J. Henderson D. 8 August 2015; by phone.

16. History and epidemiology of global smallpox eradication. Centers for Disease Control and Prevention. 1999. https://emergency.cdc.gov/agent/smallpox/training/overview/pdf/eradicationhistory .pdf (accessed 13 December 2016).

17. Seymour J. Case 1: Eradicating smallpox. Center for Global Development. http://www.cgdev.org /doc/millions/MS_case_1.pdf (accessed 13 December 2016).

18. Stolberg S. Threats and responses; New fight for an old warrior. *New York Times.* 2002. http:// www.nytimes.com/2002/12/14/us/threats-and-responses-new-fight-for-an-old-warrior.html (accessed 13 December 2016).

19. Langer. D. A. Henderson.

20. Brown B. The virus detective who discovered Ebola in 1976. BBC News. 2014. http://www.bbc .com/news/magazine-28262541 (accessed 13 December 2016).

21. Salter J. Professor Peter Piot: "As long as there is even one case left, Ebola could still reignite." *Telegraph.* 2015. http://www.telegraph.co.uk/news/worldnews/ebola/11475881/Professor-Peter -Piot-As-long-as-there-is-even-one-case-left-Ebola-could-still-reignite.html (accessed 13 December 2016).

22. These are the most recently available statistics as of this writing.

23. In 2007, Dr. Brundtland was invited to join the Elders, a group of senior former world leaders first headed by Nelson Mandela with the aim of providing solutions to some of the world's most intractable problems, with an emphasis on human rights. That same year, she was appointed as a UN special envoy on climate change to assist in negotiations with governments in securing international agreements to limit global warming. She remains a board member of the United Nations Foundation and a director of the Council of Women World Leaders, a group whose membership has expanded to nearly 40 since she first took office 34 years ago. Langton J. Norway's iron lady Gro Harlem Brundtland honoured with Zayed Future Energy Prize. *The National.* 2016. http://www.thenational.ae/uae/environment/norways-iron-lady-gro-harlem-brundtland -honoured-with-zayed-future-energy-prize#full (accessed 13 December 2016).

24. The Skoll Foundation. Gro Harlem Brundtland: I'm a lucky person. 2014. https://www.youtube .com/watch?v=3_6cL71L870 (accessed 13 December 2016).

25. Brundtland G. *Madam prime minister: A life in power and politics.* New York: Farrar, Straus and Giroux, 2002.

26. Langton. Norway's iron lady.

27. Lewington J. Lastman's on-air gaffes add to Toronto's woes. *The Globe and Mail.* 2003. http:// www.theglobeandmail.com/news/national/lastmans-on-air-gaffes-add-to-torontos-woes /article1013974/ (accessed 13 December 2016).

28. Chinoy M. SARS "stopped dead in its tracks." CNN. 2003. http://www.cnn.com/2003 /HEALTH/06/17/sars.wrapup/ (accessed 13 December 2016).

29. Ibid.

30. These factors contributed to undetected spread of the Ebola virus and impeded rapid containment. Ebola one year report. World Health Organization. 2015. http://www.who.int/csr/disease /ebola/one-year-report/factors/en/ (accessed 13 December 2016).

31. Quick J. Liu J. 7 June 2016; by phone.

32. Boseley S. World Health Organisation admits botching response to Ebola outbreak. *The Guardian.* 2014. https://www.theguardian.com/world/2014/oct/17/world-health-organisation -botched-ebola-outbreak (accessed 14 December 2016).
33. MSF international president United Nations special briefing on Ebola. Médecins Sans Frontières (MSF) International. 2014. http://www.msf.org/en/article/msf-international-president-united -nations-special-briefing-ebola (accessed 13 December 2016).
34. Miles T. WHO leadership admits failings over Ebola, promises reform. Reuters. 2015. http:// www.reuters.com/article/us-health-ebola-who-idUSKBN0NA12J20150419 (accessed 13 December 2016).
35. Onishi N. Clashes erupt as Liberia sets an Ebola quarantine. *New York Times.* 2014. http://www .nytimes.com/2014/08/21/world/africa/ebola-outbreak-liberia-quarantine.html (accessed 13 December 2016).
36. Gladstone R. Liberian leader concedes errors in response to Ebola. *New York Times.* 2015. http:// www.nytimes.com/2015/03/12/world/africa/liberian-leader-concedes-errors-in-response-to -ebola.html (accessed 13 December 2016).
37. Nyenswah T, Kateh F, Bawo L et al. Ebola and its control in Liberia, 2014–2015. Centers for Disease Control and Prevention. 2016. http://wwwnc.cdc.gov/eid/article/22/2/15-1456_article (accessed 13 December 2016).
38. Kerecman Myers D. Tolbert Nyenswah: A Liberian perspective on Ebola. Global Health NOW. 2014. https://www.globalhealthnow.org/2014-08/tolbert-nyenswah-liberian-perspective-ebola (accessed 13 December 2016).
39. Nyenswah et al. Ebola and its control.

Chapter 7. Resilient Systems, Global Security

1. Gall C. Afghans consider rebuilding Bamiyan Buddhas. *New York Times.* 2006. http://www .nytimes.com/2006/12/05/world/asia/05iht-buddhas.3793036.html?pagewanted=all (accessed 1 May 2017).
2. Dubitsky S. The health care crisis facing women under Taliban rule in Afghanistan. *Human Rights Brief* 1999; 6, 2: 10–11. https://www.wcl.american.edu/hrbrief/06/2dubitsky.pdf.
3. Golden J. Starting from zero: Dr. Ihsanullah Shahir on leadership and management in Afghan-istan. Management Sciences for Health. 2015. http://www.msh.org/news-events/stories/starting -from-zero-dr-ihsanullah-shahir-on-leadership-and-management-in (accessed 1 May 2017).
4. Rasooly M, Govindasamy P, Aqil A et al. Success in reducing maternal and child mortality in Afghanistan. *Global Public Health* 2013; 9: S29–42. DOI: 10.1080/17441692.2013.827733.
5. Akseer N, Salehi A, Hossain S et al. Achieving maternal and child health gains in Afghanistan: A countdown to 2015 country case study. *Lancet Global Health* 2016; 4: e395–413. DOI: 10.1016/ S2214-109X(16)30002-X.
6. Waldman R, Newbrander W. Afghanistan's health system: Moving forward in challenging cir-cumstances 2002–2013. *Global Public Health* 2014; 9: S1–5. DOI: 10.1080/17441692.2014.924188.
7. Rodin J. *The resilience dividend: Being strong in a world where things go wrong.* New York: Public Affairs, 2014.
8. Masten A. Ordinary magic: Resilience processes in development. *American Psychologist* 2001; 56: 227–38.
9. Garvin D, Edmondson A, Gino F. Is yours a learning organization? *Harvard Business Review* 2008; 86, 3: 109–16.
10. Quick J. Stop AIDS, stop Zika, stop them all. *Huffington Post.* 2016. http://www.huffingtonpost .com/jonathan-d-quick/stop-aids-stop-zika-stop-_b_10941172.html (accessed 7 July 2017).
11. Lynch D. How to stop an Ebola outbreak: Lessons from Nigeria And Senegal. *International Business Times.* 2014. http://www.ibtimes.com/how-stop-ebola-outbreak-lessons-nigeria-senegal -1706297 (accessed 1 May 2017).
12. Soleye was kind enough to let me share her aunt's story and our conversation with our staff on that frightening day in October 2014, in order to help me explain why I had sent Ian Sliney and his team to Liberia at their risk.
13. Lynch. How to stop.
14. Quick J. Wubneh H. March 26, 2009; in person.
15. Partnering to achieve epidemic control in Ethiopia. PEPFAR. 2015. http://www.pepfar.gov /countries/ethiopia/index.htm (accessed 1 May 2017).
16. Antiretroviral therapy coverage in sub-Saharan Africa. World Health Organization. 2017. http:// www.who.int/hiv/data/art_coverage/en/ (accessed 1 May 2017).

17. Countries offering free access to HIV treatment. World Health Organization. 2017. http://www
.who.int/hiv/countries_freeaccess.pdf (accessed 25 May 2017).

18. GDP per capita, PPP (current international $). World Bank. 2017. http://data.worldbank.org
/indicator/NY.GDP.PCAP.PP.CD?locations=ET&view=chart (accessed 25 May 2017).

19. Antiretroviral treatment wards were also separated from traditional services like antenatal care
and TB screening, which made it easy to single out and discriminate against patients seeking HIV
treatment.

20. ENHAT-CS Partners. From emergency response to a comprehensive country-owned system for
HIV care and treatment 2011–2014. Management Sciences for Health. 2012. https://www.msh
.org/sites/msh.org/files/eth_enhat_eop_finalproof_nov12.pdf (accessed 25 May 2017).

21. Stories of success from Ethiopia: The Tsadkane holy water well. I-TECH. 2014. http://news
.go2itech.org/2014/09/stories-of-success-from-ethiopia-the-tsadkane-holy-water-well/ (accessed
1 May 2017).

22. Mekonnen G. Ethiopia: One teacher can save thousands of lives. Management Sciences for Health.
2015. https://www.msh.org/news-events/stories/ethiopia-one-teacher-can-save-thousands-of-lives
(accessed 1 May 2017).

23. The new regime was not without its fundamental faults. The dictatorial administration punished
dissent and continued, from the previous administration, a track record of human-rights violations. Even so, the new administration brought with it a lot of hope, little corruption, and true
commitment to improving health and education.

24. Strategic plan for intensifying multi-sectoral HIV/AIDS response (2004–2008). International
Labour Organisation. 2004. http://www.ilo.org/wcmsp5/groups/public/—ed_protect/—
protrav/—ilo_aids/documents/legaldocument/wcms_125381.pdf (accessed 25 May 2017).

25. Countries offering free access to HIV treatment. World Health Organization. 2017. http://www
.who.int/hiv/countries_freeaccess.pdf (accessed 25 May 2017).

26. Ethiopia network for HIV/AIDS treatment, care, & support. Management Sciences for Health.
2015. https://www.msh.org/our-work/projects/ethiopia-network-for-hivaids-treatment-care
-support (accessed 1 May 2017).

27. Integration of HIV and other health services. Management Sciences for Health. 2017. https://
www.msh.org/our-work/health-areas/hiv-aids/integration-of-hiv-and-other-health-services (accessed 1 May 2017).

28. Bradley E. et al. Grand strategy and global health: the case of Ethiopia. *Global Health Governance*
2011; 5, 1: 1–11.

29. Partnering to achieve epidemic control in Ethiopia. PEPFAR. 2017. https://www.pepfar.gov
/documents/organization/199586.pdf.

30. National Network of Positive Women Ethiopia was also launched to match HIV-positive women
to treatment, palliative care, and community support services. See: ENHAT-CS Partners. From
emergency response to a comprehensive country-owned system for HIV care and treatment
2011–2014. Management Sciences for Health. 2012. https://www.msh.org/sites/msh.org/files
/eth_enhat_eop_finalproof_nov12.pdf (accessed 25 May 2017).

31. Mother Mentor/mother support group strategy for expansion of peer support for mothers
living with HIV. Management Sciences for Health. 2017. https://www.msh.org/resources
/mother-mentormother-support-group-strategy-for-expansion-of-peer-support-for-mothers
(accessed 1 May 2017).

32. The group was started because 30 to 35 percent of infants born to HIV-infected women will acquire HIV—the virus is transmitted in utero, during birth, or during breastfeeding. But many
pregnant women who are HIV positive either don't know it, do know it and don't receive ARVs
during pregnancy, or receive treatment during pregnancy and then discontinue after pregnancy.
Assessment of the care and treatment of HIV-exposed infants born at ENHAT-CS-supported
health centers. Management Sciences for Health. 2017. https://www.msh.org/resources
/%EF%BF%BCassessment-of-the-care-and-treatment-of-hiv-exposed-infants-born-at-enhat-cs
-supported (accessed 1 May 2017).

33. Jember, a Mother Mentor at a health center in the Tigray region, leads pregnant and breastfeeding women, and some of their husbands, through a year of peer-group sessions. Since September
2011, Jember and her Mother Mentor colleagues have provided support and services to almost
10,000 HIV-positive mothers. Eshetu G. So that no child be born with HIV: Ethiopia. Management Sciences for Health. 2014. https://www.msh.org/news-events/stories/so-that-no-child
-be-born-with-hiv-ethiopia (accessed 1 May 2017).

34. Kahssaye M. Ethiopian mothers' support groups mentor HIV-positive moms. Management Sciences for Health. 2013. https://www.msh.org/news-events/stories/ethiopian-mothers-support
-groups-mentor-hiv-positive-moms (accessed 1 May 2017).

35. Beaubien J. Firestone did what governments have not: Stopped Ebola in its tracks. NPR. 2014. http://www.npr.org/sections/goatsandsoda/2014/10/06/354054915/firestone-did-what -governments-have-not-stopped-ebola-in-its-tracks (accessed 1 May 2017).

36. Panoc N. How corporations helped stop the Ebola crisis. *Wilson Quarterly*. 2014. https:// wilsonquarterly.com/stories/how-corporations-helped-stop-ebola-crisis/ (accessed 1 May 2017).

37. Quick J and Fryer B. Knight A. 24 March 2017; by phone.

38. Quick J. Brilliant B. 27 October 2016; in person.

39. Lidman M. Sisters in Liberia fight Ebola. Global Sisters Report. 2014. http://globalsistersreport .org/news/ministry/sisters-liberia-fight-ebola-12196 (accessed 1 May 2017).

40. "One Health" is a whole-systems approach that unites experts from a variety of disciplines— including doctors, dentists, epidemiologists, veterinarians, environmental experts, NGOs, the private sector, and the faith community—in an effort to boost and coordinate surveillance for potentially dangerous pathogens that can mix and jump among livestock, birds, and humans. For more information, see: http://www.onehealthinitiative.com.

41. To ensure broadly shared international ownership, a core principle is that member nations take leadership roles within the GHSA. This includes rotation of the GHSA Secretariat (held in the first four years by Finland, Indonesia, South Korea, and Uganda) and contributing to develop- ment in specific action areas. See: https://www.GHSAgenda.org/.

42. The Joint External Evaluation tool published by WHO in early 2016 builds directly on WHO's own IHR assessment tools and country experience with GHSA action program as- sessments. To add an independent perspective, evaluation teams include experts from other countries as well as national professionals. After review by national health officials, the result- ing reports are made publicly available online. The tool is available at GHSAgenda.org and JeeAlliance.org.

43. Frieden T. President Obama cements global health security agenda as a national priority. Cen- ters for Disease Control and Prevention. 2016. https://blogs.cdc.gov/global/2016/11/04 /president-obama-cements-global-health-security-agenda-as-a-national-priority/ (accessed 1 May 2017).

44. Reinforcing the global nature of health security, these countries include Canada, Italy, the U.K. and the U.S., as well as scores of developing countries. More than a dozen funders including the U.S., U.K., the European Union, and the World Bank have committed support.

45. Joint external evaluation of core IHR capacities of the United States of America. World Health Organization. 2016. http://apps.who.int/iris/bitstream/10665/254701/1/WHO-WHE-CPI -2017.13-eng.pdf?ua=1 (accessed 25 May 2017).

46. The National Health Security Preparedness Index: Summary of key findings. 2017. http://nhspi .org/wp-content/uploads/2017/04/2017-NHSPI-Key-Findings.pdf. The US NHSPI was devel- oped through the initiative and support of the Robert Woods Johnson Foundation.

Chapter 8. Active Prevention, Constant Readiness

1. Mathur P. Hand hygiene: Back to the basics of infection control. *Indian Journal of Medical Re- search*. 2011; 134, 5: 611–20. DOI:10.4103/0971-5916.90985. http://www.ncbi.nlm.nih.gov/pmc /articles/PMC3249958/ (accessed 10 February 2017).

2. Situation report: Zika virus, microcephaly, Guillain-Barré syndrome. World Health Organ- ization. 2017. http://www.who.int/emergencies/zika-virus/situation-report/10-march-2017 /en/ (accessed 11 February 2017).

3. Wilder-Smith A, Gubler D, Weaver S, Monath T, Heymann D, Scott T. Epidemic arboviral diseases: Priorities for research and public health. *The Lancet Infectious Diseases* 2017; 17: e101–6.

4. Andersson N, Arostegui J, Nava-Aguilera E et al. Evidence based community mobilization for dengue prevention in Nicaragua and Mexico (Camino Verde, the Green Way): Cluster random- ized controlled trial. *British Medical Journal*. 2015; 351:h3267. DOI: 10.1136/bmj.h3267.

5. While not risk free, the managed use of DDT to prevent mosquitoes from nesting in places where people and animals live and work does not pose the same environmental and health risks posed by farmers applying large amounts on soil. Up until the early 1980s, WHO promoted indoor residual spraying of DDT for malaria control. Residual spraying involves spraying long-acting DDT on the walls of houses and animal shelters. Any malaria-carrying mosquitoes are killed when they land on these surfaces. Given concerns about health and environment, WHO stopped supporting the use of DDT to prevent malaria and focused on other prevention measures. Because research demonstrated that indoor spraying programs with DDT posed no harm to wildlife or

to humans, in 2006 WHO once again supported indoor DDT (along with 12 other pesticides) to be used in the context of integrated vector management. See: WHO gives indoor use of DDT a clean bill of health for controlling malaria. World Health Organization. 2006. http://www.who .int/mediacentre/news/releases/2006/pr50/en/ (accessed 14 April 2017).

6. McNeil D. "Big success story": Sri Lanka is declared free of malaria. *New York Times*. 2016. http://www.nytimes.com/2016/09/13/health/sri-lanka-declared-free-of-malaria.html?_r=0 (accessed 14 April 2017).

7. Elimination of malaria in the United States (1947–1951). Centers for Disease Control and Prevention. 2010. https://www.cdc.gov/malaria/about/history/elimination_us.html (accessed 13 April 2017).

8. Malaria Transmission in the United States. Centers for Disease Control and Prevention. 2015. https://www.cdc.gov/malaria/about/us_transmission.html (accessed 14 April 2017).

9. Achieving the malaria MDG target. World Health Organization/UNICEF. 2015. http://www .who.int/malaria/publications/atoz/9789241509442/en/.

10. Gething P, Casey D, Weiss D et al. Mapping *Plasmodium falciparum* mortality in Africa between 1990 and 2015. *New England Journal of Medicine*. 2016; 375: 2435–45: 10.1056/NEJMoa1606701. http://www.nejm.org/doi/full/10.1056/NEJMoa1606701#t=article.

11. Gates B, Chambers R. From aspiration to action: What will it take to end malaria? Bill & Melinda Gates Foundation/Office of the UN Secretary-General's Special Envoy for Financing the Health Millennium Development Goals for Malaria/Malaria No More. Endmalaria2040.org. 2015. http://endmalaria2040.org/assets/Aspiration-to-Action.pdf (accessed 14 April 2017).

12. End Malaria Council. Global leaders launch council to help end malaria. Cision PR Newswire. 2017. http://www.prnewswire.com/news-releases/global-leaders-launch-council-to-help-end -malaria-300393873.html (accessed 13 April 2017).

13. Wilder-Smith A et al. Epidemic arboviral diseases.

14. In chapter 11, I will go into detail about the ways scientists are developing and utilizing wonderful tools for detecting disease, such as the Global Viral Forecasting Initiative (GVFI), financed by Google and created by Nathan Wolfe.

15. About us. Wildlife Works. 2017. http://www.wildlifeworks.com/company/aboutus.php (accessed 13 April 2017).

16. Home-bushmeat crisis task force. Bushmeat Crisis Task Force. 2017. http://www.bushmeat.org/ (accessed 13 April 2017).

17. Programs and policies to do this are seeing broad success in 17 countries across four continents, according to a report from the Union of Concerned Scientists (UCS): Deforestation success stories. Union of Concerned Scientists. 2014. http://www.ucsusa.org/global_warming/solutions /stop-deforestation/deforestation-success-stories.html (accessed 14 April 2017).

18. Venter O, Koh L. Reducing emissions from deforestation and forest degradation (REDD+): Game changer or just another quick fix? *Annals of the New York Academy of Sciences* 2012; 1249: 137–50. DOI:10.1111/j.1749-6632.2011.06306.x. http://www.un-redd.org/ (accessed 12 April 2017).

19. Influenza A(H1N1) update 38. World Health Organization. 2009. http://www.who.int/csr/don /2009_05_25/en/ (accessed 14 April 2017).

20. Swine influenza statement. World Health Organization. 2009. http://www.who.int/mediacentre /news/statements/2009/h1n1_20090425/en/ (accessed 13 April 2017).

21. Report of the WHO influenza H1N1 vaccine deployment initiative. World Health Organization. 2012. http://www.who.int/influenza_vaccines_plan/resources/h1n1_deployment_report .pdf (accessed 14 April 2017).

22. Borse R, Shrestha S, Fiore A et al. Effects of vaccine program against pandemic influenza A(H1N1) virus, United States, 2009–2010. *Emerging Infectious Diseases* 2013; 19. DOI:10.3201/ eid1903.120394.

23. The unprecedented speed and scale for vaccine development and production contributed to variations in coverage. For example, among 27 European countries, coverage varied from 3 percent to 68 percent for healthcare workers and from 0 percent to 58 percent for pregnant women (the two highest risk groups). Mereckiene J, Cotter S, Weber J et al. Influenza A(H1N1) pdm09 vaccination policies and overage in Europe. *European Surveillance* 2012; 17, 4: 1–10 pii=20064. http://www.eurosurveillance.org/ViewArticle.aspx?ArticleId=20064 (accessed 15 March 2017).

24. First global estimates of 2009 H1N1 pandemic mortality released by CDC-led collaboration. Centers for Disease Control and Prevention. 2012. https://www.cdc.gov/flu/spotlights/pandemic -global-estimates.htm (accessed 14 April 2017).

25. Health and Human Services. An HHS retrospective on the 2009 H1N1 influenza pandemic to advance all hazards preparedness. Homeland Security Digital Library. 2012. http://www.hsdl .org/?view&did=714799 (accessed 14 April 2017).

26. MacKenzie D. Swine flu myth: This is just mild flu. The death rates are even lower than for normal flu. *New Scientist*. 2009. https://www.newscientist.com/article/dn18056-swine-flu-myth -this-is-just-mild-flu-the-death-rates-are-even-lower-than-for-normal-flu/ (accessed 14 April 2017).

27. Recommended vaccinations by age. Centers for Disease Control and Prevention. 2016. https:// www.cdc.gov/vaccines/vpd/vaccines-diseases.html (accessed 13 April 2017).

28. Khazeni N, Hutton DW, Garber AM, Hupert N, Owens DK. Effectiveness and cost-effectiveness of vaccination against pandemic influenza (H1N1) 2009. *Annals of Internal Medicine* 2009 Dec 15; 151(12): 829–39.

29. Fortunately, some pharmaceutical companies have large-scale production capacities, allowing them to shift from seasonal influenza to pandemic influenza production. Nonetheless, setting up a new production line and actually growing the vaccines take time.

30. Fox M. Pricey vaccines hurt poor countries, doctors group says. NBC News. 2015. http://www .nbcnews.com/health/health-news/pricey-vaccines-hurt-poor-countries-doctors-group-says -n289926 (accessed 13 April 2017).

31. Osterholm M, Kelley N, Manske J et al. The compelling need for game-changing influenza vaccines: An analysis of the influenza vaccine enterprise and recommendations for the future. Center for Infectious Disease Research and Policy. 2012. http://www.cidrap.umn.edu/sites /default/files/public/downloads/ccivi_report.pdf (accessed 14 April 2017).

32. One thing U.S. consumers can do is to apply pressure to pharmaceutical companies through their congressional representatives. Rosenthal E. The price of prevention: Vaccine costs are soaring. *New York Times*. 2014. http://www.nytimes.com/2014/07/03/health/Vaccine-Costs-Soaring -Paying-Till-It-Hurts.html?_r=0 (accessed 14 April 2017).

33. Ibid.

34. Health and Human Services. How to pay. Vaccines.gov. 2016. https://www.vaccines.gov/getting /pay/ (accessed 14 April 2017).

35. Pagliusi S, Leite L, Datla M et al. Developing Countries Vaccine Manufacturers Network: Doing good by making high-quality vaccines affordable for all. *Vaccine* 2013; 31: B176–83.

36. The Global Alliance for Vaccine and Immunization (GAVI). Alleviating system wide barriers to immunization: Issues and conclusions from the second GAVI consultation with country representatives and global partners. Norad. Oslo: 2004.

37. McLean K, Goldin S, Nannei C, Sparrow E, Torelli G. The 2015 global production capacity of seasonal and pandemic influenza vaccine. *Vaccine* 2016; 34: 5410–13.

38. Africa takes second "step" toward strengthening supply chain management. The Global Alliance for Vaccine and Immunization. 2016. http://www.gavi.org/library/news/gavi-features/2016 /africa-takes-second-step-toward-strengthening-supply-chain-management/ (accessed 14 April 2017).

39. Ibid.

40. Yogi Berra Quotes . . . Famous Quotes and Quotations. 2017. http://www.famous-quotes-and -quotations.com/yogi-berra-quotes.html (accessed 14 April 2017).

41. Epidemic Intelligence Service. Centers for Disease Control and Prevention. 2014. http://www .cdc.gov/EIS/downloads/factsheet.pdf (accessed 14 April 2017).

42. Pendergrast M. An interview with Mark Pendergrast. Mark Pendergrast. 2017. http:// markpendergrast.com/an-interview-with-mark-pendergrast (accessed 14 April 2017).

43. About ProMED-mail. International Society for Infectious Diseases. 2010. http://www .promedmail.org/aboutus/ (accessed 7 July 2017).

44. The TED Prize is awarded annually to a leader with a creative, bold wish to spark global change.

45. Global Public Health Intelligence Network. About GPHIN. Government of Canada. 2016. https://gphin.canada.ca/cepr/aboutgphin-rmispenbref.jsp?language=en_CA (accessed 16 April 2017).

46. Chapter 5: SARS: lessons from a new disease. World Health Organization. 2003. http://www .who.int/whr/2003/chapter5/en/index3.html (accessed 14 April 2017).

47. Galaz V. Pandemic 2.0: Can information technology help save the planet? *Environment Magazine*. 2009. http://www.environmentmagazine.org/Archives/Back%20Issues/November -December%202009/Pandemic-full.html (accessed 13 April 2017). See also: Quick J. Heymann D. 25 March 2008; by phone.

48. Wójcik O, Brownstein J, Chunara R, Johansson M. Public health for the people: Participatory

infectious disease surveillance in the digital age. *Emerging Themes in Epidemiology* 2014; 11: 7. http://www.ete-online.com/content/11/1/7EMERGING THEMES (accessed 14 April 2017).

49. About HealthMap. HealthMap. 2017. http://www.healthmap.org/site/about (accessed 14 April 2017).

50. Resnick G. "Flu Near You" wants to track influenza trends in U.S., save lives. Daily Beast. 2014. http://www.thedailybeast.com/articles/2014/01/12/flu-near-you-wants-to-track-influenza-trends-in-u-s-save-lives.html (accessed 14 April 2017).

51. Williams G. Larry Brilliant is humanity's best hope against the next pandemic. *Wired UK*. 2014. http://www.wired.co.uk/article/pandemic-hunter (accessed 14 April 2017).

52. Experts call showing up to work sick "presenteeism," the opposite of absenteeism, and it is an epidemic in itself. Mason M. Sniffling, sneezing and turning cubicles into sick bays. *New York Times*. 2006. http://www.nytimes.com/2006/12/26/health/26cons.html (accessed 19 April 2017).

53. Information about social distancing. Santa Clara County Health and Hospital System. http://www.cidrap.umn.edu/sites/default/files/public/php/185/185_factsheet_social_distancing.pdf (accessed 8 July 2017).

54. Earn D, He D, Loeb M et al. Effects of school closure on incidence of pandemic influenza in Alberta, Canada. *Annals of Internal Medicine* 2012; 156: 173–81. DOI: 10.7326/0003-4819-156-3-201202070-00005. http://annals.org/aim/article/1033342/effects-school-closure-incidence-pandemic-influenza-alberta-canada (accessed 14 April 2017).

55. Tognotti E. Lessons from the history of quarantine, from plague to influenza A. *Emerging Infectious Diseases* 2013; 19: 254–59. https://wwwnc.cdc.gov/eid/article/19/2/12-0312_article (accessed 14 April 2017).

56. Werner E. Do quarantines actually work? Experts question effectiveness. *PBS NewsHour*. 2014. http://www.pbs.org/newshour/rundown/quarantines-rarely-used-effectiveness-questioned/ (accessed 14 April 2017).

57. Tognotti. Lessons from the history.

58. Ibid.

59. Civil War "medicine." Civil War Trust. http://www.civilwar.org/education/pdfs/civil-was-curriculum-medicine.pdf (accessed 14 April 2017).

60. Hall J. One in seven women could die in childbirth in Ebola hit countries. *Daily Mail*. 2014. http://www.dailymail.co.uk/health/article-2829867/One-seven-pregnant-women-die-childbirth-Ebola-hit-countries-medical-facilities-overwhelmed-say-charities.html (accessed 14 April 2017).

61. Bernstein L. Ebola has crippled the health system. Now Liberians are dying of common illnesses too. *Washington Post*. 2014. https://www.washingtonpost.com/world/africa/with-ebola-crippling-the-health-system-liberians-die-of-routine-medical-problems/2014/09/20/727dcfbe-400b-11e4-b03f-de718edeb92f_story.html?utm_term=.215ee1d33c89 (accessed 14 April 2017).

62. Such exercises also help develop contingency plans for patient transport, medical supplies, sanitation, telecommunications, and other essential services. World Health Organization. See: WHO guidelines for pandemic preparedness and response in the non-health sector. World Health Organization. 2009.

63. IHR Procedures concerning public health emergencies of international concern (PHEIC). World Health Organization. 2017. http://www.who.int/ihr/procedures/pheic/en/ (accessed 14 April 2017).

64. Here's how WHO declares a PHEIC: WHO's director-general convenes with an Emergency Committee of global public-health experts who provide temporary recommendations, or health measures that should be implemented by the affected state or other states, to prevent or reduce the global spread of disease. These are recommendations but act as global reference points on which to focus efforts to contain and reduce the spread of disease. The Emergency Committee gives advice to the director-general on when a PHEIC should be declared, recommendations to members, and when the PHEIC should be terminated. At least one member of the Emergency Committee should be from the affected state party. Kreuder-Sonnen C, Hanrieder T. The WHO's new emergency powers—from SARS to Ebola. Völkerrechtsblog. 2014. http://voelkerrechtsblog.org/the-whos-new-emergency-powers-from-sars-to-ebola/ (accessed 14 April 2017).

65. The director-general can also draw global attention to an outbreak without declaring a PHEIC. Indeed, the director-general met with the Emergency Committee nine times about MERS. These meetings keep SARS on the global radar as a serious disease threat and provide advisement to WHO. Fidler D. Ebola report misses mark on international health regulations. Chatham House, The Royal Institute of International Affairs. 2015. https://www.chathamhouse.org/expert/comment/ebola-report-misses-mark-international-health-regulations# (accessed 14 April 2017).

66. Swine influenza statement. World Health Organization. 2009. http://www.who.int/mediacentre /news/statements/2009/h1n1_20090425/en/ (accessed 14 April 2017); WHO statement on the meeting of the International Health Regulations Emergency Committee concerning the international spread of wild poliovirus. World Health Organization. 2014. http://www.who.int /mediacentre/news/statements/2014/polio-20140505/en/ (accessed 14 April 2017); Statement on the 1st meeting of the IHR Emergency Committee on the 2014 Ebola outbreak in West Africa. World Health Organization. 2014. http://www.who.int/mediacentre/news/statements /2014/ebola-20140808/en/ (accessed 14 April 2017).

67. Fourth meeting of the Emergency Committee under the International Health Regulations (2005) regarding microcephaly, other neurological disorders and Zika virus. World Health Organization. 2016. http://www.who.int/mediacentre/news/statements/2016/zika-fourth-ec/en/ (accessed 14 April 2017).

68. Screening of travelers involves different combinations of immunization and travel history reviews, symptom questionnaires, temperature-taking, or other measures, depending upon the country and the specific diseases of concern. Rhymer W, Speare R. Countries' response to WHO's travel recommendations during the 2013–2016 Ebola outbreak. *Bull World Health Organization* 2017; 95, 1: 10–17. DOI: 10.2471/BLT.16.171579. Epub 18 October 2016.

69. Travelers' health. Centers for Disease Control and Prevention. 2017. https://wwwnc.cdc.gov /travel/ (accessed 14 April 2017); European Centre for Disease Prevention and Control. 2017. http://ecdc.europa.eu/en/Pages/home.aspx (accessed 13 April 2017).

70. Osterholm M. Preparing for the next pandemic. *New England Journal of Medicine* 2005; 352, 18: 1839–42.

71. "The EIS program is perennially underfunded. It was severely hampered during the Reagan administration, which ignored AIDS for years and then didn't want to talk about condoms. But it wasn't just conservative Republicans. The EIS program was nearly killed during the Clinton administration's 're-inventing government' reforms. Unfortunately, chronic under-funding is typical for public health. We prefer to throw money at individual clinical care rather than funding prevention, surveillance, and disease detection." Pendergrast. Interview with Mark Pendergrast.

Chapter 9. Fatal Fictions, Timely Truths

1. Ebola outbreak: Guinea health team killed. BBC News. 2014. http://www.bbc.com/news/world -africa-29256443 (accessed 23 March 2017).

2. Phillip A. Eight dead in attack on Ebola team in Guinea. "Killed in cold blood." *Washington Post.* 2014. https://www.washingtonpost.com/news/to-your-health/wp/2014/09/18/missing-health -workers-in-guinea-were-educating-villagers-about-ebola-when-they-were-attacked/ (accessed 23 March 2017).

3. Bavier J. Crowds attack Ebola facility, health workers in Guinea. Reuters. 2015. http://www .reuters.com/article/2015/02/14/us-health-ebola-guinea-idUSKBN0LI0G920150214 (accessed 23 March 2017).

4. Leavitt J. The public as an asset, not a problem. UPMC Center for Health Security. 2003. http:// www.upmchealthsecurity.org/our-work/events/2003_public-as-asset/Transcripts/leavitt .html (accessed 23 March 2017).

5. Sugg C. Coming of age: Communication's role in powering global health. Policy briefing. BBC. 2016. http://www.bbc.co.uk/mediaaction/publications-and-resources/policy/briefings/role-of -communication-in-global-health (accessed 23 March 2017).

6. Working Group on "Governance Dilemmas" in Bioterrorism Response. Leading during bioattacks and epidemics with the public's trust and help. *Biosecurity and Bioterrorism: Biodefense Strategy, Practice, and Science* 2004; 2(1): 25–40.

7. Covey S. *The speed of trust: The one thing that changes everything.* New York: Free Press, 2006; and Quick J. Reynolds B. 28 November 2016; by phone.

8. Kahneman D. *Thinking, fast and slow.* New York: Farrar, Straus & Giroux, 2011; and Ariely D. *Predictably irrational: The hidden forces that shape our decisions.* Revised and expanded edition. New York: HarperCollins e-Books, 2014.

9. The human brain uses more energy than any other organ. It takes up 3 percent of our body weight and uses 20 percent of our energy.

10. Peretti J. SUVs, handwash and FOMO: How the advertising industry embraced fear. *The Guardian.* 2014. https://www.theguardian.com/media/2014/jul/06/how-advertising-industry -concept-fear (accessed 23 March 2017).

11. Ibid.

12. Crowley M, Grunwald M. The Hottest Zone. *Politico*. 2014. http://www.politico.com/magazine /story/2014/10/how-the-media-stoked-ebola-panic-112095 (accessed 23 March 2017).

13. Hedgecock S. 5 crazy U.S. outbreaks of Ebola paranoia. *Forbes*. 2014. http://www.forbes.com /sites/sarahhedgecock/2014/10/29/5-crazy-u-s-outbreaks-of-ebola-paranoia/#4520340a4067 (accessed 23 March 2017).

14. Golston H. Bridal shop closes where nurse with Ebola visited. *USA Today*. 2015. https://www .usatoday.com/story/news/nation-now/2015/01/08/bridal-shop-closes-after-visit-by-ebola -nurse/21448393/# (accessed 23 March 2017).

15. McKenna M. Ebolanoia: The only thing we have to fear is Ebola fear itself. *Wired*. 2014. https:// www.wired.com/2014/10/ebolanoia/ (accessed 23 March 2017).

16. Mulholland Q. Be very afraid: How the media failed in covering Ebola. *Harvard Political Review*. 2014. http://harvardpolitics.com/covers/afraid-media-failed-coverage-ebola/ (accessed 23 March 2017).

17. American Public Health Association. Learning from the experiences of Red Cross volunteers in Guinea. 2014. https://apha.confex.com/recording/apha/142am/mp4/free/4db77adf5df9fff0d3 caf5cafe28f496/paper315977_1.mp4 (accessed 23 March 2017).

18. Lee J. *An epidemic of rumors: How stories shape our perception of disease*. Boulder, CO: Utah State University Press, 2014.

19. Hogan C. "There is no such thing as Ebola." *Washington Post*. 2014. https://www.washingtonpost .com/news/morning-mix/wp/2014/07/18/there-is-no-such-thing-as-ebola/?tid=a_inl (accessed 23 March 2017).

20. Whipps H. How smallpox changed the world. Live Science. 2008. http://www.livescience.com /7509-smallpox-changed-world.html (accessed 23 March 2017).

21. Wisconsin Historical Society. Odd Wisconsin: Smallpox outbreak of 1894 led to battles in Milwaukee streets. *Wisconsin State Journal*. 2013. http://host.madison.com/wsj/news/local/health _med_fit/odd-wisconsin-smallpox-outbreak-of-led-to-battles-in-milwaukee/article_63e02acc -649f-11e2-9692-001a4bcf887a.html (accessed 23 March 2017).

22. Ibid.

23. According to 2015 research conducted by Edelman, a global public relations firm, 50 percent of survey respondents generally distrust their governments (with strong regional variations), and 60 percent of countries now distrust the media. Trust around the world. Edelman. 2015. http:// www.edelman.com/insights/intellectual-property/2015-edelman-trust-barometer/trust -around-world/ (accessed 23 March 2017).

24. Outbreak communication: Best practices for communicating with the public during an outbreak. World Health Organization. 2004. http://www.who.int/csr/resources/publications/WHO _CDS_2005_32/en/ (accessed 23 March 2017).

25. Fryer B. Ropeik D. 12 April 2016; by phone.

26. Fischhoff B. Scientifically sound pandemic risk communication. U.S. House Science Committee briefing: Gaps in the national flu preparedness plan, social science planning and response. 2005: 2. http://www.apa.org/about/gr/science/advocacy/2005/fischhoff.pdf.

27. Elected officials and public leaders can and must learn how to communicate in a health crisis, whether it is a naturally occurring epidemic or an act of bioterror. Woe to the leader who thinks he or she will be a "natural" when people around them are sick and dying from a mysterious attacker. The CDC's Crisis and Emergency Risk Communication (CERC) training and plan for a flu pandemic is an example of an effort to communicate effectively during emergencies (https://emergency.cdc.gov /cerc/). These principles are used by public-health professionals and public-information officers to provide information that helps individuals, stakeholders, and entire communities make the best possible decisions for themselves and their loved ones. Another excellent guide is from the UPMC Center for Health Security, "How to Lead During Bioattacks with the Public's Trust and Help," which prepares leaders for the governance dilemmas they will face in a major public-health crisis: how to prevent illness, suffering, and death; how to manage trade and borders; how to uphold civil liberties; how to manage the 24/7 news cycle; and so forth. How to lead during bioattacks with the public's trust and help. UPMC Center for Biosecurity. 2004. http://www.upmchealthsecurity .org/our-work/interactives/leadership-guide/curriculum/leadership_manual.pdf (accessed 23 March 2017).

28. In addition to Hong Kong, Reynolds has acted as an international crisis communications consultant on health issues for France, Australia, Canada, former Soviet Union nations, NATO, and WHO. She wrote the book now taught in universities and other settings nationwide and internationally, *Crisis and Emergency Risk Communication*. Crisis emergency and risk communication. Centers for Disease Control and Prevention. 2014. https://emergency.cdc.gov/cerc /resources/pdf/cerc_2014edition.pdf (accessed 23 March 2017).

29. Quick J. Reynolds B. 28 November 2016; by phone. During the Ebola epidemic, Dr. Thomas Frieden, then head of the CDC, modeled Reynolds's advice. He returned from West Africa with a clear message: this is a situation; this is what we must do. He called Ebola a "tragic virus" and spelled out the action needed to stop its spread and save lives: active surveillance, rapid case investigation, emergency treatment of patients with suspected Ebola, contact tracing and follow-up, widespread infection control, and safe burials. CDC chief on West African Ebola: "We know what to do, but it's not easy." NPR. 2014. http://www.npr.org/2014/08/01/337034361/cdc-chief-on-west-african-ebola-we-know-what-to-do-but-its-not-easy (accessed 23 March 2017).

30. Crisis emergency and risk communication: Basic guide. Centers for Disease Control and Prevention. 2008. https://emergency.cdc.gov/cerc/resources/pdf/cerc_guide_basic.pdf (accessed 23 March 2017).

31. Quick J. Rohde H. 22 May 2017; email communication.

32. Outbreak of West Nile–like viral encephalitis—New York, 1999. Centers for Disease Control and Prevention. 1999. https://www.cdc.gov/mmwr/preview/mmwrhtml/mm4838a1.htm (accessed 23 March 2017).

33. American Public Health Association. Learning from the experiences.

34. Anoko J. Communication with rebellious communities during an outbreak of Ebola virus disease in Guinea: An anthropological approach. Ebola Response Anthropology Platform. 2014. http://www.ebola-anthropology.net/case_studies/communication-with-rebellious-communities-during-an-outbreak-of-ebola-virus-disease-in-guinea-an-anthropological-approach/ (accessed 23 March 2017).

35. Anoko was also practicing a form of "positive deviance," a method of changing behavior based on careful listening and then deploying successful practices learned from people themselves. Many years ago, Jerry and Monique Sternin, both nutritionists, went to Vietnam to do a field observation. They each noticed that in some communities children were starving, but in others they thrived. What made the difference? Some people inside the village already had the solution. As it turned out, the children who thrived were fed little bits of shrimp in their food, contrary to the prevailing cultural practice. All around the world, the Sternins noticed that "positive deviants" defied the cultural norms within their own communities and quietly went about disobeying the rules. The Sternins set about working at the local level to identify those positive deviants who could amplify these inherent, positive practices (as opposed to focusing on what was going wrong in the community and "fixing" it). In so doing, they found that the lives of the poor could be improved. The optimum solution, then, was to have the people who were already doing a good job of feeding their children become the mentors and leaders for the rest of the community. (For more about positive deviance, see: http://www.positivedeviance.org/about_pdi/.)

36. Hussain M. MSF says lack of public health messages on Ebola "big mistake." Reuters. 2015. http://www.reuters.com/article/us-health-ebola-msf-idUSKBN0L81QF20150204 (accessed 23 March 2017).

37. Quick J. Jalloh MB. 8 November 2016; in person.

38. About Sierra Leone. UNDP in Sierra Leone. 2016. http://www.sl.undp.org/content/sierraleone/en/home/countryinfo.html (accessed 23 March 2017).

39. 2014 Ebola outbreak in West Africa—case counts. Centers for Disease Control and Prevention. 2016. https://www.cdc.gov/vhf/ebola/outbreaks/2014-west-africa/case-counts.html (accessed 16 November 2016).

40. Lessons from the response to the Ebola virus disease outbreak in Sierra Leone May 2014–November 2015, summary report. National Ebola Response Centre. 2016. http://nerc.sl/sites/default/files/docs/EVD%20Lessons%20Learned%20Summary%20A5%20FINAL.pdf (accessed 16 November 2016).

41. Operational Manual. National Ebola Response Centre. 2014. http://nerc.sl/?q=pillarclusters (accessed 13 November 2016).

42. Mohammad B. Jalloh. Focus 1000. 2017. http://www.focus1000.org/index.php/mohammad-bailor-jalloh (accessed 23 March 2017).

43. Other members of SMAC included two other local NGOs (Goal, and Restless Development) as well as BBC Media Action and the U.S. CDC.

44. Hogan C. "There is no such thing as Ebola."

45. Surviving Ebola: Our champions fight stigma. Restless Development. 2014. http://restlessdevelopment.org/news/2014/12/09/ebola-champions-survivors (accessed 23 March 2017).

46. Get-to-zero Ebola campaign underway in Sierra Leone. Global Ebola Response. 2015. http://ebolaresponse.un.org/get-zero-ebola-campaign-underway-sierra-leone (accessed 23 March 2017).

47. Traditional healers union hold 1 day workshop to support reaching zero Ebola in Sierra Leone.

Focus 1000. 2015. http://focus1000.org/index.php/nw/119-traditional-healers-union-hold-1-day-workshop-to-support-reaching-zero-ebola-in-sierra-leone (accessed 23 March 2017).

48. Author calculation from data reported in: Ebola situation report 30 December 2015. World Health Organization. 2015. http://apps.who.int/ebola/current-situation/ebola-situation-report-30-december-2015 (accessed 7 July 2017).

49. Lessons from the response to the Ebola virus disease outbreak in Sierra Leone May 2014–November 2015, summary report. National Ebola Response Centre. 2016. http://nerc.sl/sites/default/files/docs/EVD%20Lessons%20Learned%20Summary%20A5%20FINAL.pdf (accessed 14 November 2016).

50. Goodchild van Hilten L. Should the media take more responsibility in epidemics? Elsevier Connect. 2016. https://www.elsevier.com/connect/should-the-media-take-more-responsibility-in-epidemics (accessed 23 March 2017).

51. Yan Q, Tang S, Gabriele S, Wu J. Media coverage and hospital notifications: Correlation analysis and optimal media impact duration to manage a pandemic. *Journal of Theoretical Biology* 2016; 390: 1–13.

52. Lai A, Tan T. Combating SARS and H1N1: Insights and lessons from Singapore's public health control measures. *Austrian Journal of South-East Asian Studies* 2012; 5, 1: 74–101. http://www.seas.at/aseas/5_1/ASEAS_5_1_A5.pdf.

53. Pulitzer Prize winners by year. The Pulitzer Prizes. 2015. http://www.pulitzer.org/prize-winners-by-year/2015.

54. Examples of their headlines include: Ebola turns loving care into deadly risk; Those who serve Ebola victims soldier on; Ebola's mystery: One boy lives, another dies; Ambulance work in Liberia is a busy and lonely business; How Ebola roared back; Village frozen by fear and death; Liberia's Ebola crisis puts president in harsh light; Fear of Ebola breeds a terror of physicians; Cuts at W.H.O. hurt response to Ebola crisis. *New York Times.* https://www.nytimes.com/interactive/2015/04/20/world/africa/ebola-coverage-pulitzer.html (accessed 23 March 2017).

55. Sugg. Coming of age.

56. Wilkinson S. Practice briefing: Using media and communication to respond to public health emergencies. BBC. 2016. http://www.bbc.co.uk/mediaaction/publications-and-resources/policy/practice-briefings/ebola (accessed 23 March 2017).

57. Ayres A, ed. *The wit and wisdom of Mark Twain.* New York: Harper & Row, 1987: 139. Knowingly or unknowingly, Twain was actually quoting a proverb used in an 1855 sermon by the popular London preacher Charles Haddon Spurgeon: "If you want truth to go round the world you must hire an express train to pull it; but if you want a lie to go round the world, it will fly; it is as light as a feather, and a breath will carry it. It is well said in the old Proverb, 'A lie will go round the world while truth is pulling its boots on.'" Spurgeon C. *Spurgeon's gems: Being brilliant passages from the discourses of the Rev. C. H. Spurgeon.* London: Alabaster & Passmore, 1859: 154–55.

58. Oyeyemi S, Gabarron E, Wynn R. Ebola, Twitter, and misinformation: A dangerous combination? *British Medical Journal* 2014; 349: g6178.

59. Ebola situation report 8 April 2015. World Health Organization. 2015. http://apps.who.int/ebola/current-situation/ebola-situation-report-8-april-2015 (accessed 23 March 2017).

60. Ebola: Experimental therapies and rumored remedies. World Health Organization. 2014. http://www.who.int/mediacentre/news/ebola/15-august-2014/en/ (accessed 23 March 2017).

61. Henderson M. Why millennials believe vaccines cause autism. *Forbes.* 2015. http://www.forbes.com/sites/jmaureenhenderson/2015/02/10/why-millennials-believe-vaccines-cause-autism/#66bb7b003a1d (accessed 23 March 2017).

62. Sarmah S. Fighting the endless spread of Ebola misinformation on social media. *Fast Company.* 2014. http://www.fastcompany.com/3034380/fighting-the-endless-spread-of-ebola-misinformation-on-social-media (accessed 23 March 2017).

63. Hogan. "There is no such thing as Ebola."

64. Ibid.

65. Carter M. How Twitter may have helped Nigeria contain Ebola. *British Medical Journal* 2014; 349: g6946.

66. The health communicator's social media toolkit. Centers for Disease Control and Prevention. 2011. http://www.cdc.gov/socialmedia/tools/guidelines/pdf/socialmediatoolkit_bm.pdf (accessed 23 March 2017).

67. Sarmah. Fighting the endless spread.

68. Fung I, Tse Z, Cheung C, Miu A, Fu K. Ebola and the social media. *The Lancet* 2014; 384: 2207.

69. Lu S. An epidemic of fear. *American Psychological Association* 2014; 46, 3: 46. http://www.apa.org/monitor/2015/03/fear.aspx.

70. PMC also advocates for human rights, the environment, and population control. See: https://www.populationmedia.org/.

71. Center P. Sex, soap operas, and social change: Kriss Barker teaches sabido and changes the world. GlobeNewswire News Room. 2014. https://globenewswire.com/news-release/2014/05/19/637601/10082326/en/Sex-Soap-Operas-and-Social-Change-Kriss-Barker-Teaches-Sabido-and-Changes-the-World.html (accessed 23 March 2017).

72. Gold Coast Hospital and Health Service. Cormit Avital says she thought she was bulletproof. Gold Coast Health. 2016. https://www.youtube.com/watch?v=vRsHkDWm2EM (accessed 23 March 2017).

73. Cormit Avital says she thought she was bulletproof. *ABC News*. 2016. http://www.abc.net.au/news/2016-04-06/cormit-avital-says-she-thought-she-was-bulletproof/7304378 (accessed 23 March 2017).

74. Fact sheet: Measles. World Health Organization. 2017. http://who.int/mediacentre/factsheets/fs286/en/ (accessed 31 January 2017).

75. Foppa I, Cheng P, Reynolds S et al. Deaths averted by influenza vaccination in the U.S. during the seasons 2005/06 through 2013/14. *Vaccine* 2015; 33: 3003–9.

76. Larson H, de Figueiredo A, Xiahong Z et al. The state of vaccine confidence 2016: Global insights through a 67-country survey. *EBioMedicine* 2016; 12: 295–301.

77. Poland G, Jacobson R. The re-emergence of measles in developed countries: Time to develop the next-generation measles vaccines? *Vaccine* 2012; 30: 103–4. Data for 2012–15 from www.cdc.gov/measles/cases-outbreaks.html (accessed 27 February 2017).

78. Measles Outbreaks in Europe. World Health Organization. 2011. http://www.who.int/csr/don/2011_04_21/en/ (accessed 7 July 2017). Epidemiological update on measles in EU and EEA/EFTA member states. European Centre for Disease Prevention and Control. 2011. http://ecdc.europa.eu/en/activities/sciadvice/_layouts/forms/Review_DispForm.aspx?ID=526&List=a3216f4c-f040-4f51-9f77-a96046dbfd72 (accessed 23 March 2017).

79. Measles outbreaks across Europe threaten progress of elimination. Press release. World Health Organization. 2017. http://www.euro.who.int/en/media-centre/sections/press-releases/2017/measles-outbreaks-across-europe-threaten-progress-towards-elimination (accessed 23 March 2017).

80. See: Pertussis cases by year (1922–2015). Centers for Disease Control and Prevention. 2017. https://www.cdc.gov/pertussis/surv-reporting/cases-by-year.html (accessed 7 July 2017) and Phadke V, Bednarczyk R, Salmon D, Omer S. Association between vaccine refusal and vaccine-preventable diseases in the United States. *JAMA* 2016; 315: 1149.

81. Parker L. The anti-vaccine generation: How movement against shots got its start. *National Geographic*. 2015. http://news.nationalgeographic.com/news/2015/02/150206-measles-vaccine-disney-outbreak-polio-health-science-infocus/ (accessed 23 March 2017). Two of the 14 children were too young to be vaccinated, and another had received only one of the two recommended doses, according to local health officials.

82. Henderson. Why millennials believe.

83. Nyhan B, Reifler J, Richey S. The role of social networks in influenza vaccine attitudes and intentions among college students in the southeastern United States. *Journal of Adolescent Health* 2012; 51: 302–4. http://cpj.sagepub.com/content/18/3/155.abstract?ijkey=a20de7e74fce454c6392f0fefb1ce9090c881c46&keytype2=tf_ipsecsha (accessed 23 March 2017).

84. Vaccine Confidence Project. The state of vaccine confidence. London School of Hygiene and Tropical Medicine. 2015. http://www.vaccineconfidence.org/The-State-of-Vaccine-Confidence-2015.pdf (accessed 23 March 2017).

85. Larson H. Vaccines and public behavior. 2014. https://www.youtube.com/watch?v=-94ldp9 MoMA (accessed 23 March 2017).

86. Majewski S, Afsar O. Tracking anti-vaccination sentiment in Eastern European social media networks. UNICEF. 2013. https://www.unicef.org/ceecis/Tracking_anti-vaccine_sentiment_in_Eastern_European_social_media_networks.pdf (accessed 23 March 2017).

87. U.S. Food and Drug Administration. Thimerosol and vaccines. 2017. https://www.fda.gov/biologicsbloodvaccines/safetyavailability/vaccinesafety/ucm096228 (accessed 23 Marrch 2017).

88. Deer B. Revealed: MMR research scandal. 2004. *Sunday Times*. http://briandeer.com/mmr/lancet-deer-1.htm (accessed 23 March 2017).

89. MMR timeline. *The Guardian*. 2010. https://www.theguardian.com/society/2010/jan/28/mmr-doctor-timeline (accessed 23 March 2017).

90. Flaherty DK. The vaccine-autism connection: A public health crisis caused by unethical medical practices and fraudulent science. *Annals of Pharmacotherapy* 2011; 45, 10: 1302–4. DOI:10.1345/aph.1Q318. PMID 21917556.

91. O'Neill B. The media's MMR shame. *The Guardian*. 2006. https://www.theguardian.com/commentisfree/2006/jun/16/whenjournalismkills (accessed 23 March 2017).

92. Boseley S. MMR vaccinations fall to new low. *The Guardian*. 2004. https://www.theguardian.com/uk/2004/sep/24/society.politics (accessed 23 March 2017).

93. Data from Public Health England published by the Vaccine Knowledge Project, University of Oxford. http://vk.ovg.ox.ac.uk/measles (accessed 20 February 2017).

94. Measles vaccination has saved an estimated 17.1 million lives since 2000. World Health Organization. 2015. http://www.who.int/mediacentre/news/releases/2015/measles-vaccination/en/ (accessed 23 March 2017).

95. Nyhan B, Reifler J. When corrections fail: The persistence of political misperceptions. *Political Behavior* 2010; 32, 2: 303–30. DOI: 10.1007/s11109-010-9112-2 (accessed 30 March 2010).

96. Nyhan B, Reifler J. Does correcting myths about the flu vaccine work? An experimental evaluation of the effects of corrective information. *Vaccine* 2015; 33: 459–64.

97. Mooney C. Study: You can't change an anti-vaxxer's mind. *Mother Jones*. 2014. http://www.motherjones.com/environment/2014/02/vaccine-denial-psychology-backfire-effect (accessed 23 March 2017).

98. Nyhan B. Infectious messaging. 2015. http://www.youtube.com/watch?v=JR_HZCju5Tc (accessed 23 March 2017).

99. Ibid.

100. Hayden G. Clinical review: Measles vaccine failure. *Clinical Pediatrics* 1979; 18: 155–56. http://journals.sagepub.com/doi/abs/10.1177/000992287901800308 (accessed 19 November 2016).

101. Obregon R, Waisbord S. The complexity of social mobilization in health communication: Top-down and bottom-up experiences in polio eradication. *Journal of Health Communication* 2010; 15: 25–47.

102. Vaccine Confidence Project. Dangerous liaisons confidence commentary: Blog archive. London School of Hygiene and Tropical Medicine. http://www.vaccineconfidence.org/ (accessed 19 November 2016).

103. Quick J. Larson H. 25 November 2016; by phone.

104. Ibid.

105. About us. Vaccine Confidence Project. London School of Hygiene and Tropical Medicine. http://www.vaccineconfidence.org/about/ (accessed 19 November 2016).

106. About us. Immunization Action Coalition. 2017. http://www.immunize.org/aboutus/ (accessed 19 November 2016).

107. Moms Who Vax. http://momswhovax.blogspot.com/ (accessed 19 November 2016).

108. Shellenbarger S. Most students don't know when news is fake, Stanford study finds. *Wall Street Journal*. 2016. https://www.wsj.com/articles/most-students-dont-know-when-news-is-fake-stanford-study-finds-1479752576 (accessed 19 November 2016).

109. The case for compulsory immunization may be stronger in countries and populations where mortality rates are still high and health services less available. Among European countries, mandatory immunization policies are not associated with higher immunization rates. This may reflect a dynamic in which countries are more likely to make immunization mandatory when populations are less likely to follow voluntary official advice. Compulsory vaccination and rates of coverage immunisation in Europe. ASSET Reports. 2014. http://www.asset-scienceinsociety.eu/reports/page1.html (accessed 15 April 2017).

110. Every U.S. state has an immunization requirement for public school entry. The majority of states permit only medical or religious exemptions from mandatory immunization for school entry. The exemption process varies among states, as do additional reasons for exemption. See: State school immunization requirements and vaccine exemption laws. Centers for Disease Control and Prevention. 2017. https://www.cdc.gov/phlp/docs/school-vaccinations.pdf (accessed 1 June 2017).

111. Saint-Victor D, Omer S. Vaccine refusal and the endgame: Walking the last mile first. *Philosophical Transactions of the Royal Society B: Biological Sciences* 2013; 368: 20120148.

112. Quick J. Larson H. 25 November 2016; by phone.

113. Lin L, Savoia E, Agboola F, Viswanath K. What have we learned about communication inequalities during the H1N1 pandemic: A systematic review of the literature. *BMC Public Health* 2014; 14. DOI:10.1186/1471-2458-14-484.

Chapter 10. Disruptive Innovation, Collaborative Transformation

1. Fact Sheet: Poliomyelitis. World Health Organization. 2017. http://www.who.int/mediacentre/factsheets/fs114/en/ (accessed 7 July 2017).

2. According to the Global Polio Eradication Initiative, "vulnerable" countries are Cameroon, Equatorial Guinea, Ethiopia, Iraq, Nigeria, Somalia, South Sudan, and Syria. See: Where we work. Global Polio Eradication Initiative. 2017. http://www.polioeradication.org/Keycountries.aspx (accessed 23 April 2017).

3. Oxford J. Leslie Collier obituary. *The Guardian*. 2011. https://www.theguardian.com/science/2011/may/09/leslie-collier-obituary (accessed 23 April 2017).

4. Fenner F, Henderson D, Arita I et al. Smallpox and its eradication. World Health Organization. 1988. http://www.who.int/iris/handle/10665/39485 (accessed 23 April 2017).

5. Ibid.

6. Foege W, Millar J, Lane J. Selective epidemiologic control in smallpox eradication. *American Journal of Epidemiology* 1971; 94, 4: 311–15. pmid:5110547.

7. Brittain A. How a method used to wipe out smallpox is making a comeback in the fight against Ebola. *Washington Post*. 2015. https://www.washingtonpost.com/news/worldviews/wp/2015/02/14/how-a-method-used-to-wipe-out-smallpox-is-making-a-comeback-in-the-fight-against-ebola/ (accessed 23 April 2017).

8. Schnirring L, Roos R. High effectiveness found in Guinea Ebola ring vaccination trial. Center for Infectious Disease Research and Policy. 2015. http://www.cidrap.umn.edu/news-perspective/2015/07/high-effectiveness-found-guinea-ebola-ring-vaccination-trial (accessed 23 April 2017).

9. When the 2014 Ebola outbreak occurred, there was no approved vaccine, so no one, not even health workers, could be vaccinated to prevent infection. There was no point-of-care rapid test, so people who had been exposed had to be isolated, and people traveling from affected areas could not be tested. Similarly, when the Zika virus exploded in Latin America in late 2015, there was no rapid test and no vaccine. Since the early 2000s, new preventive technologies against the night-biting *Anopheles* mosquito had dramatically reduced malaria in many countries, especially in children. Comparable progress had not been made to control the day-biting, urban-dwelling *Aedes aegypti* mosquito that carries dengue, chikungunya, Zika, and yellow fever viruses.

10. Bower J, Christensen C. Disruptive technologies: Catching the wave. *Harvard Business Review* 1995; Jan/Feb: 53–54. https://hbr.org/1995/01/disruptive-technologies-catching-the-wave.

11. In 2016, a new threat, the Zika virus, was haunting communities throughout the Western Hemisphere and beginning to threaten countries elsewhere. The disease was moving fast. As of this writing, vaccines are not yet available for Zika, dengue, MERS, and several of the other viruses of pandemic potential. An effective vaccine for several common strains of Ebola became available in 2016, too late for West Africa.

12. Fryer. B. Barouch. D. 7 September 2017; by phone.

13. Mukherjee S. The race for a Zika vaccine. *New Yorker*. 2016. http://www.newyorker.com/magazine/2016/08/22/the-race-for-a-zika-vaccine (accessed 23 April 2017).

14. Berkley S. Transcript of "HIV and flu—the vaccine strategy." TED Talk. 2010. https://www.ted.com/talks/seth_berkley_hiv_and_flu_the_vaccine_strategy/transcript?language=en (accessed 24 April 2017).

15. Lincoff N. Researchers closer now to HIV vaccine than ever before. Healthline. 2016. http://www.healthline.com/health-news/researchers-closer-now-to-hiv-vaccine-than-ever-before-072415 (accessed 24 April 2017).

16. The influenza vaccine was licensed first in 1945 for use by the U.S. military.

17. Waring B. Palese points way to universal influenza virus vaccine. *NIH Record*. 2014. https://nihrecord.nih.gov/newsletters/2014/06_20_2014/story1.htm (accessed 24 April 2017).

18. Osterweil N. Universal flu vaccine in the works. Coverage from the American Society for Microbiology (ASM). *Microbe*. 2016. http://www.medscape.com/viewarticle/865154#vp_2 (login required).

19. Osterholm M, Olshaker M. *Deadliest enemy: Our war against killer germs*. Boston: Little, Brown and Company, 2017.

20. Han B, Drake J. Future directions in analytics for infectious disease intelligence. *EMBO Reports* 2016; 17: 785–89.

21. Spraying is rather like applying a chain saw to drive nails. It comes with problems of its own: not only do insects develop resistance to the spray, but the technology is old. It requires serious investment in time, personnel, chemicals, and quality control for public spraying to be effective. See: Knapp J, Macdonald M, Malone D, Hamon N, Richardson J. Disruptive technology for vector control: the Innovative Vector Control Consortium and the U.S. Military join forces to explore transformative insecticide application technology for mosquito control programmes. *Malaria Journal* 2015; 14. DOI:10.1186/s12936-015-0907-9.

22. Wilder-Smith A, Gubler D, Weaver S et al. Epidemic arboviral diseases: Priorities for research and public health. *The Lancet*. 2016. DOI: 10.1016/S1473-3099 (16)30518–7.

23. While there is a range of options for controlling disease-carrying mosquitoes, there is still little scientific and public-health consensus about what combination of existing or to-be-developed mosquito-control methods will be the most effective, scalable, and sustainable in different settings and for different types of mosquitoes.

24. Oxitec: Innovative Insect Control. 2017. http://www.oxitec.com/ (accessed 24 April 2017).

25. Fedoroff N, Block J. Mosquito vs. mosquito in the battle over the Zika virus. *New York Times.* 2016. http://www.nytimes.com/2016/04/06/opinion/mosquito-vs-mosquito-in-the-battle-over-the-zika-virus.html (accessed 24 April 2017).

26. Deshpande A, McMahon B, Daughton A et al. Surveillance for emerging diseases with multiplexed point-of-care diagnostics. *Health Security* 2016; 14: 111–21. DOI: 10.1089/hs.2016.0005.

27. Mu X, Zhang L, Chang S, Cui W, Zheng Z. Multiplex microfluidic paper-based immunoassay for the diagnosis of hepatitis C virus infection. *Analytical Chemistry* 2015; 87: 8033. DOI: 10.1021/ac500247f.

28. Deshpande et al. Surveillance for emerging diseases.

29. Nouvellet P, Garske T, Mills H et al. The role of rapid diagnostics in managing Ebola epidemics. *Nature* 2015; 528: S109–16. http://www.nature.com/nature/journal/v528/n7580_supp_custom/full/nature16041.html?WT.ec_id=NATURE-20151203&spMailingID=50159890&spUserID=MjA1NzcwMjE4MQS2&spJobID=820348363&spReportId=ODIwMzQ4MzYzS0 (accessed 24 April 2017).

30. First antigen rapid test for Ebola through emergency assessment and eligible for procurement. World Health Organization. 2017. http://www.who.int/medicines/ebola-treatment/1st_antigen_RT_Ebola/en/ (accessed 24 April 2017).

31. In 2016, Zika was spreading unabated throughout the world, reaching over 60 countries and territories from its stronghold in Latin America. Had a rapid test for Zika been available to health officials in Brazil, they would have been able to track its arrival and institute control measures long before Zika became widespread in mosquitoes. Thus, it might not be spreading to growing numbers of countries and constituting a major global health threat.

32. President's Malaria Initiative—Tanzania: Malaria operational plan FY 2015. USAID. 2015. https://www.pmi.gov/docs/default-source/default-document-library/malaria-operational-plans/fy-15/fy-2015-tanzania-malaria-operational-plan.pdf: 14.

33. Nosal L. Point-of-care diagnostics and living "integrated innovation." Grand Challenges Canada. 2013. http://www.grandchallenges.ca/grand-challenges/point-of-care-diagnostics/ (accessed 24 April 2017).

34. Bartlett J. Patient education: Testing for HIV (beyond the basics). UpToDate. 2015. http://www.uptodate.com/contents/testing-for-hiv-beyond-the-basics (accessed 24 April 2017).

35. UNAIDS. Global AIDS update. World Health Organization. 2016. http://www.who.int/hiv/pub/arv/global-aids-update-2016-pub/en/ (accessed 24 April 2017).

36. Fedorko D, Nelson N. Performance of rapid tests for detection of avian influenza A virus types H5N1 and H9N2. *Journal of Clinical Microbiology* 2006; 44, 4: 1596–97. DOI: 10.1128/JCM.44.4.1596-1597.2006.

37. Bissonnette L, Bergeron M. Diagnosing infections—current and anticipated technologies for point-of-care diagnostics and home-based testing. *Clinical Microbiology and Infection* 2010; 16: 1044–53.

38. Global Virome Project. http://www.globalviromeproject.org/ (accessed 24 April 2017).

39. WMO factsheet: Early warning systems saves millions of lives. World Meteorological Organization. 2012. https://www.wmo.int/pages/prog/drr/events/GPDRR-IV/Documents/Fact Sheets/FS_nhews.pdf (accessed 24 April 2017).

40. Walsh B. Virus hunter. *Time.* 2011. http://content.time.com/time/magazine/article/0,9171,2097962,00.html (accessed 24 April 2017).

41. USAID PREDICT. UC Davis Veterinary Medicine. 2017. http://www.vetmed.ucdavis.edu/ohi/predict/ (accessed 24 April 2017).

42. Reducing pandemic risk, promoting global health: Executive summary. USAID. 2017. www.vetmed.ucdavis.edu/ohi/local_resources/pdfs/chapters/2_predict_executive_summary.pdf (accessed 24 April 2017).

43. In July 2006 the UN Food and Agriculture Organization (FAO), the Office International des Epizooties (World Organization for Animal Health, OIE), and the World Health Organization (WHO) launched a joint worldwide early warning and response system aimed at zoonoses and other animal diseases. See: Launch of global early warning system for animal diseases transmissible to humans. Press release. World Health Organization. http://www.who.int/mediacentre/news/new/2006/nw02/en/ (accessed 28 May 2017).

44. Quick J and Fryer B. Daszak P. 10 March 2016; in person.

45. Ibid.
46. Monaghan A, Morin C, Steinhoff D et al. On the seasonal occurrence and abundance of the Zika virus vector mosquito *Aedes aegypti* in the contiguous United States. *PLOS Currents*. 2016. DOI:10.1371/currents.outbreaks.50dfc7f46798675fc63e7d7da563da76.
47. Cary Institute of Ecosystem Studies. Global early warning system for infectious diseases: Technology possible, data-driven, and worthy of our investment. *Science Daily*. 2016. https://www .sciencedaily.com/releases/2016/05/160520101029.htm (accessed 24 April 2017).
48. Sachan D. The age of drones: What might it mean for health? *The Lancet* 2016; 387, 10030: 1803–4. DOI: 10.1016/S0140-6736(16)30361-0.
49. Stewart J. Drop blood, not bombs! *Wired*. 2016. https://www.wired.com/2016/05/zipline-drones -rwanda/ (accessed 24 April 2017).
50. Nambiar R. How Rwanda is using drones to deliver medical aid. CNBC. 2016. http://www.cnbc .com/2016/05/27/how-rwanda-is-using-drones-to-save-millions-of-lives.html (accessed 24 April 2017).
51. Between 2000 and 2016, Uganda experienced five Ebola outbreaks, including the largest before the 2014 West Africa outbreak, with just over 425 confirmed cases and 224 deaths. Outbreaks chronology: Ebola virus disease. Centers for Disease Control and Prevention. 2016. https://www .cdc.gov/vhf/ebola/outbreaks/history/chronology.html (accessed 24 April 2017).
52. ADDOs are also improving the quality, access, and affordability of services. ADDOs also distribute mosquito-repellent nets, antimalarial medicines, and condoms, and they follow HIV patients and provide referrals. In 2003, before accreditation, only 6 percent of those who asked for help with malaria were treated correctly for the drug. In 2004, after the program launched, 24 percent were treated correctly, and in 2010, the number reached 63 percent. Today, all the drug shops in Tanzania have been accredited. ADDO proved to be both scalable and self-sustaining because the public was enthusiastic, the entrepreneurial shop owners were incentivized to be accredited, tracking and monitoring became easier, and new products and services kept getting added. Rutta E, Liana J, Embrey M et al. Accrediting retail drug shops to strengthen Tanzania's public health system: An ADDO case study. *Journal of Pharmaceutical Policy and Practice* 2015; 8: 23. DOI: 10.1186/s40545-015-0044-4. eCollection 2015. Erratum in: *Journal of Pharmaceutical Policy and Practice* 2015; 8: 29.
53. Quick J. Accredited medicines shops and Ebola. 2014. https://www.youtube.com/watch?v =OwKb8cwuAyo&t=1s (accessed 23 April 2017).
54. Rutta E. et al. Accrediting retail drug shops.
55. Loryoun A. The accredited medicine stores in Liberia: Their role in the Ebola crisis. Impatient Optimists. 2015. http://www.impatientoptimists.org/Posts/2015/12/The-Accredited-Medicine -Stores-in-Liberia-Their-Role-in-the-Ebola-Crisis (accessed 4 April 2017).
56. The four high-level reports were variously led by Harvard University/London School of Hygiene and Tropical Medicine, the U.S. National Academy of Medicine, the United Nations, and the World Health Organization.
57. Chapter 5, Recommendation 2.1, NAM report, 2016.
58. A research and development blueprint for action to prevent epidemics. World Health Organization. 2017. http://www.who.int/blueprint/en/ (accessed 4 May 2017).
59. CEPI has been carefully designed with a participatory approach to priority-setting, the ability to capitalize on the speed and flexibility of the private sector, and strategic use of its own resources (already $500 million) to fill critical gaps. See: http://cepi.net.
60. Fact sheet on Canada's experimental vaccine for Ebola. Public Health Agency of Canada. 2015. http://www.phac-aspc.gc.ca/id-mi/vsv-ebov-fs-eng.php (accessed 23 April 2017).
61. McNeil D. New Ebola vaccine gives 100 percent protection. *New York Times*. 2016. https://www .nytimes.com/2016/12/22/health/ebola-vaccine.html (accessed 23 April 2017).
62. Final trial results confirm Ebola vaccine provides high protection against disease. World Health Organization. 2016. http://www.who.int/mediacentre/news/releases/2016/ebola-vaccine-results /en/ (accessed 23 April 2017).
63. Merck received a "Breakthrough Therapy Designation" from the U.S. Food and Drug Administration and PRIME status from the European Medicines Agency, which would speed regulatory review and make the vaccine widely available as soon as possible.
64. Kresge K. An interview with Mark Feinberg. *IAVI Report*. 2015. http://www.iavireport.org/index .php?option=com_content&view=article&id=1850&Itemid=884 (accessed 23 April 2017).
65. The Bill and Melinda Gates Foundation, for example, has a Grand Challenges in Global Health program that identifies breakthrough advances in health. See: http://gcgh.grandchallenges.org /grants?f[0]=field_challenge%253Afield_initiative%3A37072&f[1]=funding_year% 3A2005&items_per_page=50.

66. USAID announces initial results of Grand Challenge to combat Zika. USAID. 2016. https://www.usaid.gov/news-information/press-releases/aug-10-2016-usaid-announces-initial-results-grand-challenge-combat-zika (accessed 23 April 2017).

Chapter 11. Invest Wisely, Save Lives

1. In nominating Kim, President Obama noted, "He's worked from Asia to Africa to the Americas—from capitals to small villages. The World Bank is one of the most powerful tools we have to reduce poverty and raise standards of living around the globe, and Jim's personal experience and years of service make him an ideal candidate for this job." Three in running for World Bank job. Al Jazeera. 2012. http://www.aljazeera.com/news/americas/2012/03/201232454653902871.html (accessed 1 May 2017).
2. Before becoming World Bank president, Kim led the World Health Organization movement for universal AIDS treatment, created Harvard University's pioneering global health delivery program, and served as president of Dartmouth University. Management Sciences for Health was privileged to have his service as a member of our board of directors.
3. Kim J, Millen J, Irwin A, Gershman J. *Dying for growth: Global inequality and the health of the poor.* Monroe, ME: Common Courage Press, 2000.
4. Ebola: World Bank group mobilizes emergency funding to fight epidemic in West Africa. World Bank. 2014. http://www.worldbank.org/en/news/press-release/2014/08/04/ebola-world-bank-group-mobilizes-emergency-funding-for-guinea-liberia-and-sierra-leone-to-fight-epidemic (accessed 1 May 2017).
5. Jeff Skoll speaks with Dr. Jim Yong Kim at the Skoll World Forum 2017 #SkollWF 2017. 2017. https://www.youtube.com/watch?v=FM3_ejHNv6Y (accessed 1 May 2017).
6. World Bank group launches groundbreaking financing facility to protect poorest countries against pandemics. World Bank. 2016. http://www.worldbank.org/en/news/press-release/2016/05/21/world-bank-group-launches-groundbreaking-financing-facility-to-protect-poorest-countries-against-pandemics (accessed 1 May 2017).
7. Pandemic emergency financing facility: Frequently asked questions. World Bank. 2017. http://www.worldbank.org/en/topic/pandemics/brief/pandemic-emergency-facility-frequently-asked-questions (accessed 1 May 2017).
8. Jeff Skoll speaks with Dr. Jim Yong Kim.
9. The amount as of this writing stood at $4.3 billion. Budget. World Health Organization. 2017. http://www.who.int/about/finances-accountability/budget/en/ (accessed 1 May 2017).
10. Fink S. Cuts at W.H.O. hurt response to Ebola crisis. *New York Times.* 2014. http://www.nytimes.com/2014/09/04/world/africa/cuts-at-who-hurt-response-to-ebola-crisis.html (accessed 1 May 2017).
11. World Bank estimates Ebola could cost West Africa 32.6 billion dollars. Euronews. 2014. http://www.euronews.com/2014/10/10/world-bank-estimates-ebola-cost-in-west-africa-at-326-billion-dollars (accessed 1 May 2017).
12. According to a report published in 2014 by EcoHealthAlliance, the cost of an influenza pandemic ranges from $374 billion for a mild one to $7.3 trillion for one that's severe. That figure also accounts for a 12.6 percent loss in gross domestic product and millions of lives lost. It's a worst-case scenario, but not unimaginable, considering that the Ebola outbreak infected more than 24,000 people, and it's not even an airborne virus. See: Pike J, Bogich T, Elwood S, Finnoff D, Daszak P. Economic optimization of a global strategy to address the pandemic threat. *Proceedings of the National Academy of Sciences* 2014; 111: 18519–23.
13. The 2013–2014 national snapshot of public health preparedness. Centers for Disease Control and Prevention. 2014. https://www.cdc.gov/phpr/pubs-links/2013/ (accessed 1 May 2017).
14. One of those riders on the bill included defunding Planned Parenthood, an NGO that provides health care to women, including pregnant ones. See: Huetteman E. Funding planned parenthood, or not, may be key to keeping the government open. *New York Times.* 2016. http://www.nytimes.com/2016/09/13/us/politics/planned-parenthood-republicans-spending.html (accessed 1 May 2017).
15. Fryer B. Ariely D. 7 September 2016; by phone.
16. World economic global risks reports, annual reports from 2007 through 2017. World Economic Forum. 2017. https://www.weforum.org/reports/the-global-risks-report-2017 (accessed 1 May 2017).
17. 9–11 Commission Report. National Commission on Terrorist Attacks Upon the United States. 2004. https://www.9-11commission.gov/report/911Report.pdf.

18. Final Report of the National Commission on the Causes of the Financial and Economic Crisis in the United States. Financial Crisis Enquiry Commission. 2011. https://www.gpo.gov/fdsys/pkg/GPO-FCIC/pdf/GPO-FCIC.pdf.

19. Fewsmith J. China's response to SARS. *China Leadership Monitor*. 2003. http://www.hoover.org/sites/default/files/uploads/documents/clm7_jf.pdf (accessed 1 May 2017).

20. Bremer C. In Mexico's flu crisis, where is Calderon? Reuters UK. 2009. http://uk.reuters.com/article/uk-flu-mexico-calderon-analysis-sb-idUKTRE53S9DO20090429 (accessed 1 May 2017).

21. Bell A. Calderon's party loses Congress vote in Mexico. Reuters. 2009. http://www.reuters.com/article/us-mexico-election-idUSTRE56417W20090706 (accessed 1 May 2017).

22. Walsh K. Ebola becoming political issue. U.S. News. 2014. http://www.usnews.com/news/blogs/ken-walshs-washington/2014/10/10/ebola-becoming-political-issue (accessed 1 May 2017).

23. Webley K. The lessons from SARS. *Time*. 2009. http://content.time.com/time/health/article/0,8599,1894072,00.html (accessed 1 May 2017).

24. Ibid.

25. Weiss R. Ebola zone keeps Brussels Air lifeline after CEO's visit. Bloomberg. 2014. https://www.bloomberg.com/news/articles/2014-10-15/ebola-zone-keeps-brussels-air-lifeline-after-ceo-s-visit (accessed 1 May 2017).

26. No More Epidemics: A call to action. No More Epidemics. 2016. Nomoreepidemics.org. (accessed 15 February 2017).

27. Other kinds of partnerships, such as international foundations like Wellcome Trust and the Gates Foundation, provided funding to accelerate research and donated phones to help with on-the-ground communications. And NetHope, a nonprofit that focuses on communications solutions, Cisco, Facebook, and the UN Emergency Telecom Cluster established over 100 satellite terminals that extended coverage for voice and data services and created broadband solutions. Managing the risk and impact of future epidemics: Options for public-private cooperation. World Economic Forum. 2015. http://www3.weforum.org/docs/WEF_Managing_Risk_Epidemics_report_2015.pdf (accessed 1 May 2017).

28. Ibid.

29. Stack M, Ozawa S, Bishai D et al. Estimated economic benefits during the "decade of vaccines" include treatment savings, gains in labor productivity. *Health Affairs* 2011; 30: 1021–28.

30. Pike et al. Economic optimization.

31. The neglected dimensions of global security. National Academy of Medicine. 2016. https://www.nap.edu/catalog/21891/the-neglected-dimension-of-global-security-a-framework-to-counter (accessed 1 May 2017).

32. Return on investment for emergency preparedness study. World Food Programme. 2014. https://www.wfp.org/content/unicefwfp-return-investment-emergency-preparedness-study (accessed 1 May 2017).

33. 2016's $1.57 trillion global defence spend to kick off decade of growth, IHS Markit says. IHS Markit. 2016. http://news.ihsmarkit.com/press-release/2016s-15-trillion-global-defence-spend-kick-decade-growth-ihs-markit-says (accessed 1 May 2017).

34. Takahashi D. Worldwide game industry hits $91 billion in revenues in 2016, with mobile the clear leader. VentureBeat. 2016. https://venturebeat.com/2016/12/21/worldwide-game-industry-hits-91-billion-in-revenues-in-2016-with-mobile-the-clear-leader/ (accessed 1 May 2017).

35. Quick J. Frenk J. 2000; in person.

36. Wright S, Hanna L, Mailfert M. A wake up call: Lessons from Ebola for the world's health systems. Save the Children. 2015. https://www.savethechildren.net/sites/default/files/libraries/WAKE%20UP%20CALL%20REPORT%20PDF.pdf (accessed 29 October 2015).

37. No more epidemics: A call to action. No More Epidemics. 2016. http://nomoreepidemics.org/wp-content/uploads/2016/12/A-Call-to-Action.pdf (accessed 23 May 2016).

38. Financing global health 2012: The end of the golden age? Institute for Health Metrics and Evaluation. 2012. http://www.healthdata.org/sites/default/files/files/policy_report/2012/FGH/IHME_FGH2012_FullReport_HighResolution.pdf. (accessed 26 May 2016).

39. Røttingen J, Regmi S, Eide M et al. Mapping of available health research and development data: What's there, what's missing, and what role is there for a global observatory? *The Lancet* 2013; 382: 1286–307.

40. Within the U.S., the private sector accounts for 70 percent of medical R&D funding. Strengthening private sector R&D. Research!America. 2017. http://www.researchamerica.org/advocacy-action/issues-researchamerica-advocates/strengthening-private-sector-rd (accessed 1 May 2017).

41. Viergever R, Hendriks T. The 10 largest public and philanthropic funders of health research in

the world: What they fund and how they distribute their funds. *Health Research Policy and Systems* 2016; 14. DOI:10.1186/s12961-015-0074-z.

42. Osterholm and Olshaker. *Deadliest enemy*: 297.
43. Walsh B. A miracle within Trump's reach: Universal flu vaccine. Bloomberg. 2017. https://www .bloomberg.com/view/articles/2017-03-10/a-miracle-within-trump-s-reach-universal-flu -vaccine (accessed 1 May 2017).
44. Jeff Skoll speaks with Dr. Jim Yong Kim.
45. World Bank group launches groundbreaking financing facility to protect poorest countries against pandemics. World Bank. 2016. http://www.worldbank.org/en/news/press-release/2016 /05/21/world-bank-group-launches-groundbreaking-financing-facility-to-protect-poorest -countries-against-pandemics (accessed 1 May 2017).
46. Summers L. How finance can fight disease epidemics. *Washington Post*. 2015. https://www .washingtonpost.com/news/wonk/wp/2015/10/14/larry-summers-how-finance-can-fight -disease-epidemics// (accessed 1 May 2017).
47. Solon O. Fighting pandemics should be funded "like the military." *Wired UK*. 2016. http://www .wired.co.uk/article/pandemic-threat-wellcome-trust-zika-ebola (accessed 1 May 2017).

Chapter 12. Ring the Alarm, Rouse the Leaders

1. Brown T, Fee E. Social movements in health. *Annual Review of Public Health* 2014; 35: 385–98. DOI: 10.1146/annurev-publhealth-031912-114356.
2. Financing framework to end preventable child and maternal deaths (EPCMD). USAID. 2016. https://www.usaid.gov/cii/financing-framework-end-preventable-child-and-maternal-deaths -epcmd (accessed 22 March 2017).
3. Busby J. *Moral movements and foreign policy*. Cambridge: Cambridge University Press, 2010.
4. Berridge V. Public health activism: Lessons from history? *British Medical Journal* 2007; 335, 7633: 1310–12.
5. Dreier P. Social movements: How people make history. Mobilizing Ideas. 2012. https:// mobilizingideas.wordpress.com/2012/08/01/socialmovementshowpeoplemakehistory/ (accessed 6 March 2017).
6. Mbeki accuses CIA over Aids. BBC News. 2000. http://news.bbc.co.uk/2/hi/africa/959579.stm (accessed 22 March 2017).
7. Power S. The AIDS rebel. *New Yorker*. 2003. http://www.newyorker.com/magazine/2003/05 /19/the-aids-rebel (accessed 22 March 2017).
8. Report on the global HIV/AIDS epidemic. UNAIDS. 2000. http://data.unaids.org/pub/report /2000/2000_gr_en.pdf (accessed 22 March 2017).
9. Background material for this section is drawn from two sources: Nolen S. *28: Stories of AIDS in Africa*. London: Bloomsbury, 2009; and Power. The AIDS rebel.
10. McNeil J. A history of official government HIV/AIDS policy in South Africa. South African History Online. 2012. http://www.sahistory.org.za/topic/history-official-government-hivaids -policy-south-africa (accessed 22 March 2017).
11. AIDS was first reported in South Africa in 1982 in a homosexual man who had come from California; the first deaths were reported in 1985.
12. Himschall G. Generic antiretroviral therapy is safe and effective. World Health Organization. 2013. http://www.who.int/hiv/mediacentre/feature_story/commentary_genericARVs/en/ (accessed 22 March 2017).
13. Power. The AIDS rebel.
14. Mbali M. TAC in the history of rights-based, patient driven HIV/AIDS activism in South Africa. University of Michigan Library, Digital Collections. 2005. http://quod.lib.umich.edu /p/passages/4761530.0010.011/—tac-in-the-history-of-rights-based-patient-driven-hivaids ?rgn=main;view=fulltext (accessed 22 March 2017).
15. Cameron E. *Witness to AIDS*. London: I. B. Tauris & Co., 2007: 23.
16. Cameron's critical role in the battle for ARVs in Africa and other parts of the global south is portrayed in an award-winning documentary, *Fire in the Blood*: http://fireintheblood.com/.
17. Steyn, R. Justice Edwin Cameron: An activist. *Financial Mail*. 2014. https://archive.is/j7HiU (accessed 22 March 2017).
18. Cameron E. The deafening silence of AIDS. Harvard University. 2000. https://cdn2.sph.harvard .edu/wp-content/uploads/sites/13/2014/04/3-Cameron.pdf (accessed 22 March 2017).
19. Cameron E. Plenary presentation by Justice Edwin Cameron. ACT UP. 2000. http://www .actupny.org/reports/durban-cameron.html (accessed 22 March 2017).

20. Before Mandela finally spoke out, Cameron had begged to meet with him. "Mandela was the person who could have spoken with moral authority, with practical interventive effect on AIDS. But he didn't. He kept quiet,..." he told the PBS show *Frontline* in 2009. He recalled bitterly thinking that when the Spice Girls came to South Africa, Mandela "[spent] more time with the Spice Girls than he did on AIDS!" Though Cameron ultimately credited Mandela for finally confronting Mbeki on the issue, he believes thousands of lives might have been spared had Mandela spoken out sooner. See: The long walk of Nelson Mandela—Mandela & AIDS: Justice Edwin Cameron. *Frontline.* PBS. 2009. http://www.pbs.org/wgbh/pages/frontline/shows/mandela/aids /cameron.html (accessed 22 March 2017).

21. Cameron E. The dead hand of denialism. *Africa Action: Africa Policy e-Journal.* University of Pennsylvania African Studies Center. 2003. https://www.africa.upenn.edu/Urgent_Action/apic -90503.html (accessed 22 March 2017).

22. Ibid.

23. Quick J. Geffen N. 5 May 2016; by phone.

24. Another case successfully argued that the high prices for ARV drugs levied by Big Pharma violated regulations against excessive pricing and South Africa's guarantee of "right to life." Laverack G. Health activism. *Health Promotion International* 2012; 27, 4: 429–34. http://heapro .oxfordjournals.org/content/early/2012/08/24/heapro.das044.short (accessed 22 March 2017).

25. Quick J. Geffen N. 5 May 2016; by phone.

26. Nolen. *28: Stories of AIDS in Africa.*

27. Dugger C. Harvard study finds heavy costs for South Africa's misguided AIDS policies. *New York Times.* 2008. http://www.nytimes.com/2008/11/26/world/africa/26aids.html (accessed 7 March 2017).

28. Mbali. TAC in the history.

29. Global AIDS Update 2016. UNAIDS. 2016. http://www.unaids.org/en/resources/documents /2016/Global-AIDS-update-2016 (accessed 10 March 2017).

30. Schwartländer B, Grubb I, Perriëns J. The 10-year struggle to provide antiretroviral treatment to people with HIV in the developing world. *The Lancet* 2006; 368: 541–46.

31. Kapstein E, Busby J. *AIDS drugs for all: Social movements and market transformations.* Cambridge: Cambridge University Press, 2013.

32. Busby. *Moral movements and foreign policy.*

33. Quick J, Olawolu Moore E. Global access to essential medicines past, present and future. In: Parker R, Sommer M, eds. *Routledge handbook of global public health.* New York: Routledge, 2011.

34. Palmisano L, Vella S. A brief history of antiretroviral therapy of HIV infection: Success and challenges. *Annali dell'Istituto Superiore Di Sanita* 2011; 47, 1: 44–48. DOI: 10.4415/ ANN_11_01_10. Review.

35. Global AIDS Update 2016. UNAIDS. 2016. http://www.unaids.org/en/resources/documents /2016/Global-AIDS-update-2016 (accessed 10 March 2017).

36. Antiretroviral therapy (ART) coverage among all age groups. World Health Organization. 2015. http://www.who.int/gho/hiv/epidemic_response/ART_text/en/ (accessed 22 March 2017).

37. Bono. The good news on poverty (Yes, there's good news). TED Talk. 2013. https://www.ted .com/talks/bono_the_good_news_on_poverty_yes_there_s_good_news (accessed 22 March 2017).

38. Garrett L. *Betrayal of trust: The collapse of global public health.* New York: Hachette Books, 2000.

39. Hessou C. Ebola survivors facing stigma, unemployment, exclusion. United Nations Population Fund. 2015. http://www.unfpa.org/news/ebola-survivors-facing-stigma-unemployment-exclusion (accessed 22 March 2017).

40. Naimah J. The stigma that comes with fighting Ebola. Médecins Sans Frontières USA. 2015. http://www.doctorswithoutborders.org/article/stigma-comes-fighting-ebola (accessed 22 March 2017).

41. Fryer B. Hickox K. 13 September 2016; by phone.

42. For more on Kaci Hickox's story, see: Hickox K. Caught between civil liberties and public safety fears: Personal reflections from a healthcare provider treating Ebola. *Journal of Health and Biomedical Law* 2015; 11: 9–23. http://www.suffolk.edu/documents/LawJournals/Kaci_Hickox _Suffolk_Law_JHBL.pdf (accessed 22 March 2017). In this article, Hickox also recommends that the CDC guidelines for quarantine be clarified.

43. Schwartz I. Christie on mandatory quarantines: We can't count on a voluntary system. Real Clear Politics. 2014. http://www.realclearpolitics.com/video/2014/10/26/christie_on_mandatory _quarantines_we_cant_count_on_a_voluntary_system.html (accessed 22 March 2017).

44. Maxman A. Ebola panic looks familiar to AIDS activists. *Newsweek.* 2014. http://www.newsweek .com/2014/11/14/ebola-panic-looks-familiar-aids-activists-281545.html (accessed 10 March 2017).

45. Cohen D, Grunwald M. Jindal: Ban travel from Ebola nations. *Politico*. 2014. http://www.politico.com/story/2014/10/ebola-travel-bobby-jindal-comments-111592 (accessed 22 March 2017).

46. Crouch I, Battan C, Larson S et al. Ebola's fear factor. *New Yorker*. 2014. http://www.newyorker.com/magazine/2014/10/20/fear-equation (accessed 22 March 2017).

47. Moyer W. Kaci Hickox, rebel Ebola nurse loathed by conservatives, sues Chris Christie over quarantine. *Washington Post*. 2015. https://www.washingtonpost.com/news/morning-mix/wp/2015/10/23/kaci-hickox-rebel-ebola-nurse-loathed-by-conservatives-sues-chris-christie-over-quarantine/?utm_term=.6b06301850fd (accessed 1 July 2017). Judge Charles LaVerdiere ruled against the state of Maine's request to quarantine Hickox in her home, stating, "The State has not met its burden at this time to prove by clear and convincing evidence that limiting [Hickox's] movements to the degree requested [home-quarantine] is 'necessary to protect other individuals from the dangers of infection.'" http://www.courts.maine.gov/news_reference/high_profile/hickox/order_pending_hearing.pdf. Maine settled the lawsuit.

48. Ibid.

49. How to advocate on Ebola. National Nurses United. 2014. http://www.nationalnursesunited.org/news/entry/how-to-advocate-on-ebola-national-nurses-united/ (accessed 22 March 2017).

50. Fryer B. Hickox K. 13 September 2016; by phone.

51. "Philanthropreneur" is a term used by philanthropists who combine principles of entrepreneurship with philanthropy. See: Chandy R. Welcome to the new age of philanthropy—philanthropreneurship. *The Guardian*. 2014. https://www.theguardian.com/sustainable-business/2014/dec/08/new-age-of-philanthropy-philanthropreneurship (accessed 22 March 2017).

52. Evans H. What does it mean to be a citizen of the world? TED. 2016. https://www.ted.com/talks/hugh_evans_what_does_it_mean_to_be_a_citizen_of_the_world (accessed 22 March 2017).

53. McKinley J. Hugh Evans, 29, force behind global festival on Great Lawn. *New York Times*. 2012. http://www.nytimes.com/2012/08/23/arts/music/hugh-evans-29-force-behind-global-festival-on-great-lawn.html?_r=5&pagewanted=all (accessed 22 March 2017).

54. About GAVI, the Vaccine Alliance. GAVI. 2017. http://www.gavi.org/about/ (accessed 22 March 2017).

55. About ONE. ONE. 2017. https://www.one.org/us/about/ (accessed 22 March 2017).

56. Kreps D. Watch George W. Bush praise Bono's AIDS efforts. *Rolling Stone*. 2015. http://www.rollingstone.com/music/news/watch-george-w-bush-praise-bonos-aids-efforts-20151202 (accessed 22 March 2017).

57. Gostin LO, Tomori O, Wibulpolprasert S et al. Toward a common secure future: Four global commissions in the wake of Ebola. 2016. *PLoS Medicine* 2016: 13(5): e1002042. doi:10.1371/journal.pmed.1002042.

58. Moon S, Leigh J, Woskie L et al. Post-Ebola reforms: Ample analysis, inadequate action. *British Medical Journal* 2017; j280.

59. Global greenhouse gas emissions data. U.S. Environmental Protection Agency. 2015. https://www.epa.gov/ghgemissions/global-greenhouse-gas-emissions-data (accessed 22 March 2017).

INDEX

Page numbers in italics refer to tables and figures.